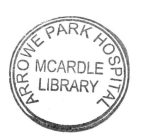
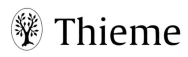

This book is dedicated to our wives, children, and parents for their support, encouragement, and love.

# Manual of Endoscopic Sinus Surgery

and its Extended Applications

Daniel Simmen, M.D.
Lecturer in Rhinology
ENT Center
The Hirslanden Clinic
Zurich, Switzerland

Nick Jones, M.D., B.D.S.,
F.R.C.S, F.R.C.S. (ORL)
Professor
Department of Otorhinolaryngology,
Head and Neck Surgery
Queens Medical Centre
University Hospital
Nottingham, United Kingdom

985 illustrations

Thieme
Stuttgart · New York

*Library of Congress Cataloging-in-Publication Data*

Simmen, D. (Daniel)
Manual of endoscopic sinus surgery and its extended applications /
Daniel Simmen, Nick Jones.
  p. ; cm.
Includes bibliographical references.
ISBN 3-13-130971-7 (alk. paper)—ISBN 1-58890-142-4 (alk. paper)
1. Paranasal sinuses—Endoscopic surgery—Handbooks, manuals,
etc.
[DNLM: 1. Paranasal Sinuses—surgery. 2. Endoscopy—methods.
3. Perioperative Care—methods.] I. Jones, Nick, 1953- II. Title.

RF421.S535 2005
617.5'23059—dc22
                                                    2004029697

Illustrators: Sandra Gubler, Heinz Ochsner

**Important note:** Medicine is an ever-changing science undergoing continual development. Research and clinical experience are continually expanding our knowledge, in particular our knowledge of proper treatment and drug therapy. Insofar as this book mentions any dosage or application, readers may rest assured that the authors, editors, and publishers have made every effort to ensure that such references are in accordance with **the state of knowledge at the time of production of the book.**

Nevertheless, this does not involve, imply, or express any guarantee or responsibility on the part of the publishers in respect to any dosage instructions and forms of applications stated in the book. **Every user is requested to examine carefully** the manufacturers' leaflets accompanying each drug and to check, if necessary in consultation with a physician or specialist, whether the dosage schedules mentioned therein or the contraindications stated by the manufacturers differ from the statements made in the present book. Such examination is particularly important with drugs that are either rarely used or have been newly released on the market. Every dosage schedule or every form of application used is entirely at the user's own risk and responsibility. The authors and publishers request every user to report to the publishers any discrepancies or inaccuracies noticed. If errors in this work are found after publication, errata will be posted at www.thieme.com on the product description page.

© 2005 Georg Thieme Verlag,
Rüdigerstrasse 14, 70469 Stuttgart, Germany
http://www.thieme.de
Thieme New York, 333 Seventh Avenue,
New York, NY 10001 USA
http://www.thieme.com

Typesetting by primustype Hurler GmbH, Notzingen
Printed in Germany by Karl Grammlich GmbH, Pliezhausen

ISBN 3-13-130971-7 (GTV)
ISBN 1-58890-142-4 (TNY)                 1 2 3 4 5 6

Some of the product names, patents, and registered designs referred to in this book are in fact registered trademarks or proprietary names even though specific reference to this fact is not always made in the text. Therefore, the appearance of a name without designation as proprietary is not to be construed as a representation by the publisher that it is in the public domain.

# Preface

# Acknowledgements

"Knowledge comes and goes, but wisdom stays"
*Alfred Lord Tennyson*

This book not only represents our individual experience, but it is the result of what we have each learnt from one another working together. We hope that it is of practical use as it is a distillation of our clinical practice. We have become more and more convinced that patient selection is one of the main keys to successful surgery, and we have tried to explain how we go about this. Much of the book focuses on how to improve the surgical approach, but we have also placed emphasis on what matters to the patient. The last sections of the book involve advanced techniques and reflect the current direction of endoscopic sinus surgery.

To Dr. Jean Shaw for her comments on the manuscript. To Dr. Bernhard Schuknecht, Neuroradiologist at the University Hospital of Zurich, for his contribution to the sections that relate to radiology.

To Prof. Peter Groscurth, Director of the Institute of Anatomy, University of Zurich, for his help in preparing the anatomical specimens. We would like to thank the departments of medical illustration at the University of Nottingham and the University of Zurich for their help.

We are grateful to our teachers, colleagues, and trainees who have all helped to educate us.

# Table of Contents

## 5    How?
### Operative Procedures: A Step-by-Step Safe and Logical Approach                                   50

## 6    An Endoscopic Tour:
### Endoscopic Examination, Anatomical Variations, and Specific Conditions                        106

## 7    The Place of Radiology                                                                        121

# 1 Principles of Practice

## ▪ Accurate Diagnosis Is the Key to Success

A good surgeon is also a good physician. The best surgical results are often obtained by optimizing medical treatment both preoperatively and postoperatively (Fig. 1.1 a, b). Optimizing medical treatment before surgery makes it less traumatic, reduces the chances of complications, and helps preserve olfactory mucosa. In order to optimize medical treatment, the surgeon needs to have an understanding of the mucosal disease. Postoperative medical treatment is frequently required to maintain the improvement that surgery produces.

The surgeon needs to have a good understanding of mucosal disease. History and examination should allow basic categorization of the disease present, but they are often insufficient to make an accurate diagnosis. It is often necessary to undertake other investigations (see Chapter 3) or to have a trial of medical treatment to clarify the underlying pathology.

Each of the clinical appearances shown in Table 1.1 can be associated with different pathological processes (Fig. 1.2 a–f). Try to arrive at a diagnosis that fits into one of the broad groups that are used for the classification of rhinosinusitis. These groups are shown in Table 1.2.

In the light of history and examination, along with the relevant special investigations, the physician can

Table 1.1 Possible clinical criteria for diagnosing rhinosinusitis on the basis of length of history and observation

| Observation | Length of history | | |
|---|---|---|---|
| | Acute < 3 weeks | Subacute > 3 weeks, < 3 months | Chronic > 3 months |
| Erythema | | | |
| Edema | | | |
| Hyperplastic mucosa | | | |
| Polyposis | | | |
| Granular mucosa | | | |
| Purulent secretion | | | |
| Dry mucosa | | | |

Table 1.2 Classification of rhinosinusitis

| Infectious | Noninfectious |
|---|---|
| Viral | *Allergic:* |
| Bacterial | Intermittent or persistent |
| Fungal | *Nonallergic:* |
| | Hormonal |
| | Drug related |
| | Vasculitis |
| | Granulomatous |
| | Autonomic |
| | Idiopathic |

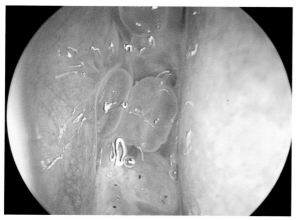
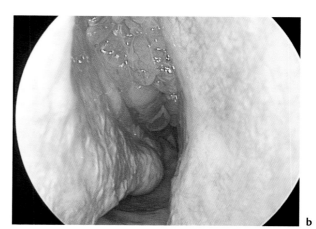

Fig. 1.1 Nasal polyps **a** before and **b** after medical treatment.

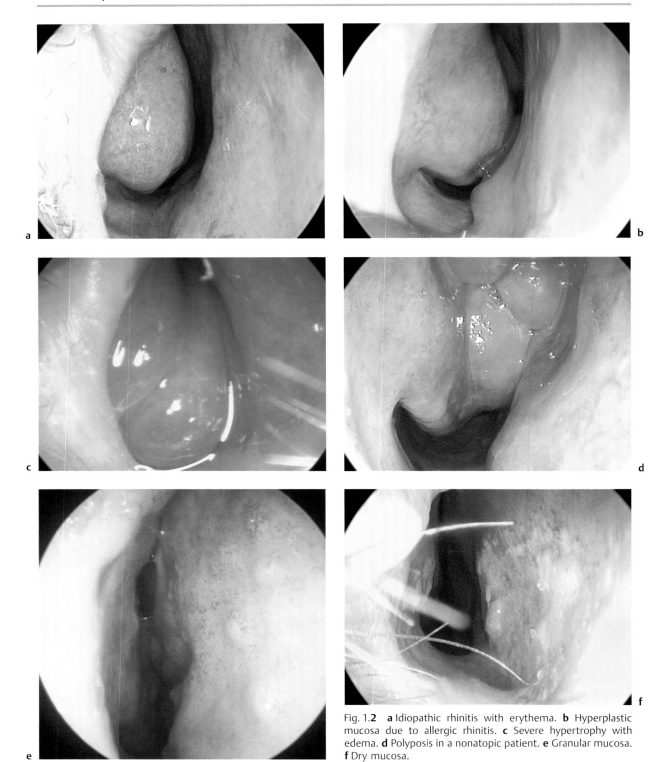

Fig. 1.2  **a** Idiopathic rhinitis with erythema. **b** Hyperplastic mucosa due to allergic rhinitis. **c** Severe hypertrophy with edema. **d** Polyposis in a nonatopic patient. **e** Granular mucosa. **f** Dry mucosa.

obtain an idea of the underlying pathology (Table 1.3; Figs. 1.3 a–d, 1.4 a–d). Based on this, medical and surgical treatment can be maximized.

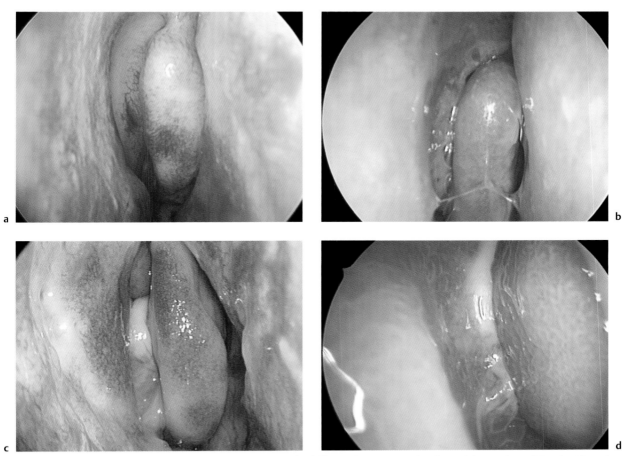

Fig. 1.**3**    **a** Normal middle meatus. **b** Serous secretions in marked allergic rhinitis. **c** Purulent bacterial secretions. **d** Purulent fungal secretions.

Table 1.**3**    Pathology of rhinosinusitis

| **Infectious** | |
| --- | --- |
| Viral | |
| Bacterial (including TB, leprosy, syphilis, etc.) | |
| Fungal | |
| **Noninfectious** | |
| Allergy | Seasonal (intermittent) |
| | Perennial (persistent) |
| Idiopathic (no systemic evidence of allergy or local infection) | |
| Rhinitis medicamentosa | Excessive use of local sympathomimetic agents |
| Hormonal | High-estrogen contraceptive pill; pregnancy |
| Autonomic | Primary symptom is rhinorrhea often reduced by ipratropium bromide; few other nasal symptoms; patients often elderly. Important not to include in idiopathic group. |
| Sarcoidosis | |
| Vasculitis | Wegener granulomatosis, systemic lupus erythematosus, overlap syndrome |
| Drug induced | Beta blockers, ACE inhibitors |

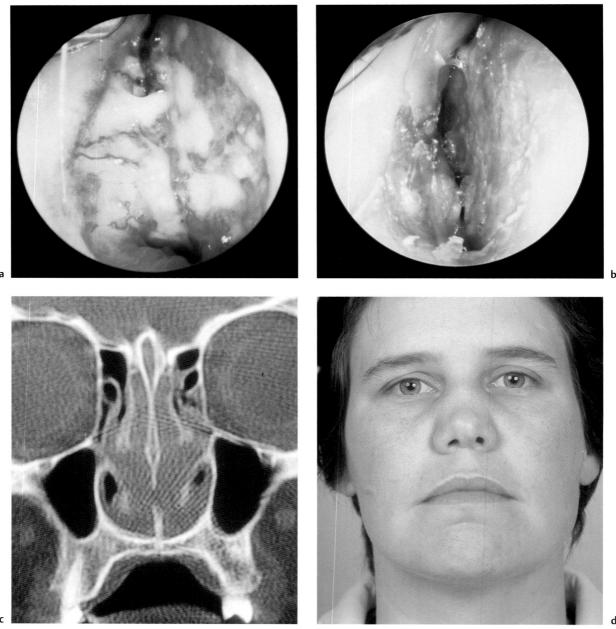

Fig. 1.**4 a**, **b** Endoscopic appearance of granulations and crusts in Wegener granulomatosis. **c** Coronal CT scan showing the mucosal changes consistent with Wegener granulomatosis; there is often bony erosion as well. **d** Collapse of the nasal dorsum often seen in nasal Wegener granulomatosis.

### ■ Focus on the Patient's Main Complaint

The patient may mention any of a large array of symptoms in nasal disease. There are **four** primary symptoms that are always worth asking about:
1  Nasal obstruction
2  Sense of smell
3  Secretions
4  Pain or pressure

It is important to rank these symptoms in their order of priority to the patient. This not only helps to make a diagnosis, but it focuses the surgeon's mind on how best to meet the patient's needs—underline the patient's main complaint.

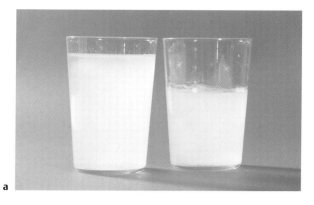

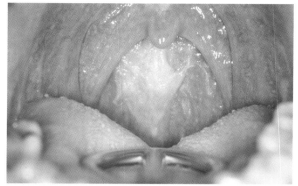

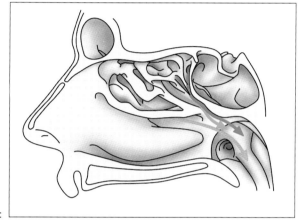

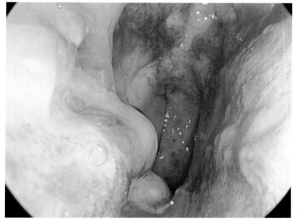

Fig. 1.**5**  **a** The amount of secretions produced per day. **b** Postnasal mucus in the pharynx. **c** Mucociliary pathways of mucus.

**d** Purulent secretions from the middle meatus tracking over clear secretions.

## ■ Dealing with the Patient's Expectations

The patient's priorities may differ from what the surgeon can achieve. For example, the patient's main concern might be their postnasal discharge, but the surgeon may only be able to improve the symptoms of obstruction with little alteration to the postnasal drip (Fig. 1.5 a–d). It is therefore vital that the surgeon is forthcoming and makes it as clear as possible to the patient which symptoms can and cannot be improved or resolved. When the physician overlooks this prior to treatment, the patient is likely to be disappointed with the outcome. Be aware that some patients may believe that even symptoms that they have not mentioned will be cured.

The patient's expectations should coincide with the surgeon's prognosis. Thus, it is worth communicating to them which specific symptoms will **not** be helped.

## ■ Optimize Medical Treatment

While it is accepted that medical treatment will complement surgery in making the mucosa as healthy as possible, it is less well recognized that it can be a useful predictor of what can be achieved by surgery. For example, in a patient with anosmia and nasal polyposis, the use of oral and topical steroids can indicate the patient's remaining olfactory potential. If the patient has no sense of smell after a course of oral steroids (Fig. 1.6 a–d), not even temporarily, then the surgeon must be very guarded in promising the patient that their sense of smell will be improved by surgery.

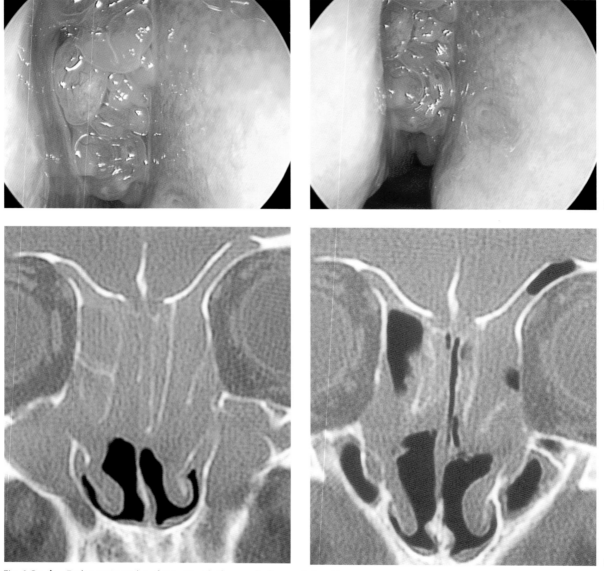

Fig. 1.**6 a**, **b**   Endoscopic and **c**, **d** CT views before and after oral steroids.

## ■ Tailor the Surgery to Fit the Extent of the Problem

There is a price to be paid for extensive tissue removal. That price may include the loss of olfactory mucosa, frontonasal stenosis, altered sensation, dryness, and an increased risk of violating the boundaries of the paranasal sinuses (Fig. 1.7 a, b).

Surgery is primarily aimed at improving ventilation of the sinuses and restoring mucociliary clearance. Removal of tissue alone does not cure mucosal disease. After a trial of full medical treatment, it is possible to see where surgery will be of most benefit. This means that it is often possible to preserve valuable tissue, such as mucosa in the olfactory cleft, that might otherwise be removed (Fig. 1.8 a–d). Far less surgery is needed if medical treatment has been successful.

## ■ Minimize Surgical Morbidity

Morbidity can be caused by poor surgical technique, but it can also arise from excessive tissue removal. Good surgical technique is based on setting explicit goals and achieving these with the minimal amount of tissue trauma.

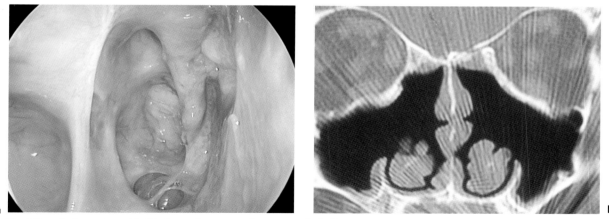

Fig. 1.**7**  **a** Endoscopic and **b** CT views after overzealous removal of olfactory mucosa.

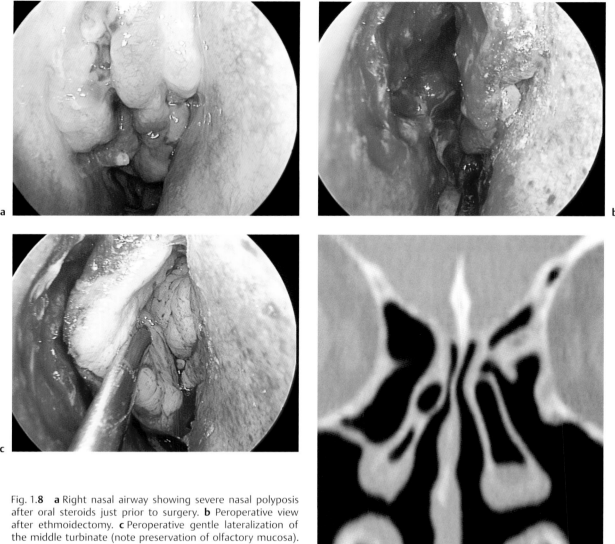

Fig. 1.**8**  **a** Right nasal airway showing severe nasal polyposis after oral steroids just prior to surgery. **b** Peroperative view after ethmoidectomy. **c** Peroperative gentle lateralization of the middle turbinate (note preservation of olfactory mucosa). **d** Postoperative CT view to show open olfactory cleft.

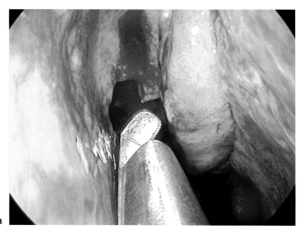
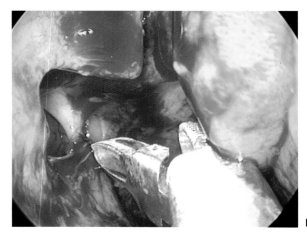

a                                                       b

Fig. 1.**9**  **a** Use of Hajek forceps to neatly remove the mucosa and bone of a right uncinate process. **b** Through-cutting forceps joining natural and accessory ostia.

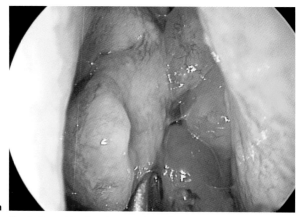
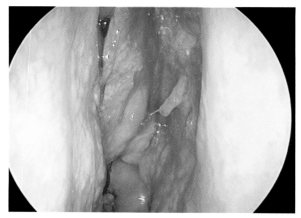

a                                                       b

Fig. 1.**10**  **a** Nasal polyps in the olfactory area medial to the middle turbinate, deliberately not removed at surgery. **b** The superior turbinate can now be seen after lateralization of the middle turbinate along with 2 months of topical nasal steroids.

### How Can This Be Achieved?

Work out what surgical steps are needed and then take them systematically. This strategy will not only avoid unnecessary tissue removal but is also very time efficient. Progress is made step by step rather than by aimlessly exploring the sinuses. You must decide which step needs to be done next and then do this as atraumatically as possible. This means:

- Punching tissue rather than tearing it.
- Preserving mucosal integrity in the frontonasal recess.
- Respecting olfactory mucosa.
- Avoiding mucosal damage to adjacent surfaces (Fig. 1.9 a, b).

The surgeon must be aware of the variations in anatomy that can occur and the potential to cause damage to the surrounding structures (see further discussion in Chapter 6).

### ■ Sense of Smell Should Be Preserved at All Costs

Surgeons unfortunately often underestimate the importance of sense of smell to the patients. It is a sense that is all too often forgotten and may escape the notice of both surgeons and patients. The reason may be that the loss of this sense often creeps up on the patient slowly or that the patient does not recognize that this loss is responsible for the reduced enjoyment of food. In any case, the rewards for patients in preserving or restoring their sense of smell are enormous.

# ◼ The Importance of Postoperative Treatment

Unfortunately, surgery on its own cannot achieve or maintain healthy nasal mucosa in most patients with noninfective rhinosinusitis. Accompanying medical treatment takes on a central role. During the operation, diseased mucosa is removed that has not recovered during preoperative medical treatment, thereby optimizing the drainage zones from the sinuses. Surgery may be able to overcome mucosa–mucosa contact and restore mucociliary clearance, remove diseased tissue, and allow access to topical nasal treatment, but surgery in and of itself cannot cure intrinsic nasal disease (Fig. 1.**10 a**, **b**).

Patients need to be made aware of the need for continuing treatment in order to achieve the best possible result and an improved quality of life. One way of getting this message across to your patients with intrinsic mucosal disease is to tell them that it is like "asthma of the nose," and they will need to keep the lining under control by regular medical treatment. This will help to prevent disappointment.

# 2 Who?
## Patient Selection

### ■ Who Will Most Likely Profit from Surgery?

In determining which patients to select for surgery, the decision must be founded on the likelihood that surgical treatment is capable of offering the desired improvement. Patients with a diagnosis of rhinosinusitis and nasal polyposis who have not become symptom-free after maximum medical treatment are most likely to profit from surgery. These patients may have had a very good response to oral steroids, but their symptoms of hyposmia and congestion may start to return, even with continued topical treatment.

The key-question is: **What symptoms does the patient have and how pronounced are they?**

In making your selection, a patient's surgical history must also be considered carefully. If the patient has had previous sinus surgery that did not help, think twice before operating again. If surgery failed the first time, why should it work the second time? It is impor-

tant to be sure that the surgery was done well the first time, that the sinus ostia are open, and that there is no residual disease.

It is common to find that patients who have had previous surgery have some mucosal thickening of the lining of their sinuses on CT in spite of the sinus ostia being open. This does not necessarily mean that they have ongoing significant sinus disease. In this situation, it is important to go over the history, examination, and response to treatment in detail before embarking on surgery again (Fig. 2.1 a, b).

### ■ Symptom-oriented Patient Selection

Other criteria in determining which patients to select are, of course, their symptoms. While surgery can provide an invaluable benefit in restoring patients' health and wellbeing, advocating surgery is not an appropriate response to all symptoms that our patients may report. **Which are the cardinal symptoms?**

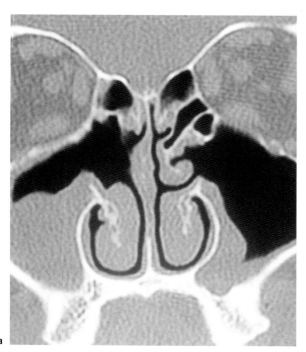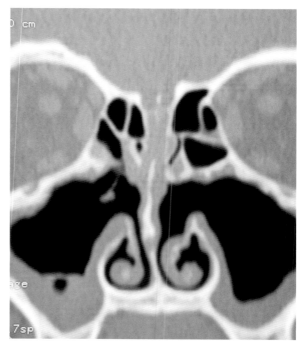

a          b

Fig. 2.**1 a, b** Typical CT images in two different patients showing changes after surgery. These mucosal changes in themselves do not mean that further surgery is warranted.

## Nasal Obstruction

This is the main reason for operating, as it is one symptom that surgery can almost be guaranteed to help (Fig. 2.**2**). However, be careful about operating on anyone whose primary symptom is not nasal obstruction—**think twice!**

Also be careful about operating on someone who complains about nasal congestion but in whom there is no objective sign of poor airflow.

## Facial Pain and Pressure

Facial pain and pressure are often wrongly attributed by patients and their primary care physicians as being due to rhinosinusitis (West and Jones, 2001).

In patients with chronic pain involving the face and/or head, it is important to see whether their symptoms are associated with, or exacerbated by, an upper respiratory tract infection and, furthermore, to see whether there is a temporal relationship with any purulent discharge. If they have no significant nasal symptoms and if their nasal endoscopy is normal, it is unlikely that their facial pain is due to rhinosinusitis. However, patients who have facial pain and purulent secretions at endoscopy do well with surgical or medical treatment, as over 80 % will be helped.

Beware if pain and pressure are the patient's main symptoms. The majority of patients with nasal polyposis have no facial pain or pressure due to rhinosinusitis unless there are purulent secretions present as well (Fahy and Jones, 2001) (Fig. 2.**3 a**, **b**).

However, if patients have symptoms of pain or pressure in addition to nasal obstruction and a loss of sense of smell, especially if the pain and pressure get worse with a cold or when flying or skiing, then you can advise the patient that these symptoms may be helped by surgery.

## Disordered Sense of Smell

The patient whose sense of smell returns after oral steroids, only to deteriorate thereafter, is the patient whose sense of smell may benefit from surgery. A patient with anosmia who has had previous surgery is unlikely to regain any sense of smell if systemic steroids have not helped (Fig. 2.**4**). However, a patient with anosmia who has not had previous surgery and did not respond to oral steroids still has a small chance of regaining their sense of smell through an ethmoidectomy and gentle liberalization of the middle turbinate. It is vital that the middle and superior turbinate are treated with absolute care in these patients when surgery is done to open the olfactory cleft (Fig. 2.**5 a–d**).

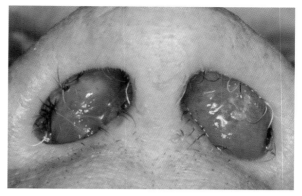

Fig. 2.**2**   Gross polyposis where the patient will appreciate the improvement in their airway after removal of the polyps.

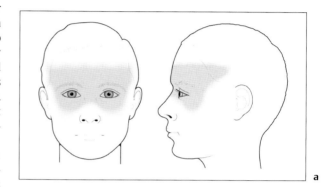

a

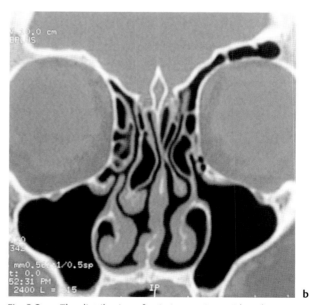

b

Fig. 2.**3**   **a** The distribution of pain in a patient with a clear airway and **b** normal CT scan in a patient whose symptoms were due to midfacial segment pain.

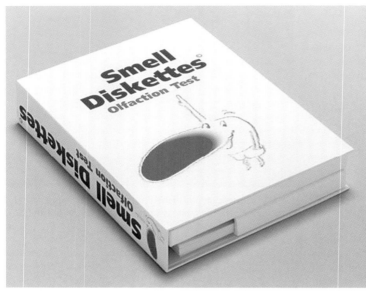
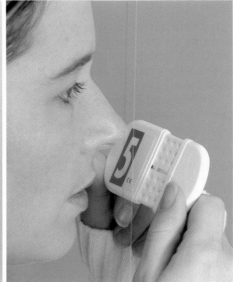

Fig. 2.**4**    A patient with anosmia would give incorrect or negative answers on the patient questionnaire for the smell-screening test.

### Anterior Rhinorrhea

Anterior rhinorrhea is usually secondary to viral or allergic rhinitis. The reason for anterior rhinorrhea in a viral rhinitis is not only an increase in mucus production but also paralysis of the cilia. The degree of cilial stasis that is needed to produce anterior purulent bacterial rhinorrhea is unusual in bacterial infections and normally only occurs in cystic fibrosis and ciliary dyskinesia.

### Posterior Rhinorrhea

As with facial pain, be very cautious about recommending surgery if posterior rhinorrhea is the patient's primary symptom (Fig. 2.**6 a**, **b**). Surgery can help reduce the discoloration of the postnasal mucus by helping drainage, but it is important not to promise the patient a "cure," as mucus secretion may be due to systemic mucosal disease. Because of this, ongoing medical treatment is often important. Patients with asthma can expect an improvement in their lower respiratory symptoms. It is also important to take time to explain to the patient the connection between the upper and lower respiratory tracts.

Normally, the paranasal sinuses produce a cupful of mucus a day, and this is swallowed along with 1.5 liters of saliva. The sensation of an increase in mucus production felt in the back of the throat is called "postnasal drip." Patients often complain of a sensation of "something" in the back of the throat that they cannot

clear and persistently attempt to clear their throat. Frequently, these symptoms are due to a hyperawareness of normal mucus. It is particularly important to warn these patients that this symptom cannot be helped by surgery. Other strategies, however, may help these patients; for example, breaking a cycle of repeated throat clearing, snorting, or hawking by swallowing ice-cold sparkling water instead.

### ■ Disease-oriented Patient Selection

Which pathological processes benefit from surgery? The symptom-oriented approach applies to the majority of patients with rhinosinusitis, whether they have polyps or not. However, there are specific diseases that deserve special mention.

### Chronic Infective Rhinosinusitis

Patients with chronic infective rhinosinusitis who have not responded to medical treatment usually benefit from surgery unless they have an immunodeficiency or a disorder of ciliary motility (Fig. 2.**7 a**, **b**).

### Aspergillosis/Fungal Disease

Patients with saprophytic fungal disease have a good prognosis with surgery (Fig. 2.**8 a–c**). Allergic fungal disease responds well to surgery in combination with topical steroids (Simmen et al., 1998). It is possible to

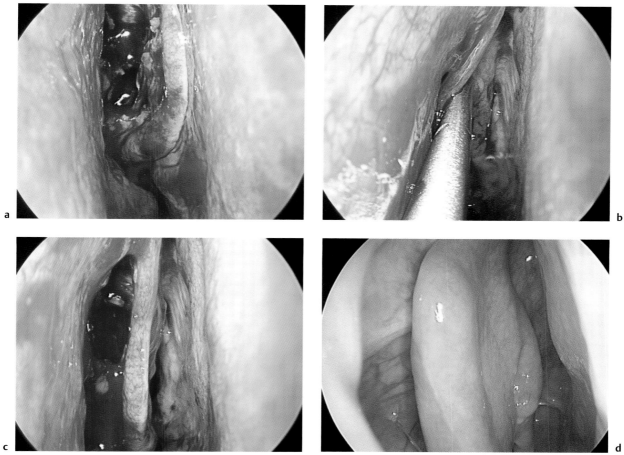

Fig. 2.**5**    **a** Peroperative right ethmoidectomy. **b** Gentle lateralization of the middle turbinate to open the olfactory cleft. **c** A lateralized middle turbinate after surgery. **d** Postoperative view of open olfactory cleft in the same patient at 6 months.

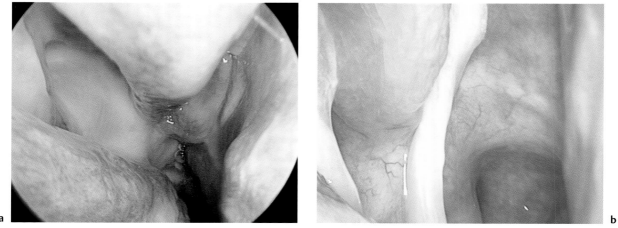

Fig. 2.**6**    **a** Clear mucus from the accessory ostia. **b** Mucus tracking back from the sphenoethmoid recess from the middle meatus.

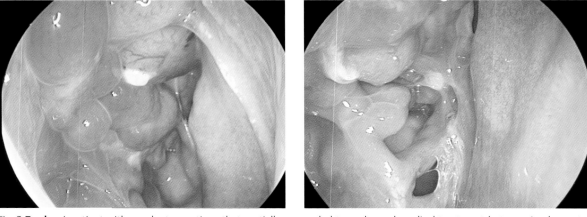

Fig. 2.**7 a**, **b**    A patient with purulent secretions that partially responded to prolonged medical treatment but remained symptomatic with middle meatal edema.

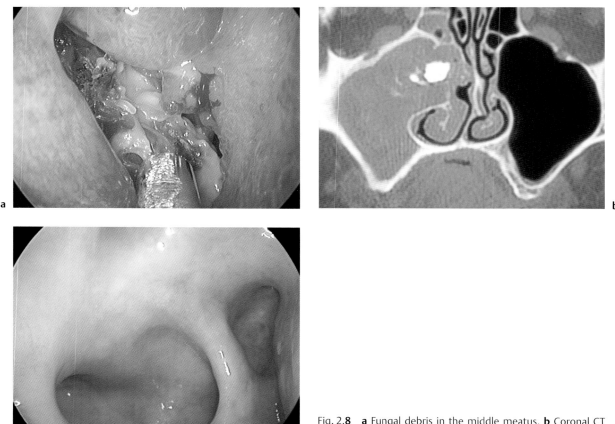

Fig. 2.**8**    **a** Fungal debris in the middle meatus. **b** Coronal CT scan with mycetoma. **c** Postoperative view after one year.

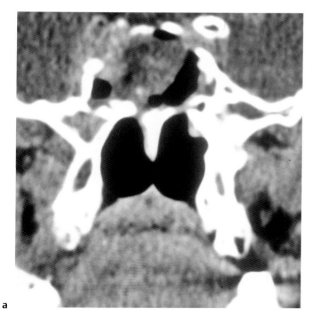

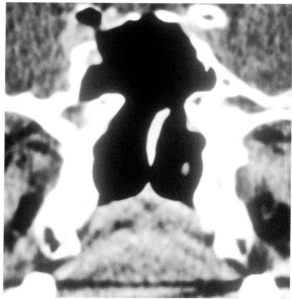

a

b

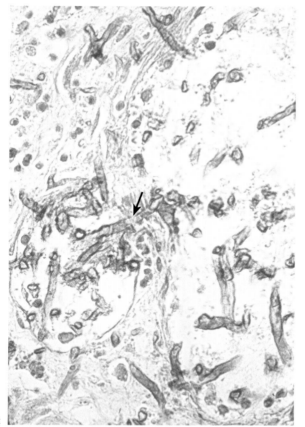

c

Fig. 2.**9**   **a** Preoperative and **b** postoperative coronal CT scans in invasive fungal sinusitis. **c** Histology showing *Aspergillus* invading a blood vessel (arrow).

reverse much of the mucosal disease and reduce the amount of surgery required by giving itraconazole for 3 weeks before surgery. A similar postoperative course will reduce the risk of recurrence. Systemic steroids are best avoided as they can transform noninvasive or allergic aspergillosis into its invasive form. Invasive fungal disease has conventionally required surgical excision accompanied by medication with amphotericin (Fig. 2.**9 a–c**). The introduction of itraconazole obviates the need for surgery in most cases of invasive aspergillosis as long as there is no blood vessel invasion. However, if the disease has invaded blood vessels and is fulminant, then wide debridement and intravenous amphotericin are mandatory.

### Maxillary Sinusitis Secondary to Dental Disease

Endonasal surgery is rarely required. If maxillary sinusitis persists in spite of good root canal or apicectomy treatment, then sinus surgery can help eradicate residual sinus disease.

### Antrochoanal Polyp

Surgery is always indicated for this type of polyp because it does not response well to medical treatment. If the whole base of the polyp in the maxillary sinus is removed, the prognosis is good; otherwise, the polyp recurs (Fig. 2.**10 a–d**).

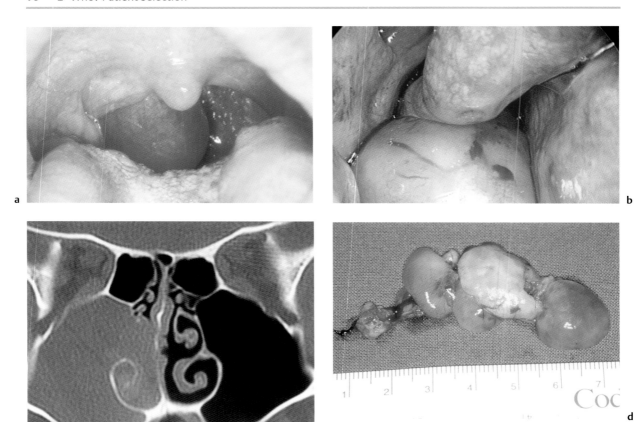

Fig. 2.**10**   **a** An antrochoanal polyp in the nasopharynx. **b** An antrochoanal polyp in the nasal airway. **c** Coronal CT scan of an antrochoanal polyp. **d** Surgical specimen of an antrochoanal polyp with its pedicle.

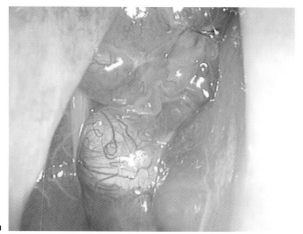

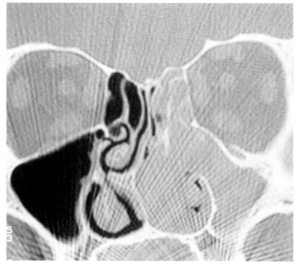

Fig. 2.**11**   **a** The endoscopic appearance of inverted papilloma is typically whiter and less translucent than inflammatory polyps. **b** CT appearance of inverted papilloma with some loss of bony definition and expansion around the soft-tissue mass.

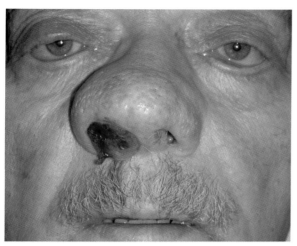

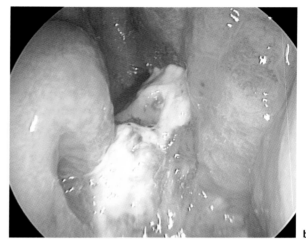

a

b

Fig. 2.**12**   **a** A unilateral nasal lesion due to adenocarcinoma. **b** Endoscopic appearance of an adeno carcinoma of the ethmoid sinuses.

## Inverted Papilloma

It is vital to send the whole specimen for histological examination, as 8–15 % of inverted papillomas are associated with malignancy or atypia. If there are no features of malignancy, the prognosis depends on removing all the diseased tissue (Fig. 2.**11 a**, **b**). If there is any atypia or malignancy, a more radical en bloc procedure is indicated.   **DVD** 14

## Unilateral Nasal Polyps Associated with Neoplasia

Surgery is necessary for biopsy and/or excision (Fig. 2.**12 a**, **b**). Any unilateral nasal polyp should be treated with suspicion, even if it looks harmless (Fig. 2.**13**). It may disguise an underlying tumor or atypical infection (Fig. 2.**14**). A biopsy should be taken in order to ensure that no infection or tumor has been overlooked.

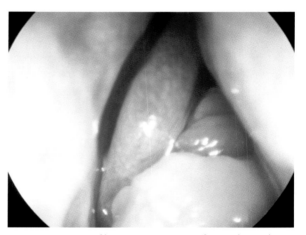

Fig. 2.**13**   A neurofibroma originating from the sphenopalatine area. A unilateral polyp may disguise an underlying tumor or atypical infection.

## Benign and Malignant Tumors

Today, many tumors can be removed endonasally. Here, the complete removal of the tumor base is critical. If this is not tumor-free, the endonasal procedure must be accompanied by an external one.

## Pediatric Rhinosinusitis

It is well recognized that adenoid hypertrophy and allergic rhinitis are common in children, as are recurrent upper respiratory tract infections (Fig. 2.**15**). The main causes of symptoms associated with rhinosinusitis in children are rhinorrhea, nasal obstruction, mouth breathing, hyponasal speech, and snoring. In children, adenoid hypertrophy reduces in size and the number

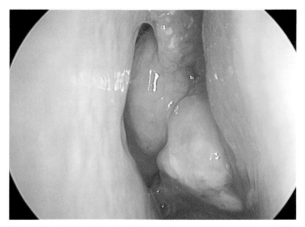

Fig. 2.**14**   A harmless-looking polyp medial to the middle turbinate and an infective-looking polyp at the origin of the turbinate—at histology an adenocarcinoma.

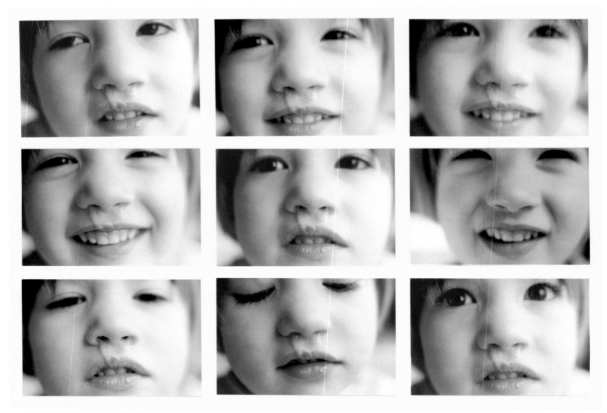

Fig. 2.**15**  Children below the age of 6 years average eight upper respiratory tract infections a year. Clear periods between infections will help distinguish upper respiratory tract infections from other causes of rhinosinusitis.

of colds decreases in frequency by the age of 8–10 years (Fig. 2.**16 a–d**).

The main treatment strategy should be conservative and not surgical. Explain to anxious parents that simple, noninvasive measures such as teaching nose-blowing, the use of saline sprays, or a trial of allergen avoidance and age-appropriate topical nasal anti-inflammatory sprays should be tried before surgery is contemplated. Because such infections are so common, antibiotics given for chronic nasal discharge often have short-lived effects.

Rhinosinusitis in children is not a surgical disease; "watchful waiting" is advised (Fig. 2.**17**). Any treatment should have safety as its first priority, as the problem usually resolves with time without intervention. It is likely that growth and maturation of the immunological response to pathogens play a major role in resolution of the disease (Jones, 1999 a; Howe and Jones, 2004).

There are few exceptions to this principle: nasal polyps (indicating possible cystic fibrosis (Fig. 2.**18 a**, **b**)) and periorbital cellulitis (Fig. 2.**19 a**, **b**). In periorbi-

tal cellulitis, an assessment of vision, parenteral antibiotics, and topical decongestants should be given. If there is concern about the possibility of a subperiosteal abscess, a CT scan should be obtained. Central signs, being unable to accurately assess vision, gross proptosis, ophthalmoplegia, deteriorating visual acuity or color vision, bilateral edema, no improvement or deterioration at 24 hours or a swinging pyrexia that does not resolve within 36 hours are all indications for a CT scan. If a subperiosteal abscess is found on CT, drainage of any pus is indicated.

### ■ Who Not to Select for Surgery

Never coerce any patient into having surgery for rhinosinusitis (Fig. 2.**20 a**, **b**). The patient has to want to proceed, knowing what can realistically be achieved and what risks are involved. At the same time, do not be forced into operating by a patient who has unrealistic expectations and whose symptoms do not correlate with clinical findings. Beware that patients often ex-

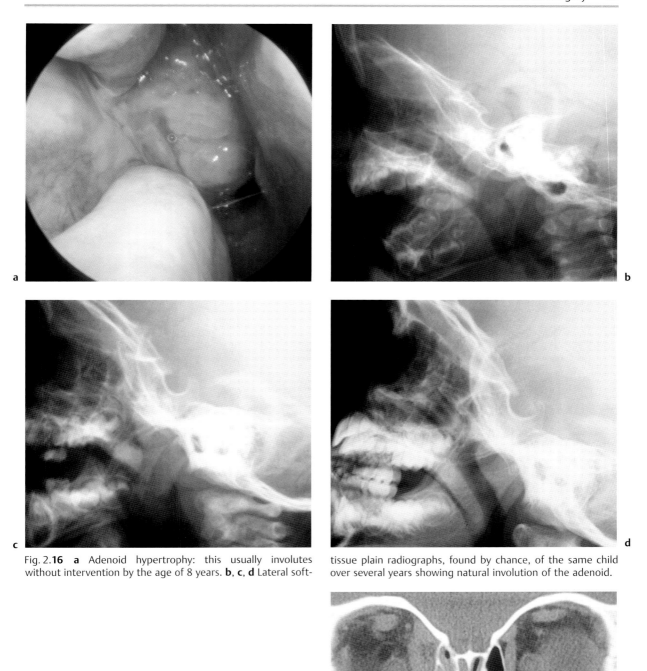

Fig. 2.**16  a** Adenoid hypertrophy: this usually involutes without intervention by the age of 8 years. **b, c, d** Lateral soft-tissue plain radiographs, found by chance, of the same child over several years showing natural involution of the adenoid.

Fig. 2.**17**  A CT scan done in an asymptomatic child having the ▷ investigation for an unrelated reason, showing coincidental mucosal changes—a common finding.

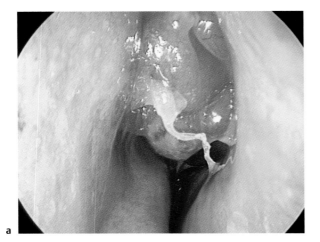

a

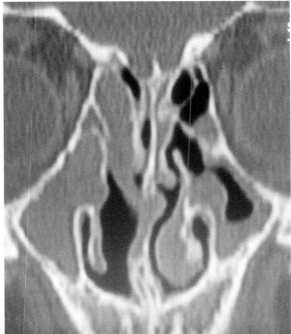

b

Fig. 2.**18**   **a** Middle meatal polyps and a smear of mucopus in a child that is consistent with cystic fibrosis. **b** Corresponding coronal CT scan.

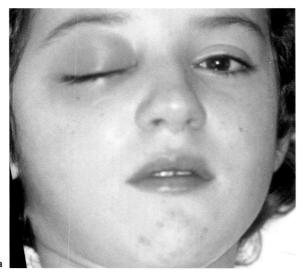

a

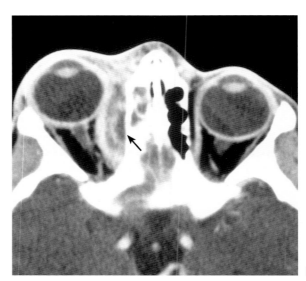

b

Fig. 2.**19**   **a** Clinical and **b** CT view showing a right periorbital abscess (arrow).

pect that all their symptoms will be cured by surgery— even those symptoms that they have not mentioned. Be sure to clarify those symptoms that may be helped and those that are unlikely to improve. Patients occasionally have sizable nasal polyps without any symptoms. Before operating, you would be well advised to manage these patients medically, delaying surgery until they develop symptoms.

### ■ Patient Expectations

Finally, we need to make sure that patients understand that it is usually not possible to cure them of their polyps forever or to eradicate all their symptoms. We explain to our patients that their symptoms are like a person trying to get from the ground floor of a skyscraper to the top floor in order get a good view. On the

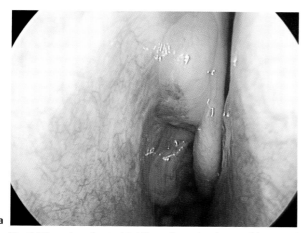
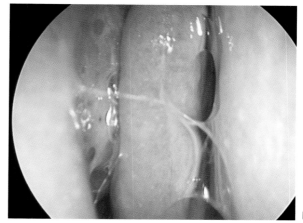

a

b

Fig. 2.**20**   **a** A patient with bilateral nasal polyps visible at endoscopy, but who is asymptomatic. **b** A patient with allergic rhinitis whose symptoms are unlikely to be helped by surgery.

ground floor, they feel blocked, with a poor sense of smell and postnasal mucus. Medical treatment can get them up a few flights of stairs, and oral steroids may get them near the top in a lift, but the lift often comes down again. Surgery together with medical treatment will help them to get a better view for a longer period, but it will not necessarily get them to the top floor (Fig. 2.**21**).

While symptoms of obstruction are often greatly improved, those of a sensation of postnasal discharge may well not be altered. Hyposmia is often improved if the mucosa in the olfactory cleft is preserved and medical treatment is continued.

Only a minority of patients with nasal polyps have symptoms of pain or pressure. If their symptoms are exacerbated by a respiratory tract infection or a change in barometric pressure, they are more likely to benefit from surgery. Be cautious if their pain or pressure does not have these features, as it may be incidental and not helped by surgery.

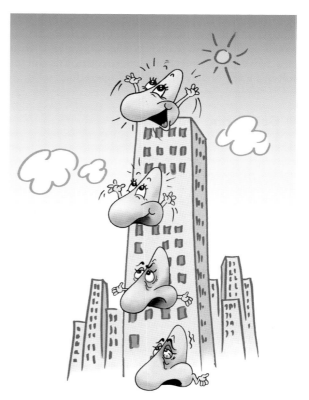

Fig. 2.**21**   Skyscraper analogy. The surgeon can use this illustration to explain symptom goals to patients.

# 3 When?
## Optimizing Diagnosis, Medical Treatment, and Timing of Surgery

The decision to operate is often made when medical treatment has failed or has only provided a small or temporary improvement in the patient's symptoms. This does not mean that medical treatment should be put to one side because it has not cured the patient. For the timing of surgery, it is important to maximize medical treatment just before operating so that the patient's mucosa is as healthy as possible. For example, ensuring that any allergic component is fully treated will minimize the amount of "hyperreactivity" of the mucosa immediately after surgery. This will reduce the amount of exudate that forms after surgery, lessen the formation of adhesions, and help the preservation of olfactory mucosa. It will also make clear to the patient that allergy is a component of their problem. In patients with an active bacterial infection, undertreating this will result in a more bloody and difficult operation.

### ■ Optimizing the Diagnosis

Making an accurate diagnosis is an important part of being in a position to optimize the preoperative medical treatment. An important part in making, or con-

firming, a diagnosis is to gauge the patient's response to medical treatment.

The diagnosis is primarily based on the patient's history, with a small but significant contribution from examination, in particular endoscopy (Fig. 3.**1a**, **b**). Radiology should be interpreted in the light of history and endoscopic findings (Fig. 3.**2**). Histology may have an invaluable role, but only in a minority of patients.

Patients may mention a whole range of nasal symptoms; rather than becoming embroiled in all of these, it is helpful to focus on the patient's four main symptoms. Beware if pain, catarrh, or postnasal mucus is the primary symptom, as in these patients surgery is unlikely to be of benefit.

### Patient History

#### Nasal Obstruction

Ask the patient whether they have unilateral obstruction or bilateral obstruction, or whether it alternates from side to side. Bilateral nasal obstruction is often associated with generalized rhinosinusitis, as is obstruction that alternates from side to side. If this is the

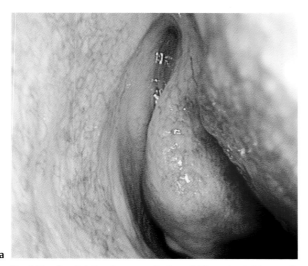
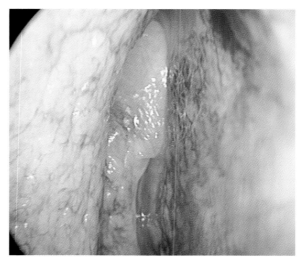

a      b

Fig. 3.**1a**, **b**   Subtle changes of ethmoiditis only visible on close-up endoscopic examination.

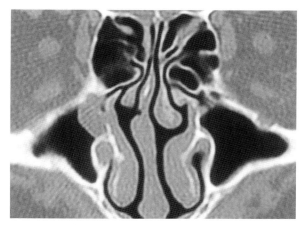

Fig. 3.**2**   Incidental mucosal changes are found in one in three asymptomatic people.

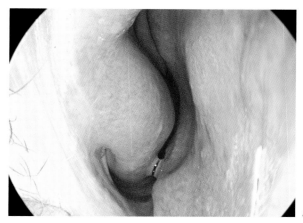

Fig. 3.**3**   **a**, **b** The inferior turbinates and **c** axial MR image showing one side congested at one point in the nasal cycle.

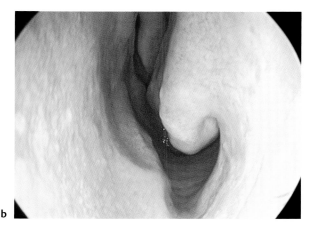

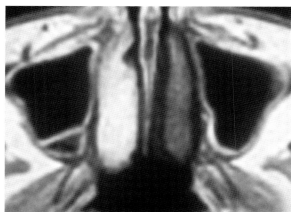

case, it is likely that the patient has generalized swelling of the nasal mucosa from any cause that can produce bilateral rhinosinusitis.

The nasal cycle happens in about 80% of patients every 3–8 hours, with one side being congested while the other is clear (Fig. 3.**3 a–c**). Any disease that causes a generalized swelling of the intranasal lining may lead to the nasal cycle being "disclosed" so that the patient notices that one side is partially blocked. In the disease-free individual, the amount of swelling of the nasal lining that occurs in the nasal cycle is usually insufficient to cause any symptoms.

If the patient has persistent unilateral nasal obstruction, the most common cause is septal deviation (Fig. 3.**4**). If there is any other pathology, such as a malignancy, there are often other associated symptoms in the history, such as a bloody mucoid discharge, loose teeth, diplopia, or distortion of the cheek (Fig. 3.**5**).

Be specific in asking the patient whether the sensation is of "blockage" or if there is a feeling that their nasal airflow is impaired. There is a subtle but important distinction between these two symptoms. Someone with an impairment in their airflow normally has a mechanical obstruction, whereas a patient who complains of "blockage" without any airflow obstruction is less likely to have intranasal pathology that will benefit from surgery. Be careful about operating on someone who has a sensation of "blockage" but whose airflow is normal, as these patients may have a feeling of pressure under the bridge of the nose, on either side of the bridge of the nose, or behind the eyes or supraorbital and infraorbital margins. This sensation of pressure is often not related to the obstruction of the ostiomeatal complex, as is implied in most orthodox texts. These patients often have a variation of a tension-type headache called midfacial segment pain that affects the midface. It gives them a feeling of blockage in this area (Jones, 2001 a) and can produce a sensation of pressure or congestion rather than pain. These symptoms usually respond to low dose amitriptyline (Fig. 3.**6**).   **DVD** 5

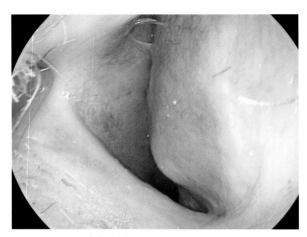

Fig. 3.**4**   A septal deviation.

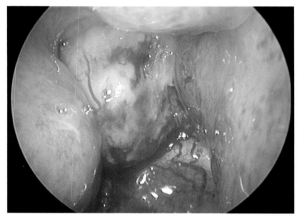

Fig. 3.**5**   A unilateral mass producing nosebleeds—an angiofibroma.

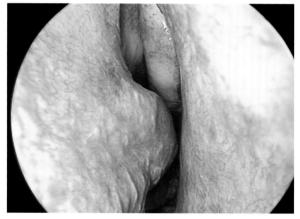

Fig. 3.**6**   A patient with symptoms of "blockage" but whose airflow and endoscopy were normal and responded to low-dose amitriptyline.

## Catarrh

The term "catarrh" means different things to different patients and you need to be quite direct in finding out what they may mean by this symptom. Ask whether it is anterior or posterior, thick or thin? Does it make them sniff, snort, or hawk?

If it is anterior, it is due either to an overproduction of mucus, such as in allergic rhinitis, or to poorly functioning cilia, such as in an upper respiratory tract infection, when the virus or bacterial toxins paralyze the cilia (Fig. 3.**7**). If it is posterior, then more detective work is needed to establish whether the patient has become hyperaware of normal mucus, or whether they really have an overproduction of mucus.

There are many reasons why the lining of the nose can produce more mucus; these essentially include all the causes of chronic rhinosinusitis. It is important that these problems are distinguished from habitual snorting or clearing of the throat. Often the snorer whose uvula is edematous complains of a sensation of "something" around the soft palate, and they may use the term "catarrh" to describe this (Fig. 3.**8**). To further complicate matters, some patients with globus pharyngeus may complain of catarrh, and they have a sensation of pooling of mucus at the level of the cricoid cartilage. Ask the patient about the color of the mucus. Is it clear, yellow, or green, or does it vary in color? Many patients who mouthbreath when they sleep wake up with some green-stained mucus that has collected in their nasopharynx or oropharynx as mucus has dried in this area and become discolored with oropharyngeal commensals (Fig. 3.**9**). It is therefore important to ask patients who complain of discolored mucus whether it is just in the morning or throughout the day. It is useful to ask them to blow their nose into a handkerchief and see whether they have any discolored mucus to confirm that is the case. If they do blow out purulent mucopus into their handkerchief, it is likely that they have a chronic infective rhinosinusitis. This is relatively unusual.

It is far more common for patients to have a hyperawareness of normal postnasal mucus and through repeated clearing of their throat or snorting to have "sensitized" these areas to the cup and a half of mucus that is normally produced from the paranasal sinuses each 24 hours. Patients with allergic rhinitis or nasal polyposis often produce a lot of yellow-stained mucus, which is due to the presence of eosinophils, and this discoloration does not necessarily mean that it is infected (Fig. 3.**10a**, **b**). In the context of the large number of people with allergic rhinitis and an increase in their production of mucus, very few complain of excessive postnasal mucus for the reasons given above.

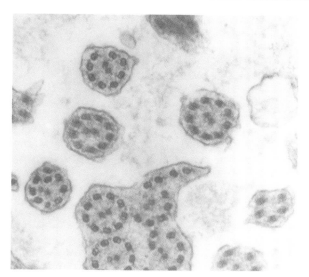

Fig. 3.**7** Fused cilia after a rhinovirus infection.

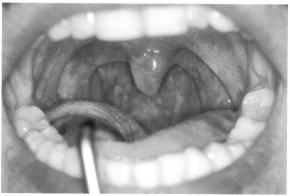

Fig. 3.**8** An edematous uvula in a patient who snorts and snores and who also has a hyperawareness of normal mucus.

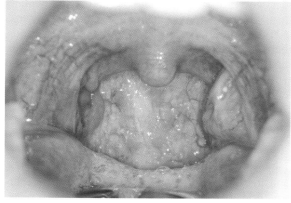

Fig. 3.**9** A snorer who mouthbreathes and has dried, discolored mucus in the morning and pharyngitis. During the day the mucus was clear, as were the sinuses.

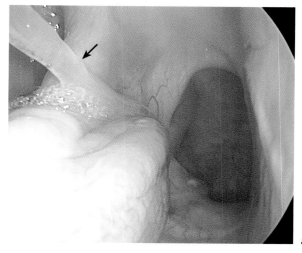

a

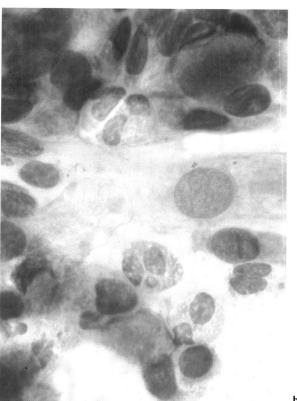

b

Fig. 3.**10** **a** Yellow stained mucus due to eosinophilia (arrow). **b** A cytological smear showing eosinophilia.

### Sneezing

Most people sneeze, but more than three sneezes together are almost pathognomonic of allergic rhinitis. If a patient sneezes a great deal in the morning, then you should be suspicious that they have an allergy to house dust mite, having been exposed to it over the previous few hours in their bedding (Fig. 3.**11 a**, **b**).

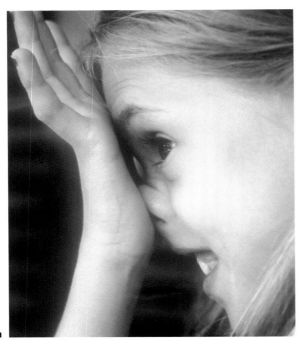
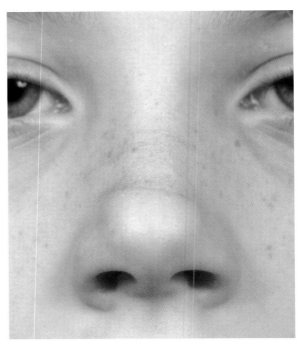

a
b

Fig. 3.**11**    **a** A nasal salute in allergic rhinitis and **b** the crease over the bridge of the nose that it creates by repeated rubbing of the nose.

Itchy and watery eyes are in keeping with an allergic rhinitis whether this is persistent or intermittent.

### Sense of Smell

Many patients complain of having a poor sense of taste, being unaware that the problem is a reduced sense of smell, which needs to be clarified (Fig. 3.**12**). The sense of taste can only discern salty, sweet, bitter, or sour. In order to taste or smell anything else, you require a functioning olfactory epithelium.

Ask the patient whether the loss of the sense of smell is total or partial. If it is total, you should enquire whether it occurred immediately after a head injury, following an influenza-like illness, or slowly in conjunction with other nasal symptoms, such as in chronic rhinosinusitis. A history of head injury must raise suspicion that the olfactory nerves were severed where they pass through the cribriform plate. If the loss followed an influenza-like illness and is absolute, then it is likely that it is secondary to a neuropathic influenza virus (Fig. 3.**13 a**, **b**).

Many patients say that their loss of sense of smell is absolute, but on closer questioning they will mention that they recently did notice a smell of burning toast, say, or some perfume. This indicates that there is some functioning olfactory mucosa (Fig. 3.**14 a**, **b**). In these patients, it is likely that they have some mucosal dis-

ease, and it is possible that their sense of smell can be improved by reversing this. A minority of patients have a distorted sense of smell and it is worth referring to a specialist text for more information on this topic (Jones and Rog, 1998).

### Pain and Pressure

Acute rhinosinusitis following an upper respiratory tract infection is extremely painful and is usually associated with pyrexia, nasal obstruction, and rhinorrhea, which is often purulent but not necessarily so.

If the acute rhinosinusitis is in the maxillary sinus, there is terrible pain in the teeth and cheek. If it is in the frontal sinus, it is usually unilateral and associated with pain in this area and extreme sensitivity of the inferior border of the supraorbital margin (Fig. 3.**15**). Patients who present with this are in extreme distress, have a temperature, and are usually toxic with beads of sweat on their temples.

Patients with acute, short-lived episodic pain on a regular basis are unlikely to have recurrent infective sinusitis. If they do, it should be associated with recurrent upper respiratory tract infections and an associated purulent discharge. If nasal endoscopy is clear when you examine these patients, you should ask them to return when they are symptomatic to ensure that they have genuine recurrent acute purulent rhinosinusitis. In many patients who have recurrent facial

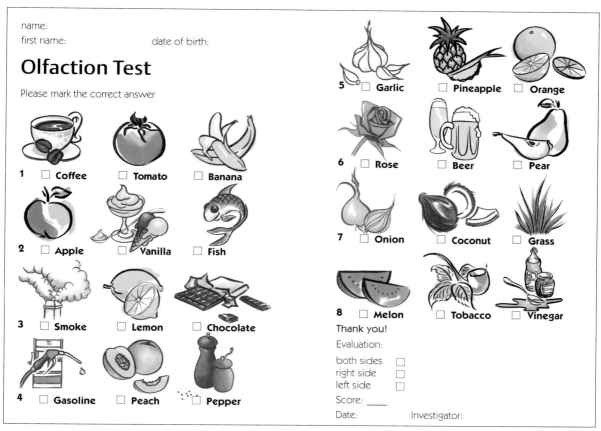

Fig. 3.**12** Smell screening test (patient questionnaire).

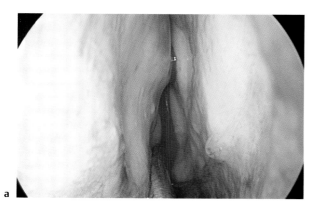

a

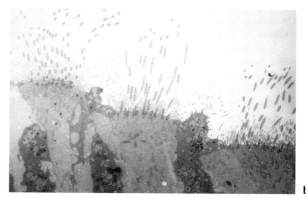

b

Fig. 3.**13** **a** The yellow color sometimes seen in functioning olfactory mucosa. The yellow color is more likely to be absent with anosmia after a neuropathic virus has damaged it. **b** Electron microscopy of olfactory mucosa.

pain it transpires that their symptoms are due to other neurological causes of facial pain. **DVD** 5

**Chronic rhinosinusitis** rarely causes pain unless it is exacerbated by an upper respiratory tract infection. Chronic rhinosinusitis can cause symptoms of pressure, but these usually coexist with other nasal symptoms, such as nasal obstruction, purulent rhinorrhea, and a disordered sense of smell.

In patients with nasal polyposis, facial pain that is due to rhinosinusitis is present only in about 12 % of patients, unless they have coexisting purulent disease, when it occurs in about 25 % of these patients (Fig. 3.**16**).

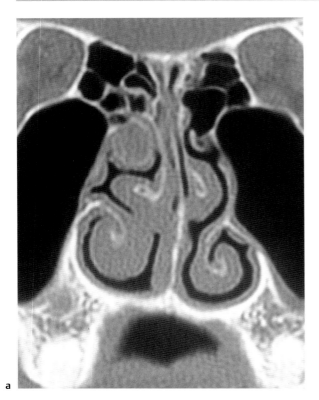

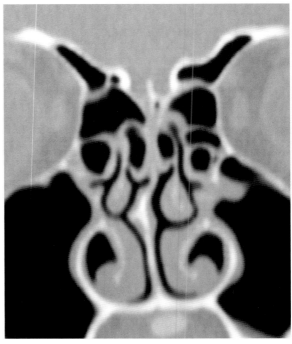

Fig. 3.**14 a**, **b**   CT scans of patients with obstruction of the olfactory cleft and hyposmia in spite of normal sinuses.

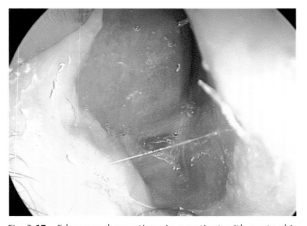

Fig. 3.**15**   Edema and secretions in a patient with acute rhinosinusitis.

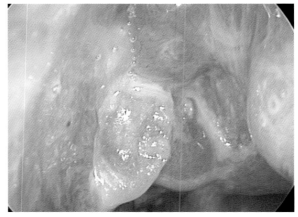

Fig. 3.**16**   Patients with polyposis who have mucopus are more likely to have coexisting symptoms of pain.

### Crusting

Crusting is a relatively uncommon symptom in patients who have not had nasal surgery. It is normally secondary to a septal perforation or a granulomatous disease, such as Wegener granulomatosis or sarcoidosis (Jennings et al., 1998; Fergie et al., 1999; Jones, 1999 b). It is a symptom that should make you take notice immediately and think of diagnoses other than allergic or infective rhinosinusitis (Fig. 3.**17 a**, **b**).

### Bleeding

Blood-stained mucus is a worrying symptom and should alert the surgeon to a possible malignancy or infective process. Many patients who are taking topical nasal steroids get some intermittent "spotting" of fresh blood when they blow their nose.

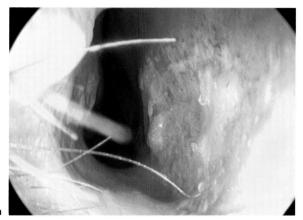

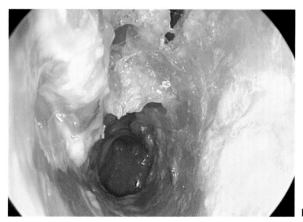

a  b

Fig. 3.**17**  **a** Dryness and crusting due to repeated nose picking. **b** The mucosal appearances seen in Wegener granulomatosis, with granulations and crusts.

### Relevant Symptoms Outside the Upper Respiratory Tract

#### Facial Swelling

Facial swelling, and in particular swelling of the cheek, is unusual with infective rhinosinusitis except where accompanied by periorbital cellulitis. The most common causes of swelling of the cheek are of dental origin (Fig. 3.**18**). In maxillary mucoceles, tumors, or where there is a dehiscence in the wall of the maxillary sinus, acute sinusitis can cause facial swelling—but this is unusual. Infective rhinosinusitis rarely causes swelling of the cheek. Many patients with midfacial segment pain (a form of tension-type headache of the midface) complain that their cheek is swollen when there is no abnormality to detect. This appears to be due to a sensory disturbance, and many of these patients also have hyperesthesia of the skin or soft tissues of the cheek or forehead. It appears that the threshold for somatosensory and nociceptive fibers is reduced in these patients.

#### Lower Respiratory Tract Problems

Does the patient have any lower respiratory tract problems? Why do we ask about this? Because the upper and lower respiratory tract are in continuity and share many common features—"The United Airways" (Fig. 3.**19**). Do they have asthma or bronchiectasis? Childhood asthma is often associated with evidence of type 1 hypersensitivity and a tendency toward intermittent rhinitis, although persistent rhinitis is also common. There may be a history of allergens exacerbating symptoms in these patients, e.g., hay fever, morning symptoms with an allergy to house dust mite, worse with pets, etc.

Patients with childhood allergic rhinitis and asthma are often atopic with positive skin-prick tests and

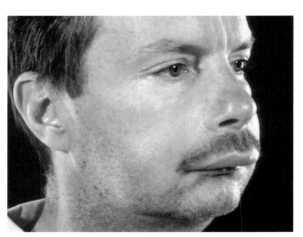

Fig. 3.**18**  A swollen cheek due to a dental infection—the most common cause.

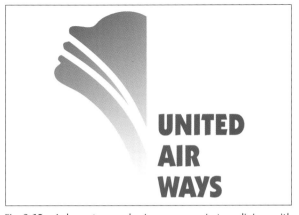

Fig. 3.**19**  A logo to emphasize one respiratory lining with nasal mucosa being in continuity with the trachea and bronchi—The United Airways. (© Erich W. Russi, Felix H. Sennhauser, Daniel B. Simmen, University of Zurich.)

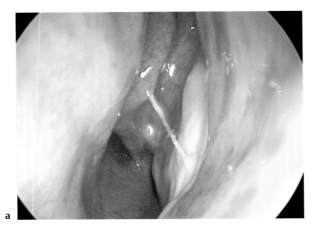

a

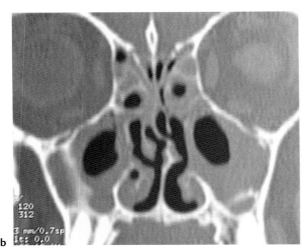

b

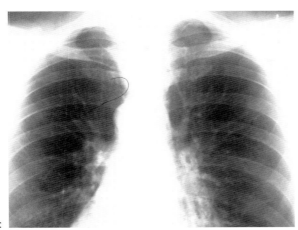

c

Fig. 3.**20**    **a** Purulent nasal secretions in a patient with ciliary dysmotility. **b** CT scan showing panrhinosinusitis in a patient with Kartagener syndrome. **c** Dextrocardia in Kartagener syndrome.

raised IgE levels and they differ from patients with late-onset asthma, who are often skin test negative and IgE negative, and who have no seasonal component or evidence of an atopic predisposition. In patients with a history of bronchiectasis, the possibility of ciliary dysmotility should be considered (Fig. 3.**20** a–c).  **DVD**  3

*Other Infections or Immunodeficiency*
Does the patient have other infections or is there any evidence of immunodeficiency? Have they had any of the following:

● Eight or more ear infections within a year?
● Two or more serious sinus infections within a year?
● Two or more months on antibiotics with little effect?
● Two or more pneumonias within one year?
● In an infant, failure to gain weight or to grow normally?
● Recurrent deep skin or organ abscesses?
● Persistent thrush in the mouth or elsewhere after the age of one year?
● A need for intravenous antibiotics to clear infections?
● Two or more deep-seated infections?
● A family history of immunodeficiency?

In these patients, the immune system must be investigated (Cooney and Jones, 2001).

**Previous Sinus Surgery**

See Chapter 2, p. 10.

**Is the Patient Systemically Well or Unwell?**

If the patient is systemically unwell and looks and feels ill, then consider connective-tissue disease and in particular vasculitis.

## Examination

Examination will provide objective information to support or cast doubt on the provisional diagnosis that may be made based on the history. Rigid nasal endoscopy is invaluable in assessing the lining of the nose and middle meatus, as well as that in the sphenoethmoid recess (Fig. 3.**21**). If nasal endoscopy is normal, the surgeon should be very wary about attributing any symptoms to rhinosinusitis. If the patient says that they are going through a good period and that this is not a representative time, then it is advisable to see them when they are symptomatic to confirm that rhinosinusitis is the cause of their problem. The majority of patients with allergic rhinitis have mucosal changes confined to the inferior turbinate, but some will have more generalized edema and this endoscopic appearance should be interpreted in light of their symptoms. Patients with late-onset asthma and rhinitis have more generalized mucosal disease affecting the lining of their nasal airway. More research is needed to improve our understanding about the pathogenesis of rhinosinusitis associated with late-onset asthma. It is important to look for the granulations associated with Wegener granulomatosis or sarcoidosis, as surgery will not help patients with these conditions. Check that there is no displacement of the orbit, which can occur with a mucocele (Beasley and Jones, 1995b; Muneer et al., 1998).

### Investigations

Skin-prick tests are helpful in determining whether someone has an allergic rhinitis and in demonstrating to them that it is their response to allergens that is partially or totally responsible for their symptoms (Fig. 3.22 a, b). This can help motivate a patient to comply with treatment and consider allergen avoidance. Total or specific IgE tests are less specific and sensitive but can help support a diagnosis in patients who are on antihistamines or steroids or in whom a skin-prick test is not helpful, e.g., in dermatographism.

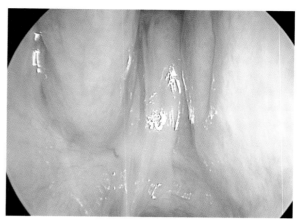

Fig. 3.**21** Nasal endoscopy showing mucopus tracking out of the sphenoid sinus.

It is helpful to use a peak flow meter for both adults and children. As many as 20% of patients with allergic rhinitis have asthma, and in some patients the coexisting asthma may not have been previously diagnosed (Fig. 3.**23**).

Immunological investigations are appropriate in patients who have the warning signs already mentioned earlier in this chapter (see p. 30). The initial in-

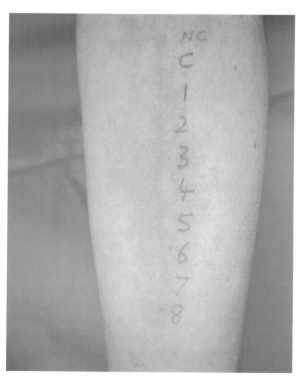

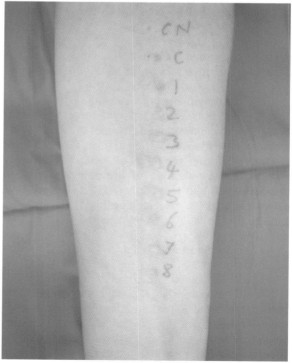

Fig. 3.**22**  **a** Skin-prick test positive to two species of house dust mite allergens. **b** Skin-prick test positive to a range of inhaled allergens.

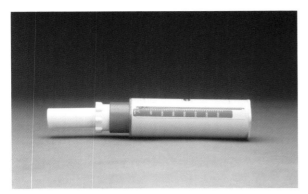

Fig. 3.**23**   A peak flow meter is useful in a rhinology clinic.

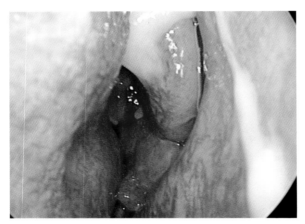

Fig. 3.**24**   Middle meatal mucopus in a patient with AIDS.

vestigations should include a full blood count and differential white cell count and total immunoglobulin levels for IgG, IgA, and IgM.

The collection of any organisms found in the nasal airway is best done using the sterile protective sheath of a large intravenous cannula in order to avoid picking up the commensals from the nasal vestibule.

Titers of specific IgGs for tetanus, Hib, and pneumococcus, and investigation of the patient's humoral response are indicated; if their IgG titers are low, patients should be vaccinated against these diseases, and the titers should then be repeated to check that they have improved.

An abnormal response needs to be discussed with an immunologist. The fasting glucose should be measured and you should consider whether an HIV test might be appropriate (Fig. 3.**24**). If these tests are normal, but in the light of the patient's progress or response to treatment there is concern about their immune function, then further investigations should be done in consultation with an immunologist.

## Response to Treatment

If the patient with purulent rhinosinusitis is not responding to the appropriate antibiotics, then the possibility of an immune deficiency, ciliary dysmotility, or an atypical infection, e.g., aspergillosis, should be considered. In general, a trial of medical treatment is almost always justified, not only for therapeutic reasons but in order to help in making a diagnosis.

## ■ Optimizing Medical Treatment

It is important to get the nasal lining as healthy as medical treatment will allow. This will not only help patients' symptoms but also minimize inflammation if surgery is required and help access and reduce intraoperative bleeding. Postoperatively, optimizing medical treatment will help maximize the benefit of any surgery. For example, opening the olfactory cleft may help improve the patient's sense of smell but it will be even better if there is no mucosal edema due to allergic rhinitis or any dryness and crusting from local staphylococcal infection and mucus stagnation.

### The Management of Allergic Rhinitis

The management of allergic rhinitis centers on allergen avoidance and compliance in the regular use of topical nasal steroids, which should be tried for at least 6 weeks in the first instance (Fig. 3.**25**). This applies to the symptom of nasal obstruction, although other symptoms such as itchy eyes and sneezing may also be helped in this way.

If the patient's primary symptoms are sneezing, itchy eyes, and clear rhinorrhea, then a nonsedative antihistamine can be given on its own or in conjunction with a topical nasal steroid for moderate or severe symptoms. Topical sodium cromoglycate works well for the symptoms of itchy eyes, but it is less effective intranasally. Topical antihistamines help some patients with sneezing and rhinorrhea, but they are not very helpful against symptoms of nasal obstruction. Ipratropium bromide can be given up to four times a day in isolation or in conjunction with these if rhinorrhea is a problem (Jones, 1999c).

Allergen avoidance has been shown to help patients who have a single allergy to house dust mite allergen. However, other allergen avoidance measures have not been shown to be helpful in clinical studies; although anecdotally they can contribute to controlling the patient's symptoms. Immunotherapy has a role to play, particularly when a single allergen, such as grass pollen, is responsible. Oral steroids can help control an acute exacerbation or help control symptoms initially while waiting for regular topical treatment and antihistamines to maintain the control of symptoms. It is important to be aware of drug interactions and side effects. Long-term intramuscular steroids should be avoided, because when side effects do occur with their use it is difficult to control them. The role of leukotriene inhibitors remains under investigation and is not yet proven.

Be aware that only 6% of patients with allergic rhinitis have hypertrophic or polypoidal mucosa, and that the majority of patients with nasal polyps do not have atopic disease. Patients with polyps and coexisting atopy usually respond well to the same treatment as those with rhinitis.

Nasal douching can be helpful particularly in patients who are troubled by mucus and crusting, but it may also have a cleansing action that helps to remove aeroallergens and cytokines (Fig. 3.26a, b).

For allergic rhinitis, the current *Allergic Rhinitis and Its Impact on Asthma* (ARIA) guidelines summarize the optimum medical treatment (Table 3.1). It is particularly important to check compliance with topical nasal steroids.

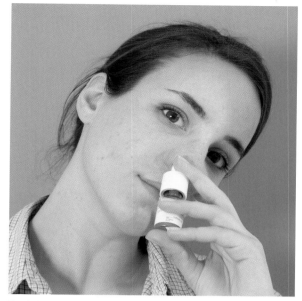

Fig. 3.**25**   Instruction on compliance and the use of topical nasal steroids is important. Use the left hand for the right nostril to avoid always hitting the same area of the septum.

## The Management of Nonallergic Rhinitis

While the pathophysiological cause of inflammation in these patients remains under dispute, the primary medical treatment is basically very similar to the treatment of allergic rhinitis, as it is anti-inflammatory. Topical and systemic steroids are used, along with nasal douching. Be careful not to overlook the patient who has overindulged in topical sympathomimetic agents and has rhinitis medicamentosa (Fig. 3.**27**). A small subset of this group has autonomic rhinitis, which is due to excessive parasympathetic stimulation. These patients are usually elderly and have clear rhinorrhea as their primary or only symptom and may respond to an ipratropium bromide spray used four times a day. Terms such as NENAR (noneosinophilic, nonallergic rhinitis) and NINAR (noninfective, nonallergic rhinitis) have been replaced by idiopathic rhinitis (Lund, 1994). The "dustbin" term of vasomotor rhinitis should be avoided and skin-prick test negative, IgE negative (and ideally nasal challenge negative) patients who have no evidence of infection

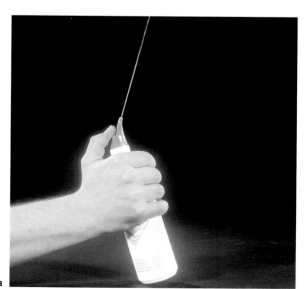

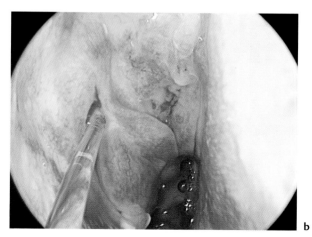

Fig. 3.**26**   **a** A proprietary saline nasal spray is convenient for douching the nose to clear stagnant mucus and debris. **b** A jet of water directed at the middle meatus.

Table 3.**1**   A summary of ARIA Guidelines. (World Health Organization Initiative Allergic Rhinitis and Its Impact on Asthma, 2001)

| |
|---|
| **Mild Intermittent** (see below for conjunctivitis)<br>Oral or intranasal $H_1$ antihistamines.<br>Intranasal decongestants ($<$ 10 days and not repeat more than twice a month).<br>Oral decongestants (not usually recommended in children).<br><br>**Moderate/Severe Intermittent** (see below for conjunctivitis)<br>Options (no preferred order):<br>• Oral or intranasal $H_1$ antihistamines.<br>• Oral $H_1$ antihistamines and decongestants.<br>• Intranasal glucocorticoids (chromones).<br>• Intramuscular injection of glucocorticoids is not usually recommended due to the possible occurrence of systemic side effects.<br><br>**Mild Persistent** (see below for conjunctivitis)<br>Options (no preferred order):<br>• As in moderate/severe intermittent, a stepwise approach is proposed. The patient should be reassessed after 2–4 weeks.<br>• If better, advised to continue. In perennial allergy, the dose may be reduced by half.<br>• If the patient has mild symptoms and is taking $H_1$ antihistamines or chromones: change to intranasal glucocorticoids. | **Moderate/Severe Persistent** (see below for conjunctivitis)<br>Intranasal glucocorticoids as first line treatment.<br>If very blocked, a short course of oral glucocorticoids may be added.<br>Alternatively, intranasal decongestants for less than 10 days.<br>If the patient does not improve:<br>• Consider the reason for failure: Inadequate compliance, nasal obstruction preventing delivery, additional nasal pathology, heavy persistent (avoidable?) allergen exposure, wrong diagnosis.<br>• Double dose of intranasal glucocorticoids if major symptom is blockage.<br>• Add $H_1$ antihistamines if major symptoms are sneezing, itching or rhinorrhea.<br>• Ipratropium bromide if the major symptom is rhinorrhea.<br>• If the patient does improve, a step-down approach should be used, but a minimal duration should be at least 3 months or for the pollen season.<br>• Referral to a specialist may be considered if the treatment is not fully effective or if after 3 months the treatment is unsuccessful.<br><br>**Management of Conjunctivitis**<br>Ocular $H_1$ antihistamines<br>Ocular chromones<br>Saline<br>Oral $H_1$ antihistamines |

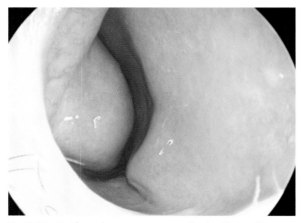

Fig. 3.**27**   Erythematous mucosa seen in rhinitis medicamentosa.

should be classified as having idiopathic rhinitis (Carney and Jones, 1996). The exception is the group with autonomic rhinitis, which has been described above.

## The Management of Infective Rhinosinusitis

Acute rhinosinusitis is usually due to *Haemophilus influenzae*, *Streptococcus pneumoniae*, and *Moraxella catarrhalis*. Where no amoxicillin-resistant *Haemophilus* exists in the local population, amoxicillin can be given along with a topical vasoconstrictor, such as 0.5% ephedrine for up to 5 days, along with a full week's course of amoxicillin and nasal douching. If *Haemophilus* resistant to amoxicillin is prevalent in the area, then an antibiotic such as amoxicillin with clavulanic acid is needed. In patients with chronic purulent rhinosinusitis, *Staphylococcus* and anaerobic organisms are more common, and it is important to give an antibiotic that will cover these. Antibiotics that cover the normal range of pathogens in chronic rhinosinusitis include amoxicillin with clavulanic acid, clindamycin, or metronidazole and a second- or third-generation cephalosporin. These antibiotics need to be given for up to 2 weeks to eradicate infection. Patients should be warned that their stool may become loose, and they should stop taking the antibiotics if they get diarrhea to avoid developing pseudomembranous colitis. Women should be warned that they may get vaginal thrush, for which an antifungal pessary may be necessary. Those on the contraceptive pill should take extra precautions over the following month.

In unilateral purulent disease, atypical infections such as aspergillosis should be borne in mind.

In general medicine, there is concern about giving steroids at the same time as antibiotics where there is purulent disease because of concern about immunosuppression. This does not appear to be an issue in rhinology, and it is often helpful to give antibiotics and topical or even systemic steroids unless the patient is systemically unwell or they have aspergillosis or the complications of infective rhinosinusitis.

Topical and systemic steroids are the mainstay of medical treatment in patients with chronic rhinosinusitis of all causes because the underlying mucosal pathology has a large inflammatory component and steroids reduce this. We advocate short but high-dose courses of systemic steroids when their use is indicated.

## The Management of Fungal Rhinosinusitis

In purulent rhinosinusitis that does not respond to two or more courses of antibiotics, the possibility of *Aspergillus* infection should be investigated (Fig. 3.**28 a**, **b**). The diagnosis of fungal disease centers on culture, skin-prick tests, CT scans, and titers of *Aspergillus* precipitins. Systemic antifungal treatment is indicated in fungal polyposis as it can dramatically reduce the amount of surgery needed. Invasive fungal disease requires long courses of itraconazole, unless the disease is of the acute fulminant type with blood vessel invasion, when intravenous amphotericin is needed. It is important to distinguish chronic expanding fungal disease that can erode bone and expand into neighboring areas from chronic invasive aspergillosis that leads not only to bone loss on CT but, most importantly, to penetration of soft tissues. Itraconazole has revolutionized the treatment of this condition. A 6- to 12-week course of itraconazole can be given before undertaking surgery. This will localize the disease and not only make surgery easier but allow more mucosa to be preserved. A 6-week postoperative course also reduces recurrence rates. It is important to monitor liver function and morning cortisol before and after one month of treatment with itraconazole, and liver function monthly thereafter.

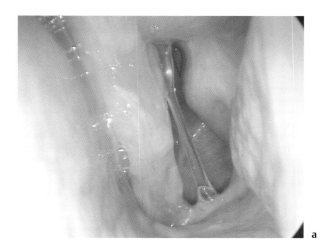

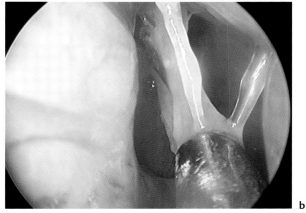

Fig. 3.**28 a**, **b**    Tenacious green discharge seen in aspergillosis.

## The Management of Chronic Rhinosinusitis with Polyposis

Polyps are not in themselves a diagnosis but a sign of inflamed mucosa, and patients who fall into this clinical category are usually managed in the same way as patients with chronic rhinosinusitis. Treat any bacterial infection if there are any purulent secretions (Fig. 3.**29 a**, **b**). Prescribe topical nasal steroids; if these fail, oral steroids should be tried unless there are contraindications. In patients with gross polyposis, we often give oral steroids initially, not only to help the patient immediately but also to see "how far up the skyscraper they can go" (see Fig. 3.**30**).

### The Use of Systemic Steroids

Systemic steroids are normally reserved for patients with rhinosinusitis and polyposis, although they can help those patients with allergic rhinitis who are resistant to other forms of treatment. We give only short courses of oral steroids so as to minimize side effects.

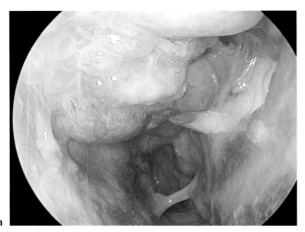
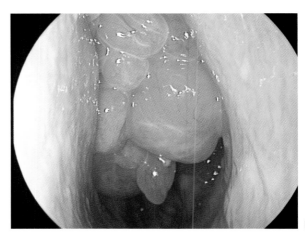

a                                                                                                         b

Fig. 3.**29 a, b**    A patient with recurrent polyposis after previous surgery who had a coexisting infection and responded to antibacterial treatment and topical nasal steroids.

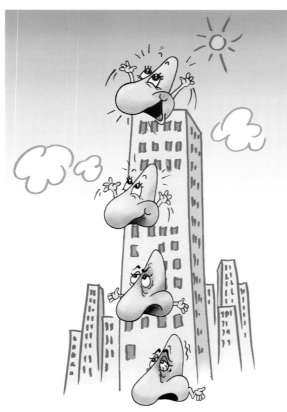

Fig 3.**30**    Skyscraper illustrating levels of treatment success. We use this illustration when discussing treatment options with patients.

The reason for using oral steroids in nasal polyposis is to reverse mucosal changes when other measures have failed (Fig. 3.31 a, b). Normally, topical nasal steroids, along with allergen avoidance and antihistamines, will control symptoms. However, a small group does have symptoms such as mucosal edema that persist even when they have complied with treatment for over 8 weeks. This is more common in nonallergic patients, particularly those with late-onset asthma. Under these circumstances, oral steroids may reverse the mucosal edema, but the degree of success varies, as does the duration of the improvement.

The reasons for using oral steroids in rhinosinusitis with nasal polyposis are:
• To reduce polyp bulk, allowing access for topical steroids
• To determine the extent of the "olfactory reserve"
• To preoperatively help reduce mucosal inflammation

In the majority of patients, the effect of a trial of oral steroids lasts only a few weeks and, in spite of maintenance treatment with topical steroids, their symptoms return. In these patients, surgery may help if obstruction or hyposmia are their main symptoms, although it is vital that the patient is aware that surgery is not a "cure" for their mucosal disease. If surgery is planned, a further course of preoperative steroids will reduce bleeding and the amount of surgery required. By allowing more mucosa to be preserved, particularly in the olfactory cleft, adhesions will be minimized and postoperative recovery will be improved as ciliary recovery will be better.

A dose of 40–70 mg (depending on body mass) of prednisolone with breakfast for 4–7 days is recommended as a means of maximizing the anti-inflammatory component of medical treatment of nasal polyposis in patients with marked allergic rhinitis or nonallergic rhinitis when other treatments have failed or in the immediate preoperative period.

It is important to check that there are no contraindications (diabetes, cardiac disease, gastric or duodenal

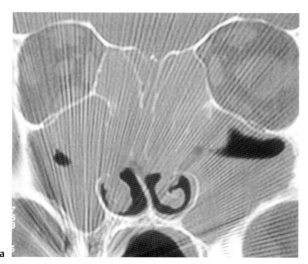

a

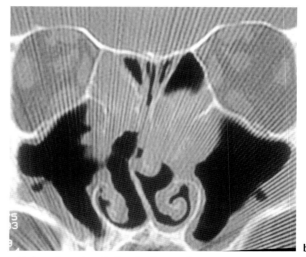

b

Fig. 3.**31 a**, **b**   CT scans showing the effect of a course of oral steroids in polyposis. **a** Before **b** afterwards.

ulcers, osteoporosis, etc.). Patients should be warned of the potential side effects: patients sometimes become excited or very active, some become depressed; the steroids should be stopped if they cause indigestion or stomach pain. The possibility of rare complications, such as ischemia of the femoral head or vertebral collapse, should be mentioned (Fig. 3.**32**).

## Optimizing the Timing of Surgery

It is important not only to maximize preoperative medical treatment in order to see how much the patient's disease can be reversed by medical means. It is worth continuing this treatment right up to the time of their potential surgery. This makes the surgery easier and reduces peroperative bleeding, which helps visibility and reduces the risk of peroperative complications (Fig. 3.**33 a**, **b**). It reduces the chance of adhesions forming and helps the surgeon to preserve mucosa. This is particularly important in the olfactory area, where it is vital to preserve as much olfactory mucosa as possible (Fig. 3.**34 a**, **b**). Having failed to fully control the patient's disease with medical treatment does not mean that you should give it up at the point where you list them for surgery.

Maximum medical treatment often demonstrates to the patient and the surgeon the amount of olfactory reserve or potential there is available. However, all too often the benefit of systemic steroids on the patient's ability to smell is short-lived. The surgeon is then in a good position to explain to the patient that they need surgery in conjunction with medical treatment to provide benefit in the long term (Fig. 3.**35**). If the patient's sense of smell fails to return after a course of steroids and they have had previous nasal surgery, it may mean

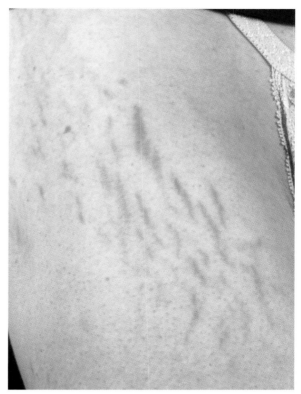

Fig. 3.**32**   Striae of the thigh after oral steroids and excessive betamethasone nose drops.

that their olfactory mucosa has already been removed, so that it is then advisable to be cautious about saying whether further surgery will help their sense of smell.

If a patient has severe nasal polyps, particularly medial to the middle turbinate, it is worth giving them a preoperative course of oral steroids to reduce the

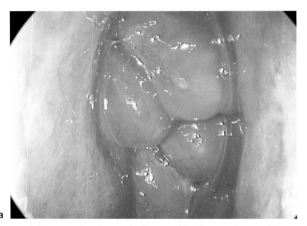
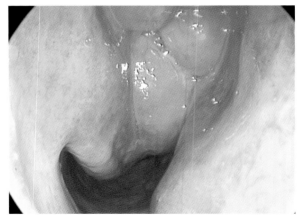

a    b

Fig. 3.**33**   Nasal polyps **a** before and **b** after oral steroids, just prior to surgery.

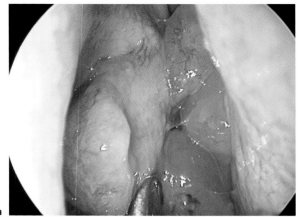
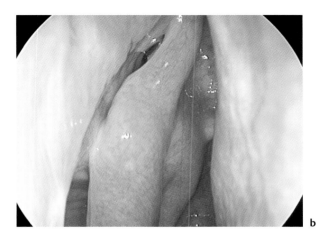

a    b

Fig. 3.**34**   Polyps in the olfactory cleft **a** before and **b** after surgery. The polyps were not removed medial to the middle turbinate. They have responded to the cleft being opened and topical nasal steroids.

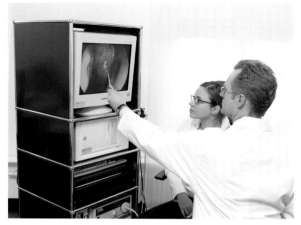

Fig. 3.**35**   It is vital to explain to the patient what can realistically be achieved.

amount of mucosal swelling, as long as there are no contraindications (Fig. 3.**36 a–d**). This will enable the surgeon to preserve as much olfactory mucosa as possible.

A full-thickness loss of mucosa results in healing by secondary intention and crusting that lasts up to one year before mucosa with cilia regenerates (Fig. 3.**37**). If the mucosa is relatively healthy at the time, it is easier to preserve the mucosa and remove the bone that will allow the sinuses to be opened, albeit with the mucosa that overlies these segments of bone. The purpose of surgery is not to denude the bone of mucosa. Exposed bone can cause a severe, nasty, dull, nagging ache due to osteitis (akin to a "dry socket" after a dental extraction) with pain lasting 10 days—another reason for preserving mucosa. It takes up to 3 months for cilia to return to partially denuded mucosa, and the patient will have to continue douching over this period to minimize crusting and mucus stagnation.

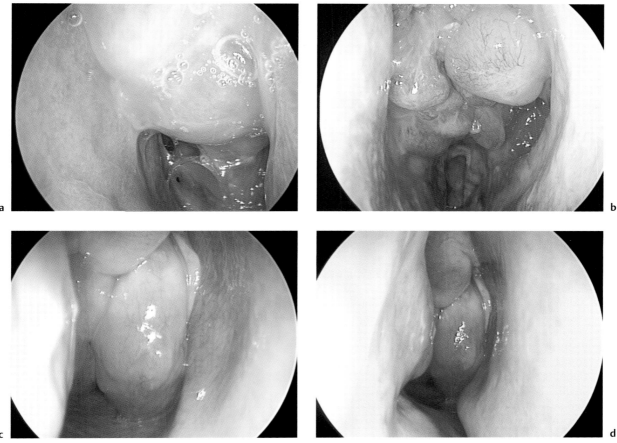

Fig. 3.**36 a, b**  The effect of preoperative oral steroids. With less inflamed polyps the bleeding and the potential for compli- cations is reduced because of improved visibility. **c, d** A dif- ferent case before and after oral steroids.

It is wise not to embark on surgery when a patient has developed, or has just had, an upper respiratory tract infection, as the amount of bleeding will be increased and the risk of developing a chest infection will be increased as well.

In summary, we would advise operating on patients when their nasal mucosa is as healthy as it is possible to get it by medical means.

**Remember:**
- Any surgeon can operate; a good surgeon operates on the right patient at the right time.
- Only operate when it is likely to result in substantial benefit to the patient.

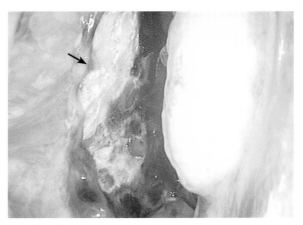

Fig. 3.**37**  Crusting over an area of exposed bone (arrow) where the full thickness of mucosa has been lost.

# 4 Why?
## Goals of Surgery in Patients with Rhinosinusitis

### ■ Why Surgery Can Help the Diseased Mucosa

Surgery in patients with rhinosinusitis can have several goals. These goals very much depend on the nature of the underlying pathology (Table 4.1; Fig. 4.1 a, b):
- Opening sinus ostia to help restore mucociliary function.
- Removing diseased tissue to relieve the symptoms of nasal obstruction.
- Aiding the delivery and distribution of topical nasal treatment to any diseased mucosa, and in particular to the paranasal sinuses.
- Reducing the surface area from which diseased mucosa arise, e.g., polyposis.
- Opening the olfactory cleft to improve sense of smell.
- Removal of diseased tissue in benign nasal lesions (the treatment of inverted papilloma needs qualifying).
- Removal of foreign material from the sinuses: e.g., a dental root in the maxillary sinus, saprophytic aspergillosis.
- Reducing mucosa–mucosa contact: this is thought by some to be a factor in the etiology of polyposis. Removing contact areas also improves mucociliary clearance.

- Removal of bony anatomical variations causing obstruction of the airway, e.g., a very large concha bullosa.

However, it is important to emphasize that many nasal and paranasal sinus conditions are due to mucosal disease that is associated with the upregulation and production of inflammatory mediators or a reduced immunity. There may be a genetic predisposition, e.g., atopy and allergic rhinitis, or in a few cases an inherited immunodeficiency; but in many there are inflammatory changes that are poorly understood, e.g., late-onset asthma and polyposis.

### ■ Rationale and Goals of Surgery in Specific Conditions

The reasons for surgery in specific conditions other than rhinosinusitis are more straightforward and are discussed below.

#### Unknown Pathology/Biopsy
- Histology is vital in order to make the right treatment plan (Diamantopopolous and Jones, 2000) (Fig. 4.2 a, b).

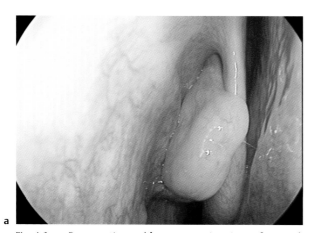
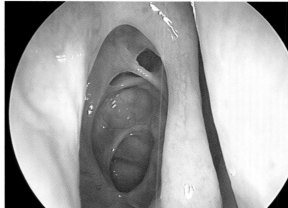

a          b

Fig. 4.1 **a** Preoperative and **b** postoperative views after a sphenoethmoidectomy—this illustrates many of the goals listed.

Table 4.**1**    Goals of surgery in chronic rhinosinusitis

| Pathology | Goals | Realistic expectations for each symptom category |
|---|---|---|
| Chronic bacterial rhinosinusitis (resistant to medical treatment) | Improve mucociliary clearance and sinus aeration; allow douching (Stammberger, 1986) | • *Obstruction:* Help<br>• *Smell:* Partial loss is often helped<br>• *Mucus:* Mucky. It becomes clear but may not cease<br>• *Pressure or pain:* Can be helped if there is a good association with the above symptoms, if there are exacerbations with purulent episodes, and if the pain is better when the mucus is no longer purulent after antibiotics |
| Recurrent acute bacterial rhinosinusitis (check if genuine, best to witness at least one episode and confirm with endoscope) | Improve mucociliary clearance and sinus aeration and alter the environment to make it less favorable for pathogens | • *Obstruction:* Not an associated symptom<br>• *Smell:* Not an associated symptom<br>• *Mucus:* Not an associated symptom<br>• *Pressure or pain:* Can be helped, but be cautious, as many types of facial pain and pressure are not due to rhinosinusitis. It is best to have good objective evidence at endoscopy or CT (even then, 1 in 3 of asymptomatic people have changes on CT) |
| Fungal rhinosinusitis (mycetoma, non-allergic, non-invasive form of aspergillosis) | Improve mucociliary clearance and sinus aeration and alter the environment to make it unsuitable for pathogens. | • *Obstruction:* If polyposis, surgery will help<br>• *Smell:* If associated with polyposis, will help<br>• *Mucus:* One of the few conditions where surgery does usually reduce mucus production<br>• *Pressure or pain:* It is unusual for pain or pressure to be a feature of any form of fungal infection |
| Idiopathic polyposis ("simple" inflammatory) | Debulk the diseased mucosa; reduce the mucosal surface area; aid access for douching and topical nasal treatment | • *Obstruction:* Improvement, average return of symptoms 6 years<br>• *Smell:* Normally quoted as 70% better, but often does not persist for > 6 months in spite of topical treatment. With opening of the olfactory cleft (see text), the results are better<br>• *Mucus:* Disappointing<br>• *Pressure or pain:* Infrequently associated with polyposis |
| Polyposis associated with late-onset asthma | Reduce the mucosal surface area; reduce mucosa–mucosa contact; restore mucociliary clearance; aid access for topical nasal treatment | • *Obstruction:* Helps<br>• *Smell:* Usually quoted as 70% better but often for < 6 months. If the ethmoid sinuses are removed to allow lateralization of the middle turbinate, the improvement is superior in quality and length of time<br>• *Mucus:* Inconsistent<br>• *Pressure or pain:* Rarely a symptom |
| Polyposis associated with asthma and aspirin sensitivity | Debulk disease and reduce the surface area from which polyps can originate | • *Obstruction:* Helps, but symptoms are often only better for 12–48 months<br>• *Smell:* Disappointing<br>• *Mucus:* Disappointing<br>• *Pressure or pain:* Rarely a symptom |
| Polyposis associated with purulent disease | Restore mucociliary clearance, reduce the mucosal surface area, aerate sinuses | • *Obstruction:* Good<br>• *Smell:* Good<br>• *Mucus:* Good<br>• *Pressure or pain:* Good |
| Polyposis associated with cystic fibrosis | Debulk diseased tissue; reduce the mucosal surface area; restore mucociliary clearance; aid access for douching and topical nasal treatment | • *Obstruction:* Good, but often not > 12 months<br>• *Smell:* Poor<br>• *Mucus:* No improvement—needs regular douching<br>• *Pressure or pain:* Rarely a symptom in this condition |

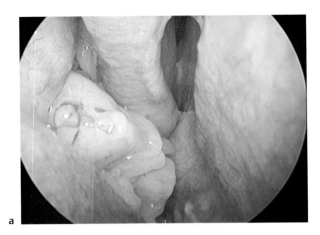

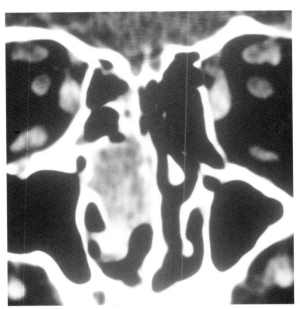

Fig. 4.**2**   **a** A harmless-looking polyp in the right middle meatus. **b** A CT image of the harmless looking polyp in **a**, which proved to be an adenocarcinoma.

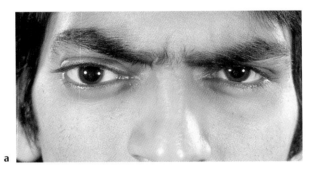

Fig. 4.**3**   **a** Clinical and **b** CT views showing a right frontal mucocele.

- Endoscopic access and visibility are often best (Howard and Lund, 1993).
- Studying the CT image helps to define the site for biopsy.
- Inflammatory polyps occur around a malignant lesion—avoid sampling only these.
- Endoscopic biopsy is associated with less morbidity than an external approach in some circumstances, e.g., the pterygopalatine fossa or orbit.
- An exception is an angiofibroma, as its MRI features are diagnostic.

## Mucoceles

- The primary goal is marsupialization and not enucleation.
- Wide drainage with preservation of mucosa around the lumen. (Fig. 4.3 a, b).
- If accessible, endoscopic drainage provides less morbidity (Kennedy, 1994).   **DVD** 10

## Antrochoanal Polyp

Remove the entire polyp along with its stalk and base (Fig. 4.4 a, b).

## Benign and Malignant Tumors

- Ensure total resection is achievable endoscopically, or warn the patient if an external approach may be needed (Fig. 4.5 a–4.7 b).
- Endoscopic postoperative monitoring helps to detect any recurrence.

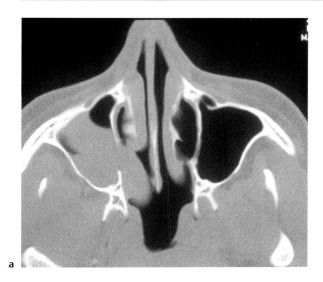

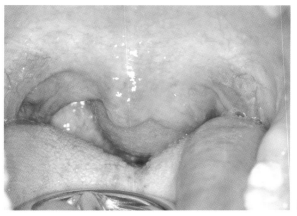

Fig. 4.**4**   **a** Axial CT scan and **b** an endoscopic view of an antrochoanal polyp that has extended into the nasopharynx and oropharynx.

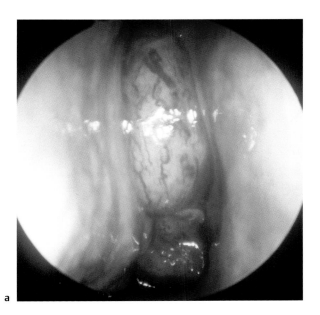

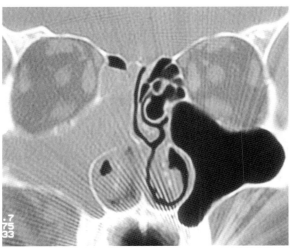

Fig. 4.**5 a**, **b**   Adenoameloblastoma that originated from the maxilla, for which a lateral rhinotomy may be needed to complete the resection.

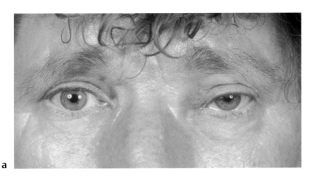

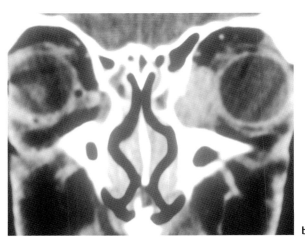

Fig. 4.**6 a**, **b**   Lymphoma of the left orbit that also produced a nasal polyp. A biopsy of this helped make the diagnosis.

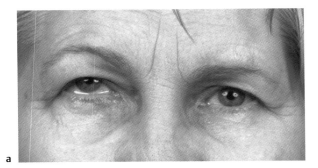

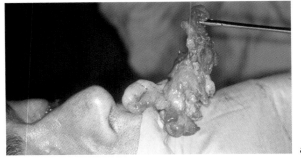

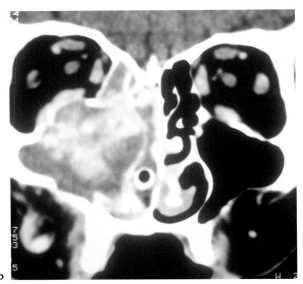

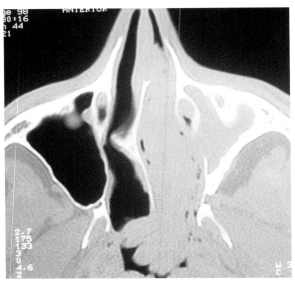

Fig. 4.**7 a** Facial appearance and **b** CT findings in an amelanotic melanoma of the right paranasal sinuses that presented with epiphora and epistaxis.

Fig. 4.**8 a** Peroperative and **b** CT views of an inverted papilloma—it should be checked for any evidence of atypia or malignancy.

## Inverted Papilloma

- The key goal is to remove all macroscopic disease.
- This tissue must be examined for atypia or malignancy. Malignant transformation is rare if there is no evidence of atypia or malignancy in the resected tissue (Fig. 4.**8 a, b**).
- You need to inform the patient if external access may be needed, e.g., disease within the frontal sinus. **DVD** 14

## Periorbital Abscess

- Drainage of pus defined on CT (Fig. 4.**9 a, b**).

## Barotrauma

- Ventilate the sinus and preserve mucosa at all cost.

## Choanal Atresia

- Endoscopes aid access and visibility to allow an adequate airway.
- Cause as little trauma as possible to the mucosa (Fig. 4.**10 a, b**).

## Epistaxis

- Localizing the site of bleeding is of the utmost importance.
- Avoid packing as this causes trauma to the nasal mucosa, making it difficult to find the site (Fig. 4.**11 a, b**).
- A primary aim is to occlude the vessel near its distal site. **DVD** 13

## Distal Nasolacrimal Duct Obstruction

- A dacryocystorhinostomy creates a nasal fistula or rhinostomy in distal nasolacrimal duct obstruction (Fig. 4.**12 a–c**).

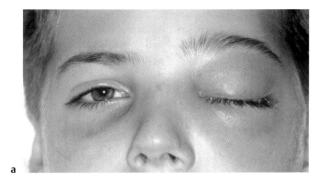
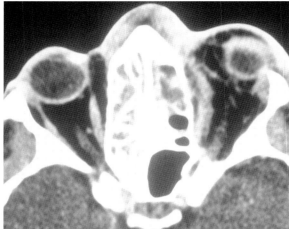

Fig. 4.**9**    **a** A left periorbital abscess, also shown on axial CT (**b**).

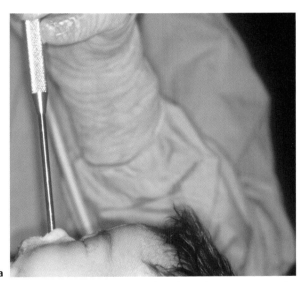
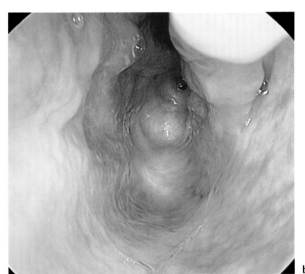

Fig. 4.**10 a**, **b**    Surgical view of left choanal atresia in a newborn child with bilateral atresia

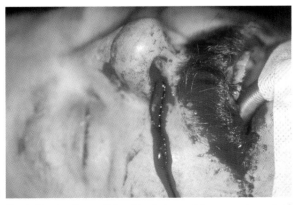
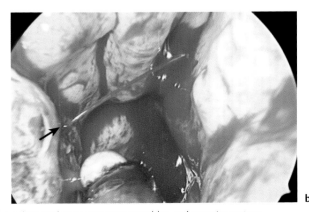

Fig. 4.**11 a**, **b**    Torrential epistaxis (arrow) from one branch of the sphenopalatine artery stopped by endoscopic cautery.

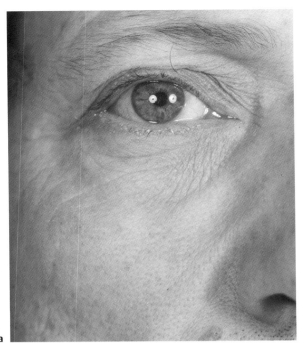

a

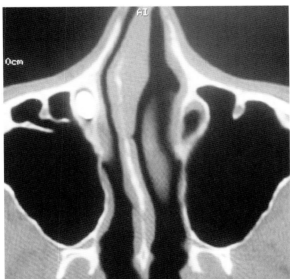

b

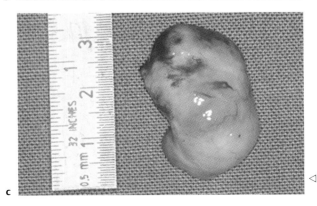

c

- A dacryocystorhinostomy is less effective in the presence of coexisting proximal obstruction.
- A dacryocystorhinostomy may help functional outflow obstruction, but with mixed results.   **DVD** 18

### Repair of Dural and Skull Base Defects

- Confirm that it is a true CSF leak (beta-2-transferrin) (Fig. 4.**13 a–c**).
- Precisely localize the defect.
- Endoscopic multilayered occlusion gives best results.
- Tell patients with defects of the frontal sinus that an external approach may be required.
- Not suitable if associated with malignancy.
- High-pressure leaks also need a shunt.   **DVD** 15

### Pituitary Surgery

- To provide access and visibility for tumor removal. **DVD** 17

### Decompression of the Orbit

- The orbit may require decompression for cosmetic reasons.
- Decompress the orbital contents for corneal exposure, pain, or compromised optic nerve function (Fig. 4.**14 a**, **b**).
- Helps in dysthyroid eye disease with reducing vision when steroids and radiotherapy fail.

### Decompression of the Optic Nerve

- Early in the presence of reduced vision after trauma to the optic nerve.
- Visual evoked potentials are important as a useful objective test in lightly anesthetized or unconscious patients (Jones, 1997) (Fig. 4.**15 a–c**).

### ■ Quality of Life

Chronic rhinosinusitis has a significant adverse effect on patients' perception of quality of life (Gliklich and Metson, 1995). Over the last few years, there has been an increasing realization that improving nasal symptoms has a dramatic effect on patients' enjoyment of life that goes far beyond the nose (Fig. 4.**16**). Discussion of this issue is also important in convincing healthcare providers that sinus surgery is of great value.

◁ Fig. 4.**12 a–c**   Epiphora due to a dacryolith in the nasolacrimal sac.

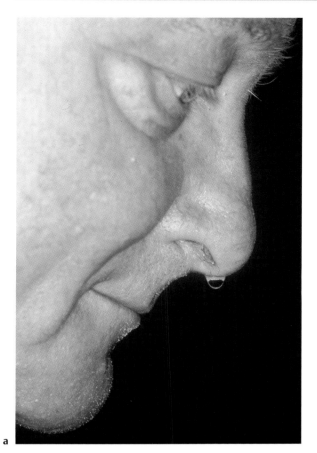

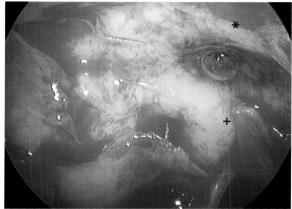

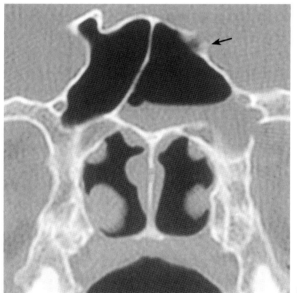

Fig. 4.**13**  **a** Clear unilateral rhinorrhea due to a CSF leak. **b** Endoscopic view of the left sphenoid sinus showing a CSF leak from the sphenoid sinus between the optic nerve (∗) and carotid artery (+). **c** Axial CT scan showing the same defect (arrow) as in **b** with a fluid level of CSF.

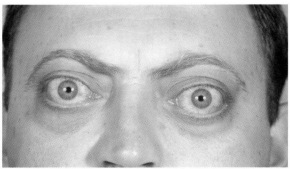

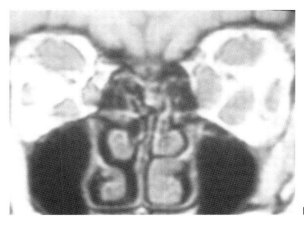

Fig. 4.**14**  **a** Bilateral proptosis in dysthyroid eye disease at danger from corneal ulceration. **b** Coronal MR image showing muscle hypertrophy due to dysthyroid eye disease.

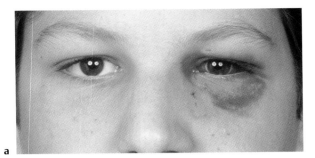

a

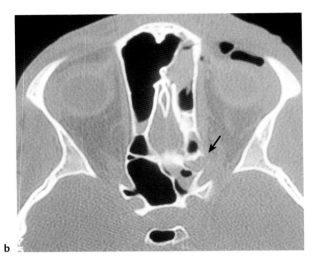

b

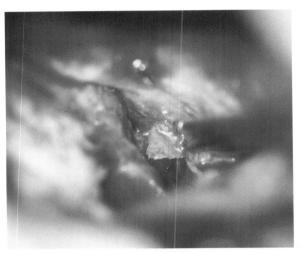

c

Fig. 4.**15**   **a** Left enophthalmos, periorbital ecchymosis, and subconjunctival hemorrhage secondary to a fracture of the medial wall of the orbit. **b** An axial CT scan showing disruption of the medial wall of the orbit toward its apex (arrow). **c** Peroperative endoscopic view showing the bony spicule that was pressing on the optic nerve.

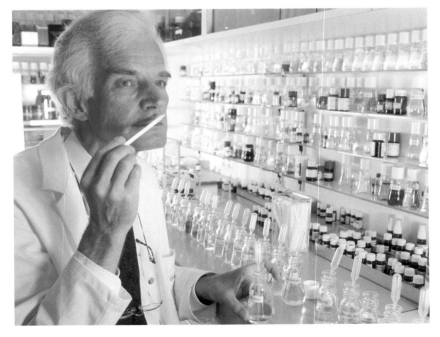

Fig. 4.**16**   A smell scientist testing new odors.

Endoscopic sinus surgery for chronic sinusitis results in an improvement in a general indicator of health, namely the SF-36 "Health Survey Questionnaire," as well as in disease-related symptoms (Winstead and Barnett, 1998). The greatest negative general health impact of chronic rhinosinusitis in the study by Winstead and Barnett was on bodily pain, social functioning, and vitality when compared with a control group. These criteria were improved 12 months after surgery, along with physical functioning, mental health, and emotional status. Endoscopic sinus surgery has also been shown to improve pulmonary function in patients with asthma and chronic rhinosinusitis (Ikeda et al., 1999), with an improvement in their average peak expiratory flow and a reduction in their need for corticosteroids.

In spite of these positive studies, we need to improve our understanding of the pathophysiology of rhinological conditions, their definition, and the staging procedures, and to validate all of these in order for us to improve the way we compare treatment strategies.

# 5 How?
## Operative Procedures: A Step-by-Step Safe and Logical Approach

This chapter focuses on technique. As the chapter progresses, so does the complexity of the procedures described, but throughout we emphasize the need to consider whether the surgeon really needs to do more or not. The format is deliberately didactic in order to make clear to the reader the exact extent of each procedure (Fig. 5.1). **DVD** 8

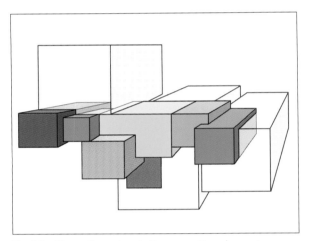

Fig. 5.1 Three-dimensional diagrammatic scheme to represent the anatomical compartments and the surgical steps possible in endoscopic sinus surgery.

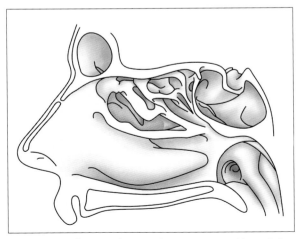

Fig. 5.2 Line diagram showing the area removed in an infundibulotomy (uncinectomy).

## ■ Procedures

**Terminology of procedures:**
- Infundibulotomy (uncinectomy) ■
  ± Maxillary sinusotomy (I, II, III) ■
- Partial anterior ethmoidectomy ■ ■
- Frontoethmoidectomy ■ ■ ■
  ± Frontal sinusotomy (I, II, III) ■
- Sphenoethmoidectomy ■ ■ ■
  ± Sphenoid sinusotomy (I, II, III) ■
- Frontosphenoethmoidectomy ■ ■ ■ ■
  ± Maxillary sinusotomy (I, II, III) ■
  ± Frontal sinusotomy (I, II, III) ■
  ± Sphenoid sinusotomy (I, II, III) ■
- Sphenoid sinusotomy (I, II, III) ■

## ■ Infundibulotomy (Uncinectomy) ■
### ± Maxillary Sinusotomy (I, II, III) ■
**DVD** 6, 7, 8

### Terminology and Classification

**Infundibulotomy:** Removal of the uncinate process with preservation of the mucosa around the natural maxillary ostium (Fig. 5.2). The upper part of the uncinate process is left intact if it is attached to the skull base or middle turbinate, in order to avoid any instrumentation near the frontal recess.

It often seems easier to continue rather than to stop, but ask yourself why you should do any more surgery. Doing unnecessary surgery increases not only bleeding but the risk of complications such as adhesion formation, causing a CSF leak and, in particular, damaging the frontal recess. This is a good example of "less is more."

**Maxillary sinusotomy I:** The natural maxillary ostium is enlarged posteriorly to a limited extent, and no more than 1 cm. If there is an accessory ostium, this is joined to the natural ostium (Fig. 5.3).

**Maxillary sinusotomy II:** Open the antrostomy to a diameter of approximately 2 cm, opening it posteriorly and inferiorly (Fig. 5.4).

**Maxillary sinusotomy III:** The antrostomy is extended close to the level of the posterior wall of the maxillary antrum and anterior to the lacrimal sac and inferiorly to the base of the inferior turbinate (Fig. 5.5).

## Indications

- An infundibulotomy as a sole procedure is done for isolated purulent maxillary sinusitis.
- An infundibulotomy is the key first step in most procedures for chronic rhinosinusitis.
- Join accessory anterior or posterior fontanelles as they are said to run the risk of producing a circular motion of mucus from one ostium to the other, thus providing a never-ending cycle that is prone to infection (Fig. 5.**6 a–c**).
- In cystic fibrosis, a wide ostium may help local irrigation and the mechanical clearance of retained secretions.
- There is some evidence that a type II maxillary sinusotomy helps atopic patients as a type I maxillary sinusotomy is prone to closing from mucosal hypertrophy (Davis et al., 1991).
- If there is maxillary sinus pathology that requires more access (type III maxillary sinusotomy): e.g., an antrochoanal polyp, where it is important to remove the base of the retention cyst, otherwise it will reform.
- A mycetoma (Fig. 5.**7 a**, **b**), foreign body, or persistent maxillary sinus problems secondary to dental problems that have received treatment, and also in polypoid maxillary disease.
- If there are extensive polyps within the maxillary sinus we would recommend using a microdebrider or through-cutting forceps to debulk these and not to strip the mucosa as to remove it would result in healing by secondary intention with long-term crusting or pooling of pus.
- In patients who are to undergo extensive ethmoid surgery or surgery geared to improving their sense of smell, it is necessary to open the maxillary ostium inferiorly so that when the middle turbinate is lateralized to open the olfactory cleft it is still possible for the sinus to drain and for the surgeon to obtain access to be able to inspect it (Fig. 5.**8 a**, **b**). Note that in patients who need to have their olfactory cleft opened, the maxillary sinusotomy should extend below the inferior edge of the middle turbinate so that it remains patent.

## Anatomy

The uncinate process is shaped like a rudder (Fig. 5.**9**); its superior extension can do one of the following:
- Merge with an agger nasi air cell or the lateral nasal wall to form a blind-ended pocket called the sulcus terminalis.
- Insert into the skull base, forming an overhang that can limit anterior access to the frontal recess.
- Insert into the middle turbinate and form a web that guards the frontal recess.

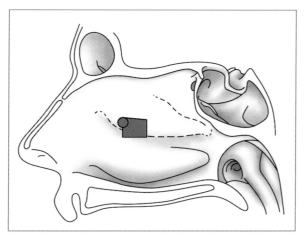

Fig. 5.**3** Line diagram showing the area of bone and mucosa to be removed in a maxillary sinusotomy type I.

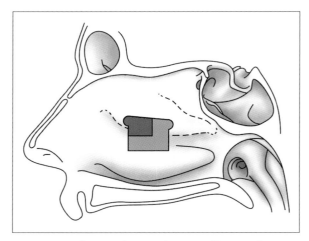

Fig. 5.**4** Line diagram showing the area of bone and mucosa to be removed in a maxillary sinusotomy type II.

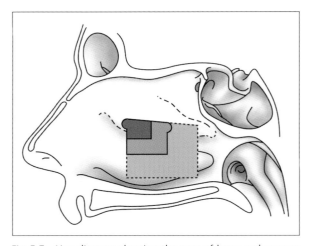

Fig. 5.**5** Line diagram showing the area of bone and mucosa to be removed in a maxillary sinusotomy type III.

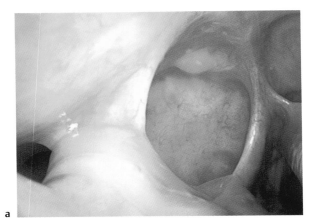

Fig. 5.**6**   **a** Endoscopic view of circulating mucus between an incomplete opening of the anterior natural ostium and a large posterior ostium. **b** The coronal CT scans show the obstructed natural anterior ostium and **c** the wider posterior ostium, away from the natural ostium.

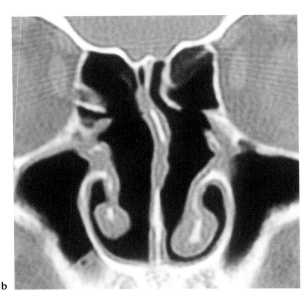

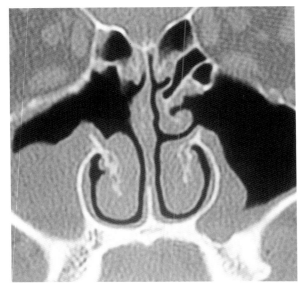

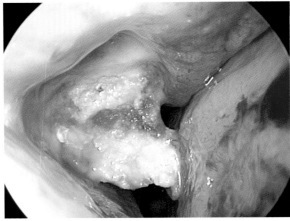

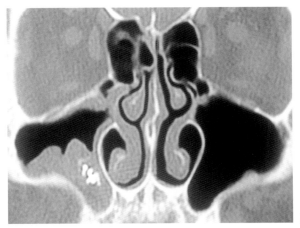

Fig. 5.**7**   **a** Endoscopic view of a mycetoma in the right maxillary sinus. **b** Coronal CT scan of the patient.

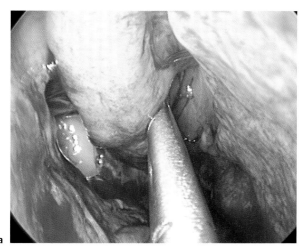
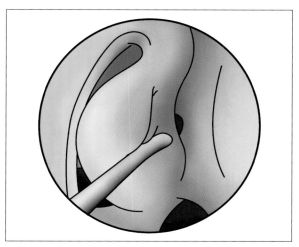

a  b

Fig. 5.**8**  **a** The maxillary sinusotomy is extended below the margin of the middle turbinate to help ensure that mucociliary clearance can take place. **b** A line diagram of **a**.

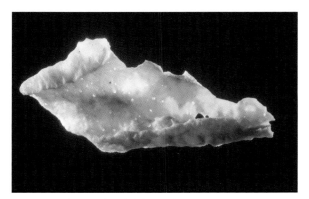

Fig. 5.**9**  A disarticulated right uncinate process.

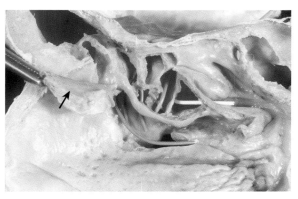

Fig. 5.**10**  The uncinate process (arrow) has been lifted forward to reveal the natural ostium of the maxillary sinus. The green wire is in the position of the infundibulum of the anterior ethmoid sinuses.

The uncinate process "guards" the natural maxillary ostium to form a slitlike corridor to it, the infundibulum ethmoidale (Fig. 5.**10**). The entrance to this corridor is the hiatus semilunaris (anterior), a crescent-shaped space at the posterior edge of the uncinate process (Fig. 5.**11**). The uncinate process is made up of very thin bone that attaches anteriorly to the bone adjacent to the nasolacrimal duct, so it is important not to come too far forward when removing the uncinate process. It extends upward to insert into the lateral nasal wall in approximately 70 % of patients and into the skull base or the middle turbinate in the remaining 30 %. The insertion of the uncinate process determines whether the frontal sinus drains directly into the middle meatus (type A) or into the infundibulum ethmoidale lateral to the uncinate process (type B) (Fig. 5.**12**).

The uncinate process is normally in a sagittal plane, although polyps in the infundibulum can push its post-

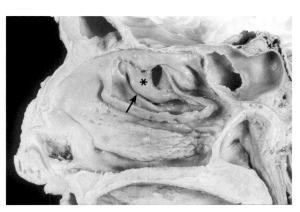

Fig. 5.**11**  A window has been made in the middle turbinate to reveal the edge of the uncinate process (arrow), the hiatus semilunaris, and the ethmoid bulla ( * ).

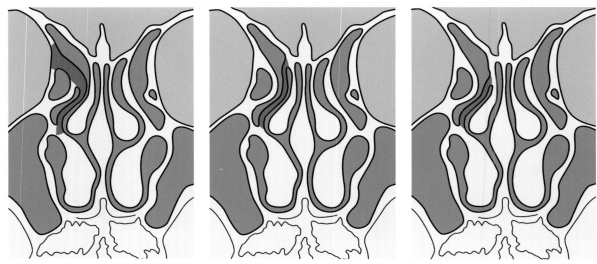

Fig. 5.**12**   This shows a type A uncinate process (left), where the frontal sinus drains directly into the middle meatus, and types B1 (center),where the uncinate process attaches to the skull base, and B2 (right), where the uncinate process attaches to the middle turbinate. Both B1 and B2 have the frontal sinus draining into the infundibulum ethmoidale.

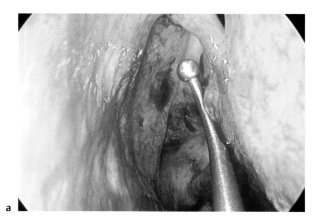

a

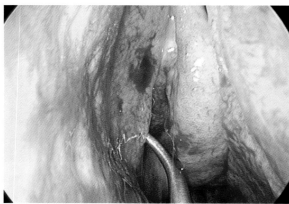

b

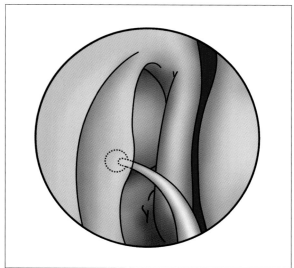

c

Fig. 5.**13 a–c**   Palpating around the edge of the uncinate process with a ball probe.

erior edge medially. In less than 1 % of healthy individuals, it can be paradoxical, curving forward on itself. It rarely contains a pneumatized cell. It is very thin and any incision through it only needs to be about 1 mm; any more and it could go through other structures that are more lateral to it. These may be anterior ethmoid air cells, but in many patients there are no cells between it and the orbit. Inferiorly, it is attached to the base of the inferior turbinate, and together these fill most of the bony defect of the medial wall of the maxillary sinus. The remainder of the medial wall of the maxillary sinus has no bone and is made up of mucosa. It forms the anterior and posterior fontanelles. It is possible to ballotte these areas that consist solely of mucosa with a curved, olive-ended sucker to help locate them. An anterior branch of the sphenopalatine artery runs in the medial wall of the maxillary sinus and is sufficiently large that opening the maxillary ostium posteriorly to within 0.5 cm of the posterior wall of the maxillary sinus will lead to bleeding.

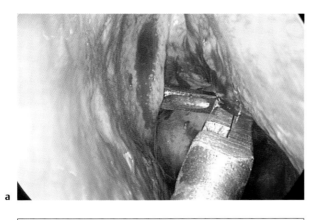
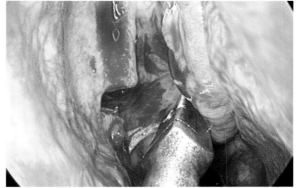

a

b

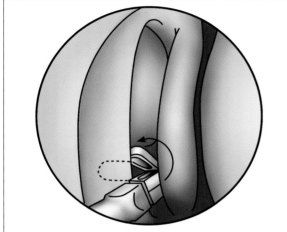
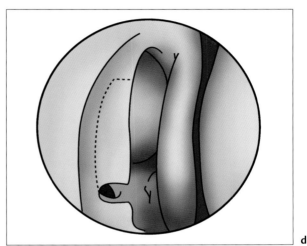

c

d

Fig. 5.**14 a–d**   The backbiter is fed around the edge of the uncinate process and an inferior horizontal bite is taken.

## Surgical Technique

It is best to assess the endoscopic findings and coronal CT images together in order to work out the position and insertion of the uncinate process before starting surgery. We recommend using a 0° endoscope for almost every procedure outside the frontal sinus. The optics of the 0° endoscope give minimal distortion and this reduces the likelihood of the surgeon losing their orientation. Check that the maxillary sinus is not hypoplastic and whether there is a large infraorbital cell (Haller cell) present, as this may alter your approach. An infraorbital cell is an inferiorly placed anterior ethmoidal air cell that is attached to the floor of the orbit in the roof of the maxillary sinus.

With a hypoplastic maxillary sinus you must stay low toward the base of the inferior turbinate in order to avoid entering the orbit. With an infraorbital cell you need to particularly check, when undertaking a middle meatal antrostomy, that you have opened the maxillary ostium widely, and not simply entered the infraorbital cell. Occasionally the lateral wall is dehiscent and then the orbit is easily entered. Under these

circumstances, it is particularly helpful to ballotte the closed eye while endoscopically inspecting the area to see whether the orbital contents prolapse into the nasal airway. It is important to do this at the beginning of surgery if there has been previous surgery.

The uncinate process is defined endoscopically by palpating it laterally with the side of a Freer's elevator or a ball probe (Fig. 5.**13 a–c**). It is mobile, unlike the rigid anterior lacrimal crest. A curved seeker can be used to gently palpate the posterior edge of the uncinate process and then be passed around its inferior edge anteriorly to feel the site of the natural ostium.

There are several ways to do an uncinectomy. For the inexperienced surgeon, a retrograde approach is safer and runs less risk of inadvertently entering the orbit. A closed Rhinoforce Stammberger antrum punch (back-biter) is advanced into the middle meatus behind the posterior edge of the uncinate process and then rotated so that the "finger" of the back-biter opens upward. This finger can then be fed into the infundibulum and the back-biter rotated so that it lies horizontally (Fig. 5.**14 a–d**).

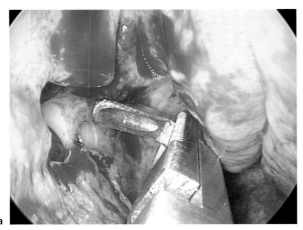
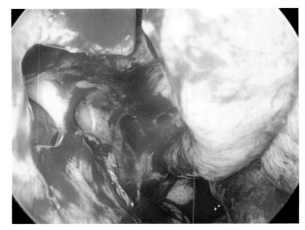

a                                                                                                                                    b

Fig. 5.**15 a**, **b**    The backbiter can be used to reduce the uncinate process, with multiple segments being removed.

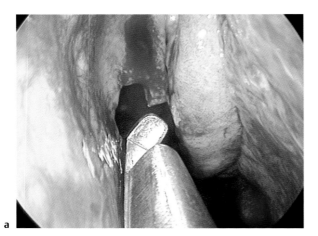
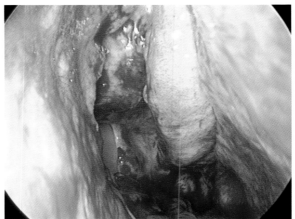

a                                                                                                                                    c

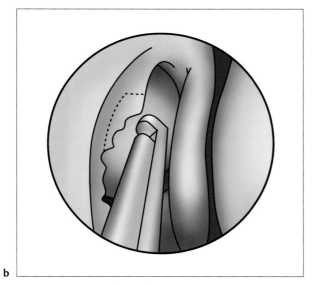

b

Fig. 5.**16 a–c**    A Hajek punch being used to remove the uncinate process.

It is best to take the first bite as low as possible near the base of the uncinate process. When the back-biters are closed they should not meet any significant bony resistance as the uncinate process is thin. If anything more than minimal resistance is met, then the back-biters should not be closed as the nasolacrimal duct may be damaged. Back-biters can take more than one bite at a time without having to be cleaned. The back-biters can then be fed upward to take a bite higher up (Fig. 5.**15 a**, **b**), thus creating a "door" of the uncinate process that can be opened or folded forward on its anterior hinge. The door of the uncinate process can then be removed using through cutters, a Hajek punch or one of the microdebriders that can "digest" bone (Fig. 5.**16 a–c**).

An alternative is to remove just the inferior strip with the back-biters and then use the 45° through cutters to nibble away upward at the uncinate process incrementally. If an infundibulectomy is all that is indicated, there is no need to follow it up to the middle turbinate or skull base if it is attached there.

The more experienced surgeon may perform an un-cinectomy by palpating the lateral wall in order to define the position of the anterior lacrimal crest, which is totally rigid unlike the uncinate process, which gives way to some extent. A sickle knife or a Freer's elevator is used to incise the uncinate process near its top edge and then to run it down in a sagittal plane, being careful not to go through it more than 1 mm, and then extend the incision inferiorly (Fig. 5.**17 a, b**).

On the patient's right side a "C" shape of mucosa and uncinate is incised, and on the other side the shape is reversed. While the incision is being made, the shoulder of the sickle knife can be used to mobilize the uncinate process medially. The initial incision can be started half way up and then extended in either direction (Fig. 5.**18 a–d**). The sickle knife is used to medialize the uncinate process in order to reveal the infundibulum; the natural ostium may also be seen. The line diagrams illustrate one way of making this incision. The remaining superior attachment can be cut with Zurich scissors or Rhinoforce Blakesley (through-cutting) forceps and the same is done at its inferior attachment (Fig. 5.**19 a–h**). With this maneuver, this segment of the uncinate process can be removed without tearing any mucosa.

Often there are tags of mucosa that need to be trimmed with through-cutting forceps or a microde-brider. If the sickle knife comes up against hard bone then this is likely to be the anterior lacrimal crest, meaning that the incision has been started too far anteriorly. Whichever method is used, as soon as the sickle knife has gone through the uncinate process, it should be medialized so that the operator can check the position of the uncinate process and the depth of the incision. It is best to use through-cutting forceps or scissors to cut mucosal tags, as to grasp them with forceps and pull runs the risk of tearing the mucosa off the lateral wall. When this happens, it can come off the lateral wall like steamed wallpaper being pulled. This would run the risk of causing stenosis of the frontonasal recess. If forceps are the only instrument available, then they should be rotated laterally toward the lateral wall in order to minimize the chance of peeling the mucosa off the lateral nasal wall.

Remember that while the uncinate process inserts into the lamina papyracea or lateral nasal wall in 70% of patients, in the other 30% of patients it is attached to the skull base or middle turbinate, and under these circumstances it will extend up to the "armpit" where the middle turbinate attaches to the lateral nasal wall and guards the frontal recess. It is unnecessary to remove the uncinate process this high up in these circumstances, unless there is good reason for operating in the frontal recess area.

Whichever method is used, there is usually a small "stub" of uncinate process remaining at its inferior at-

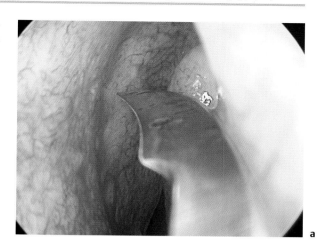
a

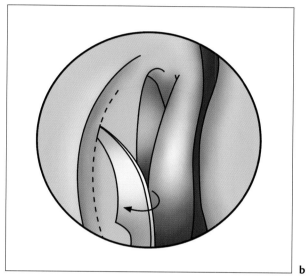
b

Fig. 5.**17 a, b**  The sickle knife is used with caution, incising only 1 mm—which is all that is needed to go through the uncinate process—and is kept in the sagittal plane as much as possible.

tachment just medial to and below the natural maxillary ostia (Fig. 5.**19 g, h**). This little piece of bone is best dissected out with the end of a fine ball probe and the mucosal remnants shaved off or trimmed with side-biting forceps.

The natural ostium can usually be visualized, but if not it can be palpated gently with a ball probe, a curette, or an olive-ended right-angled sucker unattached to the suction tube (Fig. 5.**20 a–f**). When this is done, minimal pressure should be required and it is important to direct the end of the seeker downward and laterally and to search for it from the level of the attachment of the inferior turbinate so as to minimize the chance of inadvertently entering the orbit. If the maxillary ostium cannot be seen it is likely that an insufficient amount of uncinate process has been removed; this can be

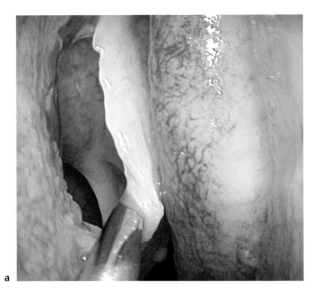

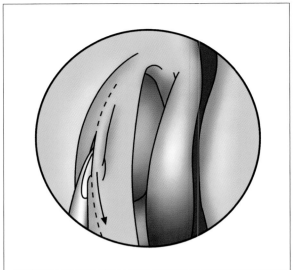

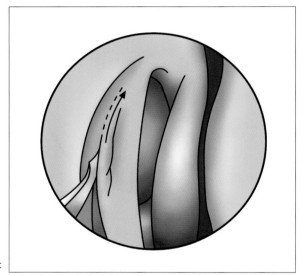

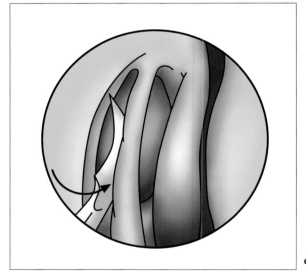

Fig. 5.**18**  **a** A right uncinectomy with the uncinate process medialized to reveal the natural maxillary ostium. **b** One method for doing an uncinectomy is to initially incise downward with a sickle knife. **c** Next turn the sickle knife around and incise in the opposite direction. **d** The uncinate process is then medialized to help define its remaining superior or inferior attachments.

trimmed either with back-biting forceps or with side-biting forceps until it is visible. Sometimes palpating the lateral nasal wall will produce a bubble out of the ostium that will locate its position.

In an infundibulotomy, where there is no reason to enlarge the natural ostium, it is important not to scuff the mucosa on the posteroinferior aspect of the natural maxillary ostium, as mucociliary clearance passes around this aspect along the lateral wall of the nose under the ethmoid bulla. Unless there are good reasons for opening the maxillary ostium it is best left

alone as opening it runs the risk of causing scar tissue around its margin that may interfere with mucociliary clearance.  **DVD** 6, 7, 8

## Alternative Surgical Techniques

Occasionally, in a very narrow nose, where access is restricted by a narrow pyriform aperture, finding the maxillary ostia can be difficult, particularly if there is active purulent disease and a great deal of bleeding with any instrumentation in the middle meatus. While

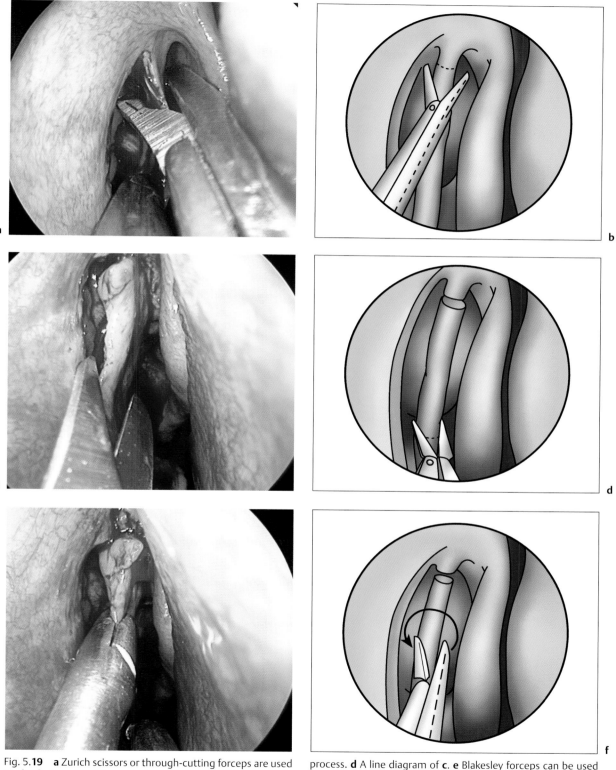

Fig. 5.**19**　**a** Zurich scissors or through-cutting forceps are used to divide any remaining superior attachment of the uncinate process. **b** A line diagram of **a**. **c** Zurich scissors are used to divide any remaining inferior attachment of the uncinate process. **d** A line diagram of **c**. **e** Blakesley forceps can be used to grasp the uncinate and rotate it laterally to free any remaining attachment. **f** A line diagram of **e**.

Fig. 5.**19 g, h**　▷

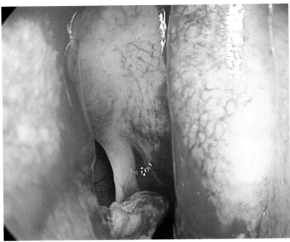

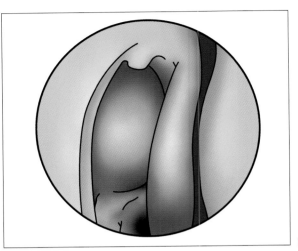

Fig. 5.**19**   **g** The natural maxillary ostium is exposed and a small part of the uncinate process is left attached both superiorly and inferiorly. **h** A line diagram of **g**.

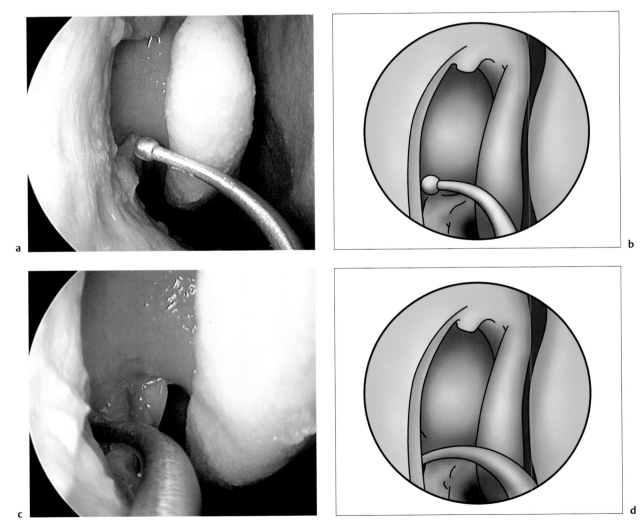

Fig. 5.**20 a–f**   The ball probe is used to palpate in order to locate the position of the natural ostium. Only use it as a probe and direct it downward away from the orbit.

Fig. 5.**20 e, f**   ▷

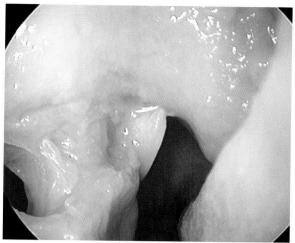

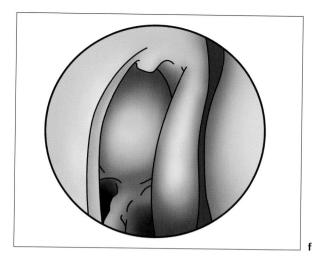

e

Fig. 5.**20 e, f**

f

the surgeon is advised not to continue if they cannot see adequately, it is unusual not to be able to gain sufficient control with local vasoconstrictors to make it possible to undertake a middle meatal antrostomy.

The "lazy" way of undertaking a middle meatal antrostomy is reserved for difficult situations when the natural ostium cannot be identified. A right-angled, olive-ended sucker not attached to the suction is used to palpate the posterior fontanelle. This area has no bone and the mucosa "gives" easily with little pressure. It is important to palpate where the inferior turbinate comes off the lateral wall and to point the curved sucker downward and laterally at 45° from the horizontal plane. When the area of the posterior fontanelle is identified, the sucker can be used to enter the maxillary sinus. This is best done relatively abruptly (as long as there is no evidence of a hypoplastic maxillary antrum on CT) so that mucosa on the medial wall of the maxillary sinus is punctured neatly and not torn off the medial bony wall of the antrum.

The sucker is then pushed and pulled forward a little to open a false ostium that is akin to a posterior fontanelle. A back-biter is inserted in this hole, having been introduced posterior to its position, and its jaws are opened widely so as to engage both the lining of the medial wall of the maxillary sinus and the mucosa of the lateral wall of the nose. Multiple bites are then taken to widen this and to come forward and join up the maxillary ostium. The uncinate process can be taken up with these bites and, as this is a crude way of undertaking an uncinectomy along with a middle meatal antrostomy, it can salvage a difficult situation.

It is important not to come too far anteriorly, in order to avoid the nasolacrimal system, but it is important to remove the uncinate process, because to leave most of it in position above the maxillary ostium encourages the formation of polyps in this crevice.

In a minority of revision cases there is so much thick osteitic bone that an anterior approach is best. This involves making an incision just anterior to the lacrimal crest and raising the mucosa posteriorly to reveal the uncinate process as it joins the lacrimal crest. The most medial lip of the lacrimal crest needs to be drilled away in order to improve visibility and access (Fig. 5.**21 a, b**).

### Maxillary Sinusotomy (I, II, III)

First of all, the natural ostium is identified. In a type I sinusotomy (Fig. 5.**22 a, b**), it is opened posteriorly to a limited extent (< 1 cm diameter) with through-cutting instruments. In a type II, it is opened further posteriorly and inferiorly (< 2 cm diameter) (Fig. 5.**23 a, b**).

A type III involves wide exposure opening of the ostium in all directions. It is possible to open it: anteriorly to the lacrimal crest; inferiorly to the base of the inferior turbinate; superiorly to the orbit; and posteriorly, level with the posterior wall of the maxillary sinus (Fig. 5.**24 a, b**). If the sinusotomy extends to within 0.5 cm of the posterior wall, a branch of the sphenopalatine artery often requires cautery.

When opening the maxillary ostium it is important not to grab and pull on any loose pieces of mucosa that line the maxillary sinus as this often leads to the whole lining starting to strip off its wall like a pig's bladder. These loose tags are best left alone or sheared with through-cutting forceps or a shaver. The most useful instruments for opening a maxillary ostium are the straight, through-cutting forceps; the movable jaw of the forceps is placed in the antrum and the bone can be nibbled away in a controlled fashion (Fig. 5.**25 a, b**).

Anteriorly, back-biters should be used carefully in order to avoid damaging the nasolacrimal sac. If any resistance is felt, the operator should stop, as it is likely

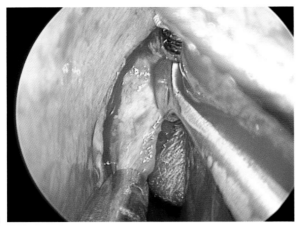
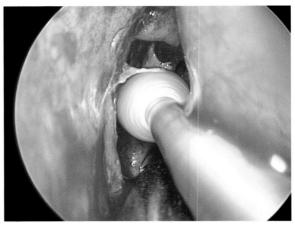

a

b

Fig. 5.**21**    **a** In a revision case where the landmarks for the uncinate process have been lost, the hard white bone of the lacrimal
crest is exposed. **b** The lacrimal crest is reduced with a coarse diamond burr to help expose and define the uncinate process.

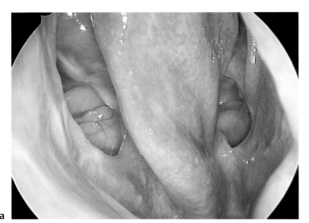
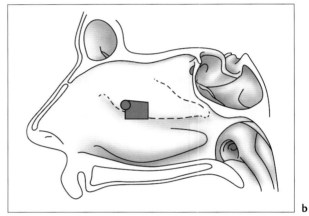

a

b

Fig. 5.**22 a**, **b**    A type I sinusotomy can be opened posteriorly to a limited extent with through-cutting instruments.

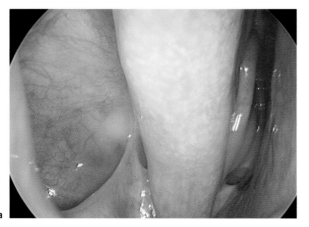
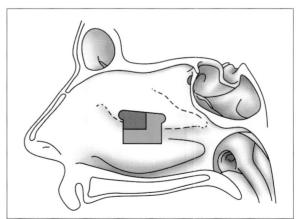

a

b

Fig. 5.**23 a**, **b**    A type II sinusotomy is done if it is thought that the middle turbinate may lateralize.

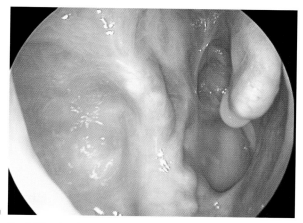
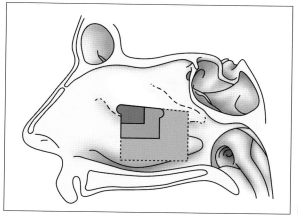

a                                                                                                              b

Fig. 5.**24 a, b**    A type III sinusotomy is done if the middle turbinate is deliberately lateralized at the end of the procedure in order to open up the olfactory cleft.

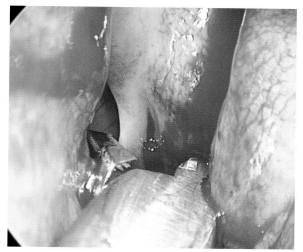
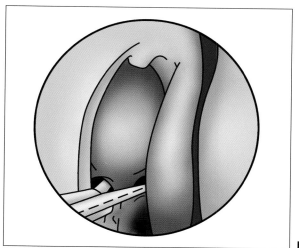

a                                                                                                              b

Fig. 5.**25**    **a** Endoscopic view and **b** line diagram of the natural ostium being joined to a posterior accessory ostium using through-cutting forceps.

that the nasolacrimal apparatus will be damaged. Superiorly, there may be a low anterior ethmoidal air cell based on the lamina papyracea or roof of the maxillary sinus. The extent of this should be estimated from the CT scan and if a large antrostomy is to be undertaken this can be palpated with a curved sucker and opened using the side of 45° Blakesley forceps while the assistant is observing the eye.

## Useful Instruments

A ball probe helps to define the posterior edge of the uncinate process if there is doubt about its position and can normally be passed around the edge and the position of the maxillary ostium felt. Rhinoforce Stammberger antrum punches (back-biters) are thin and easily passed into the middle meatus with the jaws closed

before the jaw is opened and rotated into the infundibulum. Forty-five degree, through-cutting punches are useful to incrementally remove the uncinate process. A ball probe is useful to dissect out the inferior remnant of the uncinate process (Fig. 5.**26 a**, **b**).

Powered instrumentation can also be used to tidy up the remaining tags of soft tissue. The straight, through-cutting punch is ideal for the controlled removal of the medial wall of the maxillary sinus posteriorly. The Stammberger side-biting antrum punch forceps (side-biters) are useful in opening the maxillary ostium inferiorly (Fig. 5.**27 a–d**). As these bite into the base of the inferior turbinate, this can cause more bleeding; occasionally they can bite through the whole section, through the roof of the inferior meatus, but this does not appear to cause any problem (Fig. 5.**28 a**, **b**).

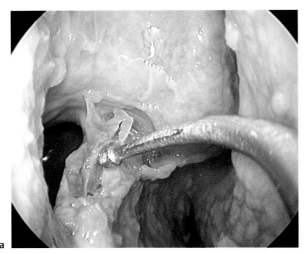
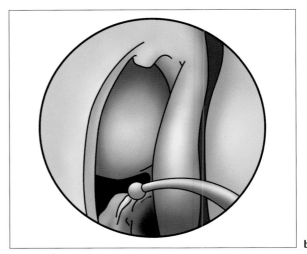

a

b

Fig. 5.**26 a, b**   A ball probe is used to remove the small inferior remnant of the uncinate process.

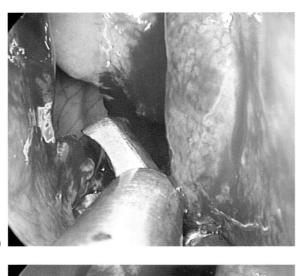
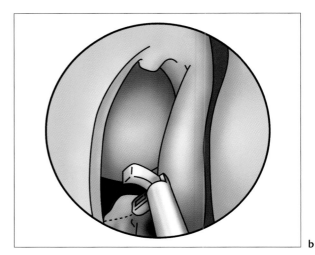

a

b

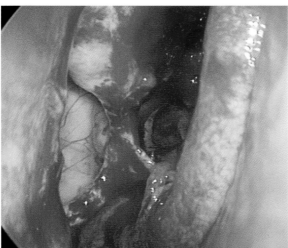
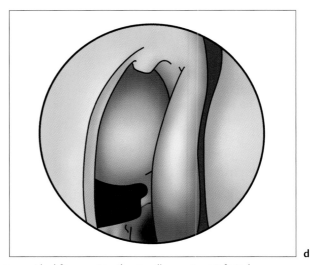

c

d

Fig. 5.**27 a–d**   The Stammberger side-biting antrum punch forceps are ideal for opening the maxillary ostium inferiorly.

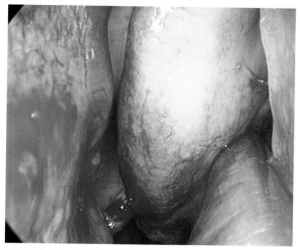

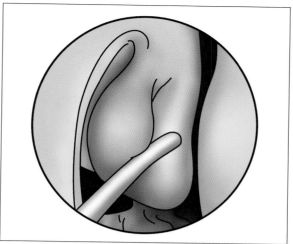

Fig. 5.**28 a, b**  The size of the sinusotomy is checked to see that it extends below the rim of the inferior turbinate if it is planned that it needs to be lateralized.

## ■ Partial Anterior Ethmoidectomy ■ ■

### Terminology and Classification

Partial anterior ethmoidectomy involves an infundibulotomy including a partial resection of the anterior ethmoid air cells. The infundibulotomy can be extended to open the anterior ethmoidal cells, to the basal lamella, and to open the agger nasi air cells, but not to open them entirely as this would mean instrumenting the frontal recess. A key point is to avoid instrumenting the frontal recess as this runs the risk of causing stenosis (Fig. 5.**29**).  **DVD** 7, 8

### Indications

- This is done for isolated anterior ethmoid and or maxillary sinus/frontal sinus disease that has not responded to maximum medical treatment.
- It is worth limiting surgery to the anterior ethmoid sinuses before entering the frontal recess, because this is often all that is necessary. As soon as you instrument the frontal recess you greatly increase the risk of causing iatrogenic disease (Kennedy, 1992).
- If surgical treatment to the anterior ethmoid sinuses is followed by medical treatment, the frontal sinus usually clears without any further intervention.

Surgery can be limited to the anterior ethmoid air cells when disease is localized to this area, such as in limited inflammatory polyps, inverted papilloma, or fungal disease (Fig. 5.**30**).

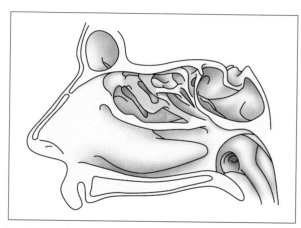

Fig. 5.**29**  A line diagram showing the extent of a partial anterior ethmoidectomy.

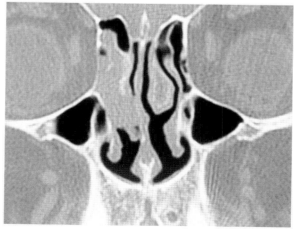

Fig. 5.**30**  Very localized inverted papilloma, localized to the anterior ethmoid sinuses.

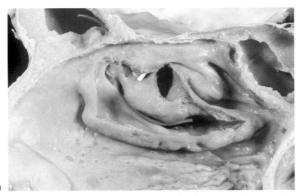
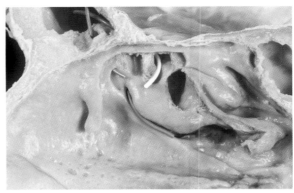

a

b

Fig. 5.**31 a**, **b**   The green wire lies in the hiatus semilunaris; the blue wire is in a bulla frontalis whose roof has been opened in the specimen in **b**. The red wire is in the frontal sinus that drains above the uncinate process—type A. The white wire marks the suprabullar recess area, and behind the bulla lie the retrobullar recess and the basal lamella.

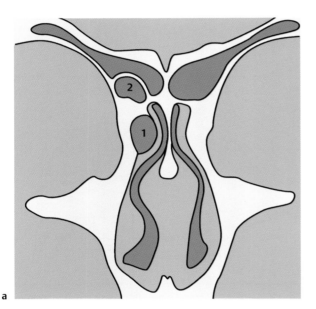

a

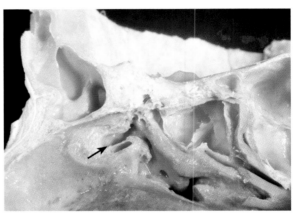

b

Fig. 5.**32**   **a** A line diagram of an agger nasi cell (1) with a bulla frontalis (2) extending into the frontal sinus. **b** The uncinate process and middle turbinate have been removed to reveal an agger nasi cell (arrow) as the most anterior cell in lateral nasal wall.

## Anatomy

The ethmoid bulla is a consistent landmark unless the patient has had previous surgery. Its ostium normally opens posteriorly or medially. It can be attached to the skull base. If it is not attached to the skull base, a suprabullar recess is formed and the anterior ethmoid artery is often found in this area. The space that forms behind the ethmoid bulla is called the retrobullar recess. The posterior wall of the retrobullar recess is made up of the basal lamella of the middle turbinate (Fig. 5.**31 a**, **b**).

The anterior cells are separated from the posterior ones by a condensation of bone called the basal lamella. The basal lamella is formed as an almost vertical wall in the coronal plane behind the ethmoid bulla. The posterior root of the middle turbinate merges with the basal lamella.

The number and size of the remaining anterior ethmoidal air cells vary according to the degree of pneumatization of the air cells. In about 8 % of individuals the cells extend forward to the extent that they lie medial to the position of the lacrimal sac, and these are called lacrimal cells. If they are large, they can form a prominence of the lateral nasal wall where the anterior end of the middle turbinate is attached (Fig. 5.**32 a**, **b**). The height and position of the agger nasi cells has been classified by Bent et al. (1994). Agger nasi cells are present in the majority of patients, but their size and position vary. If they are large they "push" the frontal recess medially and posteriorly next to the middle turbinate.

Other anterior ethmoid cells vary and can be attached laterally to the lamina papyracea or to the skull base. A cell that is based on the floor of the orbit or the roof of the maxillary sinus is called a Haller cell (Fig. 5.**33**).

## Surgical Technique

Once an uncinectomy has been done and the natural ostium has been identified, the ethmoid sinuses may be opened. It is safe to remove the sinuses that lie in a sagittal plane medial to the medial wall of the maxillary sinus (N.B.: The orbits are not two cones with their long axes in the sagittal plane, but they face slightly laterally with their medial walls lying parallel to the sagittal plane (see Fig. 12.**6**).). The bulla can be punctured with straight forceps, and as they are withdrawn their jaws can be opened to help visualize the inside of the bulla (Fig. 5.**34a–d**). The bulla can then be opened with through-cutting forceps of various angles, but it is important to leave, and define, the top of its anterior wall as a landmark (Fig. 5.**35a–d**). The ethmoid bulla is resected until the retrobullar space and basal lamella are clearly defined (Fig. 5.**36a**, **b**). There should be a few remaining anterior ethmoid cells left in an anterior ethmoidectomy if the frontal recess is to avoid instru-

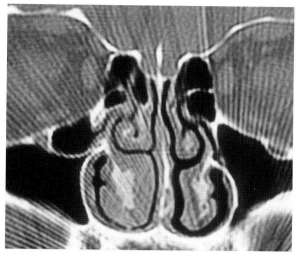

Fig. 5.**33**   A coronal CT scan showing a right inferior orbital or Haller cell.

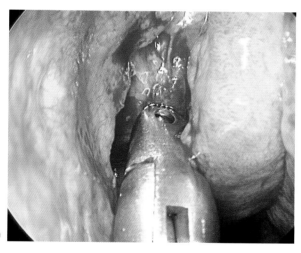
a

b

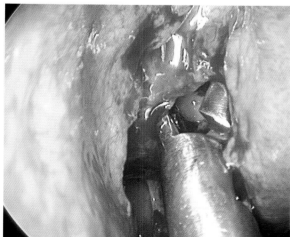
c

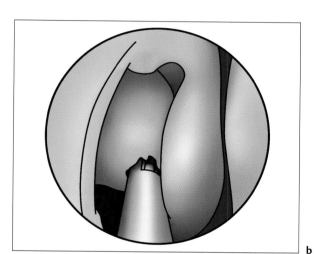
d

Fig. 5.**34a–d**   Straight Blakesley forceps are used to enter the bulla, being careful not to angle it laterally toward the orbit.

The forceps are opened before withdrawing them to help expose the inside of the bulla.

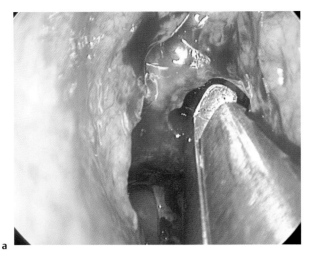

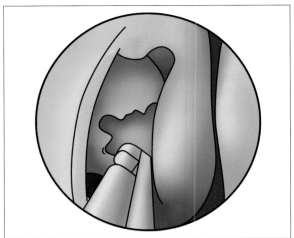

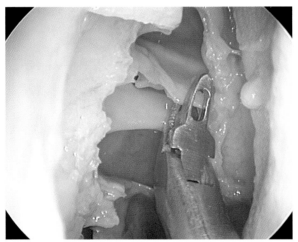

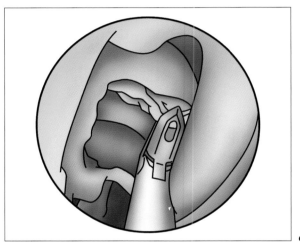

Fig. 5.**35 a–d**   A Hajek punch or through-cutting forceps are used to open the ethmoid bulla more widely, but it is important to leave its upper limit as this is a useful landmark to help localize the frontal recess.

mentation. These air cells lie on the lamina papyracea, and surgically it is safest to stay in a plane medial to the sinusotomy when looking for them. Check the CT before operating in this area. If there is any doubt, ask your assistant to observe the eye for any movement that would indicate that the orbit has been entered.

Hajek forceps are a good instrument for opening air cells because they can only be used if there is space for the posterior beak of the instrument to be inserted. Hajeks are precise and also minimize tearing of tissue. If 45° forceps are used to remove ethmoidal air cells on the lamina papyracea, it is best to use the side of the forceps for opening and removing them to limit the possibility of going into the orbit with the sharp ends of the forceps. A blunt, unattached olive-ended sucker is a useful probe to gently palpate for the presence of residual cells. As mentioned for an anterior ethmoidectomy, the frontal recess should not be instru-

mented unless there is a good reason for doing so. It is often tempting, as part of an "anatomical exercise," to continue to find the frontal recess; but it may be the worst thing you do for the patient as you then run the risk of causing stenosis. Dealing surgically with ethmoid disease along with medical treatment is usually enough to lead to an improvement in frontal sinus disease (see Fig. 5.**37**).  **DVD** 7, 8

## Alternative Surgical Techniques

It is possible to do this procedure using one of the microdebriders that can "digest" bone. If this technique is used it should be done with extreme care as it is easy to enter the orbit or skull base. The microdebriders are useful for tidying loose tags of mucosa and they avoid the temptation of pulling them, which will often result in leaving denuded bone.

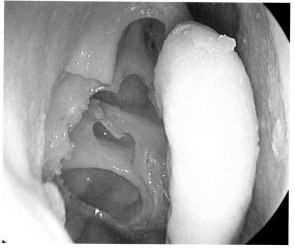

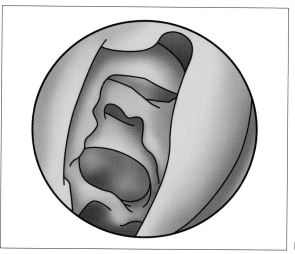

Fig. 5.**36a, b**   The anterior ethmoid sinuses have been opened. There is a remnant of the uncinate process and the antero-superior wall of the ethmoid bulla that is a useful landmark.

Note that there has been no instrumentation of the frontal recess.

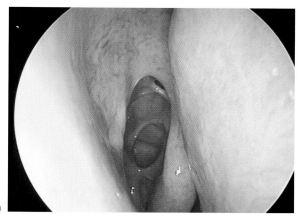

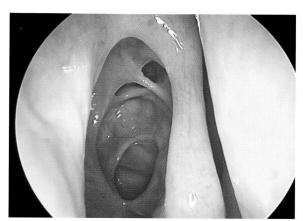

Fig. 5.**37a, b**   The postoperative appearance of a partial anterior ethmoidectomy for limited, but medically unresponsive, inflammatory disease.

## Frontoethmoidectomy ▪ ▪ ▪ ± Frontal Sinusotomy (I, II, III) ▪

### Terminology and Classification

**Frontoethmoidectomy:** This procedure involves opening of the frontal recess together with an anterior ethmoidectomy (previously described) (Fig. 5.**38**). This is only achievable with knowledge of the detailed anatomy in the area and it requires enlargement of the frontal recess with mucosal preservation at all cost.

**Frontal sinusotomy I:** No instrumentation of the frontal recess is required when the uncinate process is attached to the skull base or middle turbinate; when the uncinate process has been removed, the recess is open unless there are large agger nasi air cells, a bulla frontalis, or a supraorbital cell (Fig. 5.**39**).

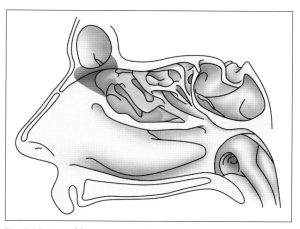

Fig. 5.**38**   In addition to an infundibulotomy and anterior ethmoidectomy, the frontal recess is opened.

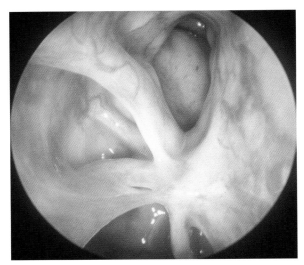

Fig. 5.**39**   Postoperative view of type I frontal sinusotomy.

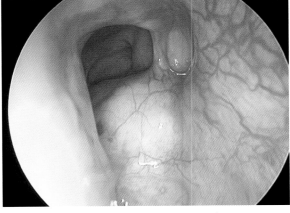

Fig. 5.**40**   Postoperative view of type II frontal sinusotomy.

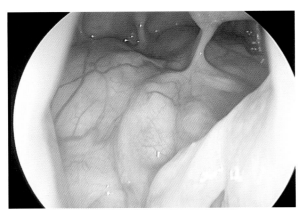

Fig. 5.**41**   Postoperative view of type III frontal sinusotomy.

**Frontal sinusotomy II:** Enlarging the frontal recess by the submucosal removal of agger nasi air cells, bulla frontalis, or a supraorbital cell (Fig. 5.**40**)

**Frontal sinusotomy III:** Extended enlargement with removal of the frontonasal spine or "beak" (Fig. 5.**41**). **DVD** 7, 8

### Indications

The primary indication for having a good reason to instrument the frontal recess is when:

- Maximum medical treatment has failed to help frontal sinus symptoms.
- A partial anterior ethmoidectomy has not succeeded.

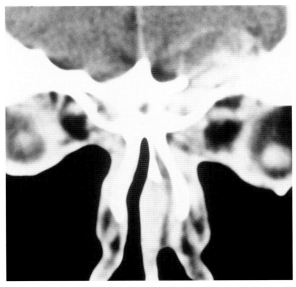

a

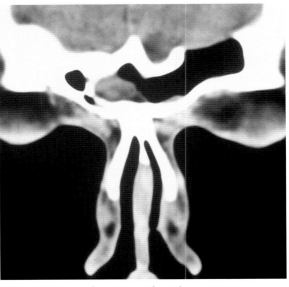

b

Fig. 5.**42**   **a** Preoperative CT scan of aspergillosis of the frontal sinus and **b** CT scan after a type II frontal sinusotomy.

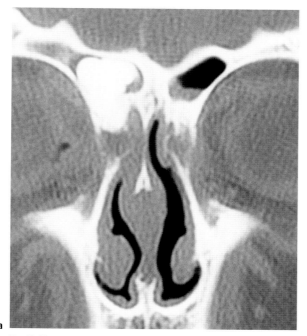

a

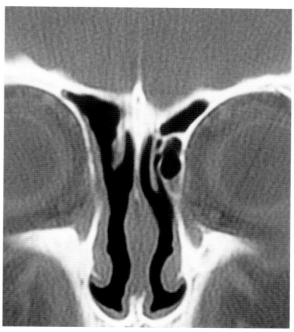

b

Fig. 5.**43**   **a** Preoperative CT scan of an osteoma in the frontal recess and **b** CT scan after a type II frontal sinusotomy.

It is important that the periodicity of frontal symptoms is associated with upper respiratory tract infections or changes in barometric pressure, or that symptoms are associated with a purulent discharge.

Opacification of the frontal recess on its own is not a reason to instrument the frontal recess, as it will often resolve with an anterior ethmoidectomy and medical treatment.

There are few other reasons for operating on the frontal recess before trying a partial anterior ethmoidectomy. These include: the presence of fungal disease in the frontal sinus (Fig. 5.**42 a, b**); barotrauma, mucocele, or osteoma causing obstruction with evidence of mucosal disease (Fig. 5.**43 a, b**); or other pathology in this area that requires wide exposure for access.

The normal frontal recess is narrow and tenuous (this raises questions about the role of anatomical variations in the pathogenesis of rhinitis). The prevalence of such "variations" and anatomical "restrictions" appears to be no more greater in a control population than in patients with proven rhinosinusitis (Jones et al., 1997 a). It seems likely that the primary problem is the mucosal pathology, and this is the reason why one individual will have chronic rhinosinusitis and another will not.

## Anatomy

To understand the frontal recess, you need first of all to know the different relationships of the uncinate process and then the variation in pneumatization of the air cells that extend into it.

Access to the frontal recess may be altered by the attachment of the uncinate process. If the uncinate process is attached to the lamina papyracea, the agger nasi air cells, or the lateral wall, it will not get in the way of the frontal recess (type A, where the uncinate process attaches to the lateral nasal wall so the frontal sinus drains into the middle meatus) (Fig. 5.**44 a–d**). The "dead end" between the uncinate process and the lateral nasal wall is called the "terminal recess" (Fig. 5.**45 a, b**). If the posterior edge of the uncinate process is followed superiorly, this will lead to the recessus terminalis, a blind ended alley between the uncinate process and the lateral wall of the nose.

Alternatively, the uncinate process can attach to the skull base or middle turbinate and limit anterior access as it forms a web that gets in the way of an anterior approach. In type B1, the uncinate process attaches to the skull base (Fig. 5.**46 a, b**). In type B2, the uncinate process attaches to the middle turbinate (Fig. 5.**47 a, b**). In these patients the frontal sinus drains directly into the ethmoid infundibulum (Fig. 5.**48 a, b**).

The variability of the anterior ethmoid air cells makes them a fascinating subject on their own (Fig. 5.**49 a, b**–5.**57 a, b**). In over 94% of people there

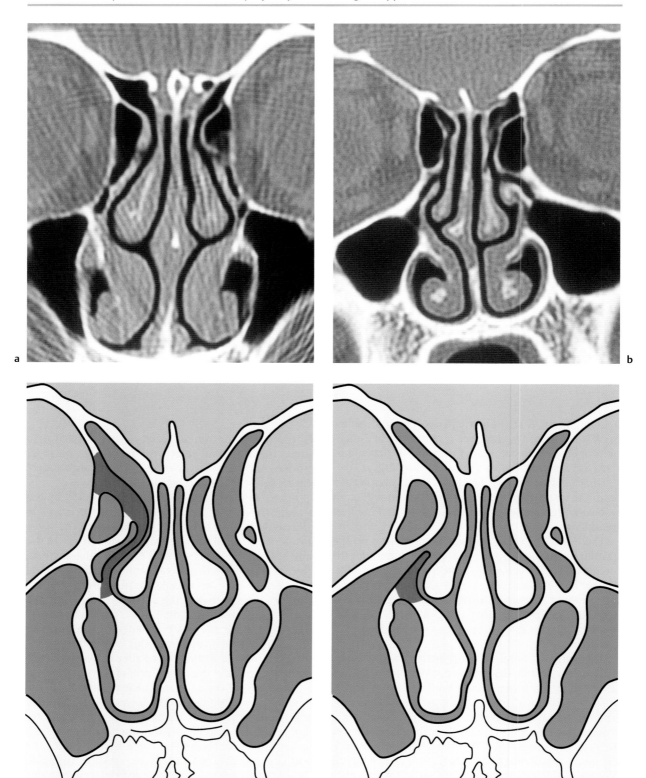

Fig. 5.**44 a**, **b**   Coronal CT scans showing a type A insertion of the uncinate process to the lateral nasal wall. Find it by following its posterior free edge. **c**, **d** Line diagrams to show the different appearances on sequential coronal CT cuts of a type A uncinate process.

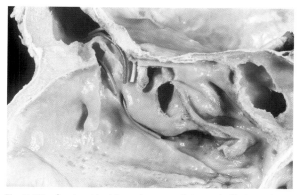
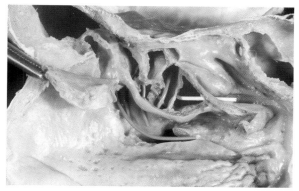

Fig. 5.**45 a, b**   In **a** the blue wire extends into a bulla frontalis. In **b** the terminal recess is revealed by a green wire when the uncinate process is folded back.

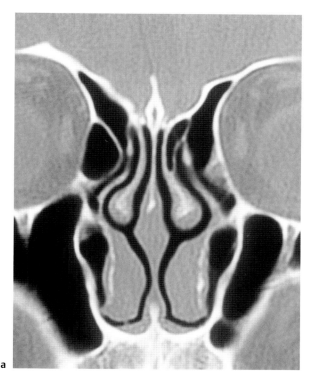
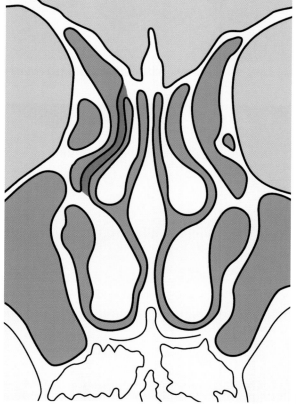

Fig. 5.**46 a, b**   In type B1 the uncinate process attaches to the skull base.

are anterior ethmoid air cells over the lacrimal bone or adjacent to the anterior aspect of the middle turbinate; these are called agger nasi air cells. A high anterior ethmoidal cell that has pneumatized into the frontal bone is called the bulla frontalis and this can displace the frontal recess posteriorly (Fig. 5.50 a, b).

The bulla frontalis can be so large that it can mimic the frontal sinus, almost forming a sinus within a sinus (Fig. 5.51 a, b).

Not infrequently a supraorbital cell, a posterior cell in the anterior ethmoid complex that is well pneumatized, can extend laterally into the frontal bone over

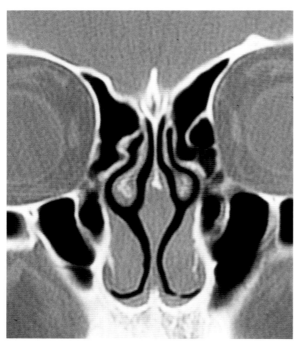
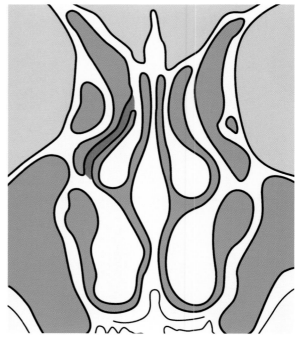

Fig. 5.**47 a**, **b**  In type B2 the uncinate process attaches to the middle turbinate.

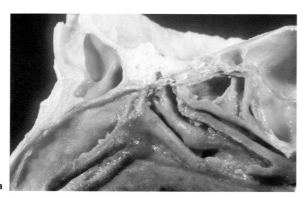
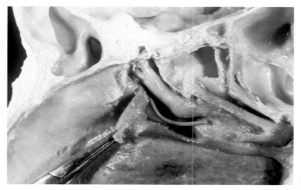

Fig. 5.**48 a**, **b**  In these specimens the frontal sinus can be seen directly draining into the ethmoid infundibulum (green wire)—type B1.

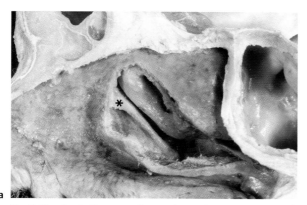
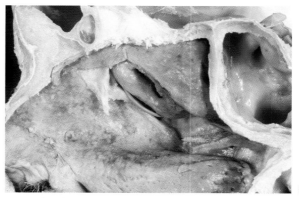

Fig. 5.**49 a**, **b**  In these specimens the uncinate process is curling medially (∗) to join the middle turbinate, which has been resected in **b** to allow the frontal sinus to be seen to drain directly into the ethmoid infundibulum (green wire)—type B2.

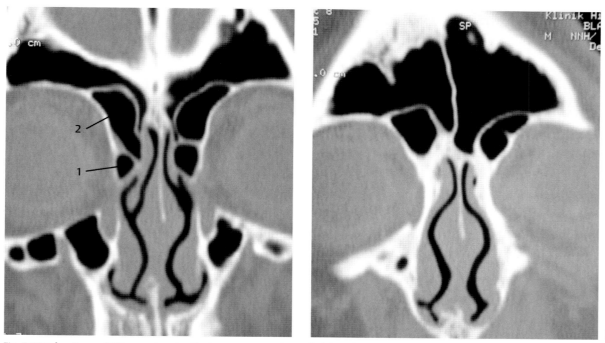

a                                                                          b

Fig. 5.**50 a, b**    Coronal CT scans showing the lower agger nasi air cells (1), with the bulla frontalis (2) extending above them into the frontal sinus.

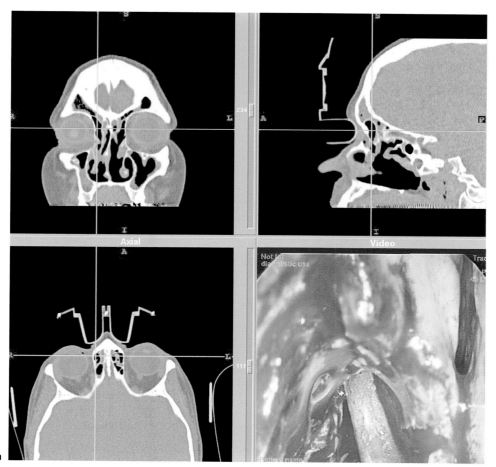

a

Fig. 5.**51**    **a** Coronal, axial, and sagittal scans taken during computer-aided surgery, showing a pneumatized bulla frontalis extending into the frontal sinus, which helps to distinguish it in this case.

Fig. 5.**51**    **b**    ▷

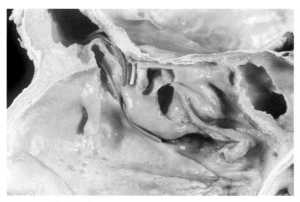

Fig. 5.**51**   **b** The blue wire is in a bulla frontalis and the red wire is in the frontal recess and sinus.

the orbit and also narrow the frontal recess by pushing it forward (Figs. 5.**52 a**, **b**, 5.**53 a**, **b**, 5.**54 a–c**). Occasionally air cells exist within the frontal sinus itself, with the ostia of these cells draining within the frontal sinus (Fig. 5.**55**). Another variation is the intersinus septal cell that may extend into the crista galli; this cell often drains into the frontal recess area (Fig. 5.**56 a**, **b**).

To explain the variations that can occur, you need to imagine different shapes and sizes of party balloons that are blown up to encroach on or extend through the channel of the frontal recess. Imagine the pneumatized ethmoid cells, agger nasi, bulla frontalis, or a supraorbital cell as balloons that can expand to narrow access to the frontal recess that forms a medial crevice between these and the middle turbinate (Fig. 5.**57 a**, **b**).

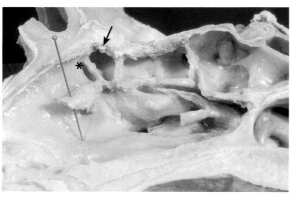

a

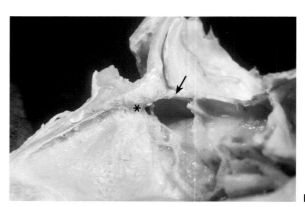

b

Fig. 5.**52 a**, **b**   A large supraorbital extension (arrow) just behind the opening of the frontal recess (∗). The frontal recess is very narrow and is positioned anteriorly because of the large supraorbital cell.

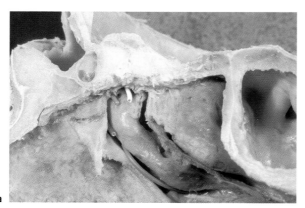

a

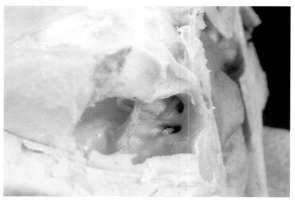

b

Fig. 5.**53**   **a** The red and blue wires both enter the right frontal sinus; the white wire goes into a supraorbital cell. **b** A view from above shows the red and blue wires entering the frontal sinus; note that the roof of this area has been removed so they can be seen.

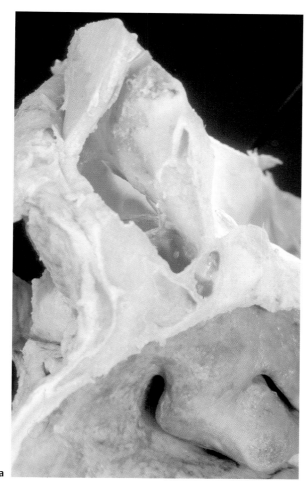

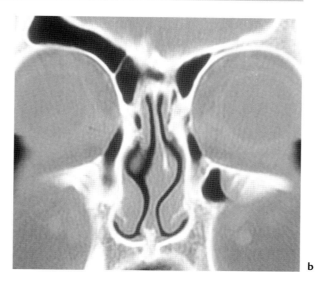

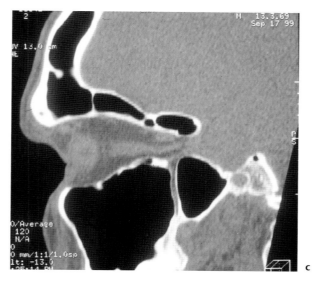

Fig. 5.**54**   **a** Light within a large supraorbital cell to help it be seen riding up into the frontal sinus. The supraorbital cell extends up into the frontal sinus posterior to the frontal recess. **b**, **c** Coronal (**b**) and sagittal (**c**) CT images showing how a supraorbital cell can extend over the skull base.

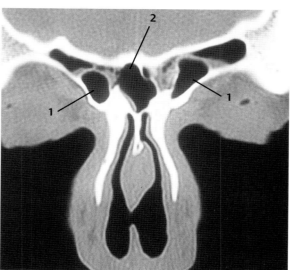

Fig. 5.**55**   A coronal CT scan showing bilateral bulla frontalis ▷ (1) and an intersinus septal cell (2) in between.

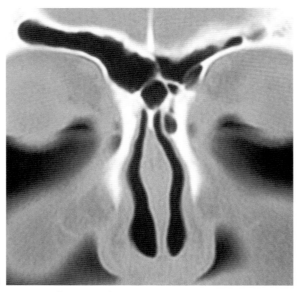
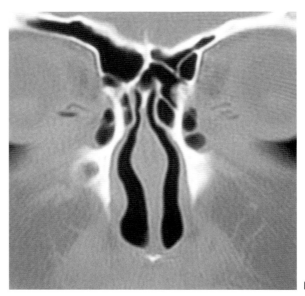

a

b

Fig. 5.**56 a**, **b**    Coronal CT scans showing an intersinus septal cell that is draining to the left.

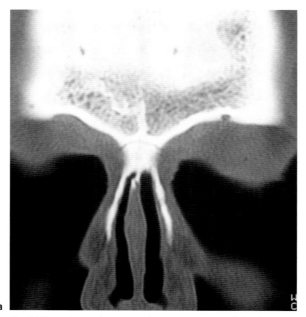
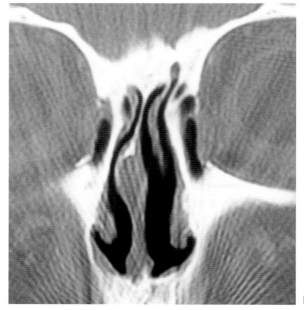

a

b

Fig. 5.**57**    **a** Coronal CT scan showing agenesis of the frontal sinus. **b** Minimal pneumatization on the left into the frontal/ethmoid bone.

## Surgical Technique

The surgeon must have a good reason for operating in this area. The landmarks that will help you are the remains of the uncinate process, the remainder of the anterior wall of the ethmoid bulla, and a knowledge of the air cells from the CT scan.

Follow the superior remnant of the uncinate process upward with a 45° through-cutting forceps. Now is the time to change to a 45° endoscope to examine the area and obtain an overview. Uncapped agger nasi cells, the terminal recess, and the ethmoid bulla form domes that are joined together. It often appears that this is all there is and they might fool you into thinking that one of them is a small frontal sinus. Careful palpation, not prodding, with a ball probe next to the middle turbinate will reveal a crevice between the middle turbinate and the uncapped cells (Fig. 5.**58 a–o**). The aim is to open this crevice, which will turn out to be the pathway to

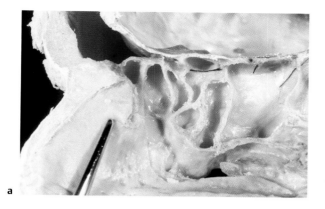

the frontal recess and the frontal sinus, by "deflating" the cells. This is best done by passing the ball probe well above their domes and gently lateralizing them. The shaft of a Kuhn curette also works well. If visibility is good, it may be possible to do this by submucosal dissection. Fragments of bone should then be removed, taking care not to grab the mucosa as you want to leave the whole circumference of mucosa in order to avoid stenosis. If the bone is thick, then the end of a Kuhn curette is ideal for this maneuver. These domes are sequentially uncapped to reveal the next tier (Figs. 5.**59**a–j, 5.**60**a, b).

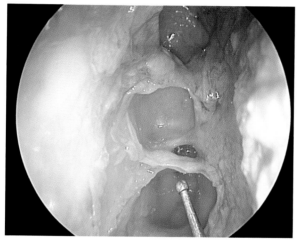

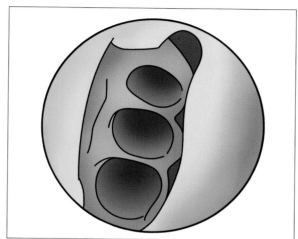

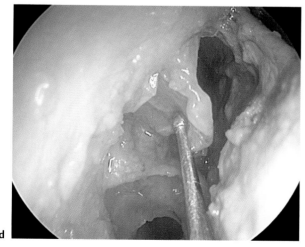

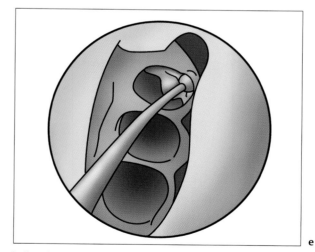

Fig. 5.**58**  **a** A sagittal section showing multiple air cells along the skull base; their variety is endless. **b**–**o** Sequential dissection of an agger nasi air cell using submucosal dissection with a ball probe. This strategy "deflates" these air cells to help open up access to the frontal recess.              Fig. 5.**58**f–o ▷

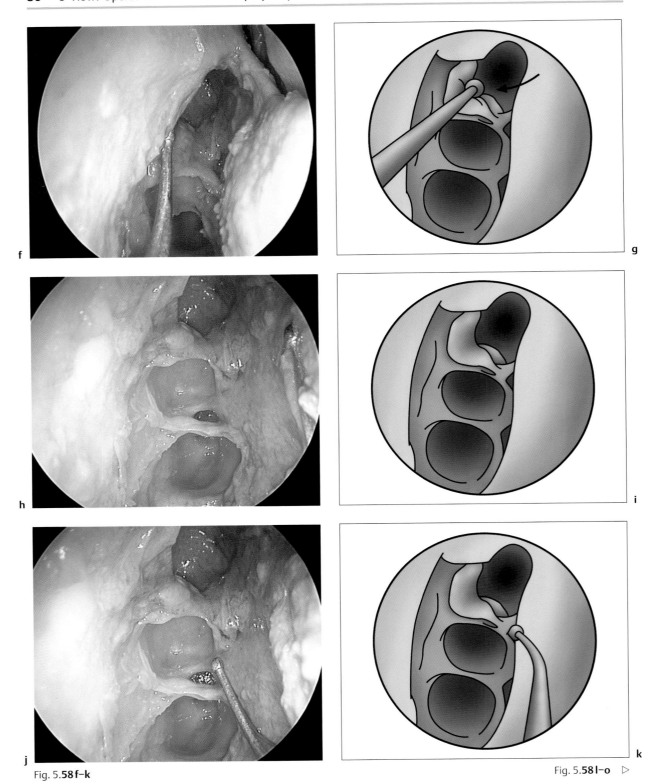

f

g

h

i

j

k

Fig. 5.**58 f–k**

Fig. 5.**58 l–o**  ▷

The deflated mucosa is then draped over the lateral nasal wall. You can tell whether you have removed the most anterior cells by feeling the beak of the frontal bone with the Kuhn curette, as it is extremely thick. By uncapping of the remnant of the ethmoid bulla, the suprabullar recess is exposed and this often contains the

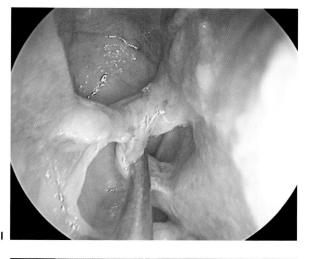

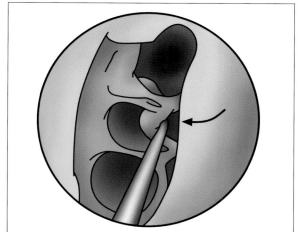

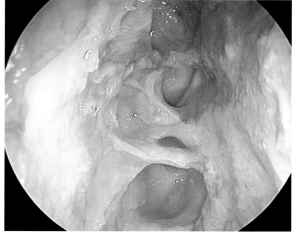

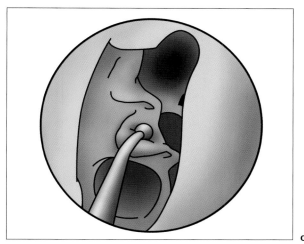

Fig. 5.**58 l–o**

anterior ethmoidal artery and in front of it a supraorbital cell if one is present. The suprabullar cell lies behind the frontal recess and can easily be mistaken for it. Once this is completed, you have done a type II frontal sinusotomy. You should now ask yourself whether you have opened the frontal recess. You can confirm that you have by:

- A ball probe, a Kuhn curette, or a curved sucker passing freely high up into the frontal sinus.
- Registering the angle and length of this ball probe on the maxillary spine and repositioning it external to the nose.
- Transillumination, with the endoscope high up in the frontal recess.
- Seeing the **convex** posterior wall of the frontal sinus along with the spacious cavern of the sinus.

In order to make sure that you have entered the frontal recess and are into the frontal sinus, grip the shaft of the ball probe between the thumb and the index finger next to the nasal spine, noting the angle of the instrument at the same time. The instrument is then withdrawn and placed alongside the outside of the nose, placing it at the same angle with the pinch grip placed alongside the nasal spine. If the end of the ball probe is then higher than the eyebrow line, it is likely that the instrument is in the frontal sinus. If it is around or just above the medial canthus, then it is likely that the ball probe is not within the frontal recess but is within an agger nasi air cell. If the handle of the ball probe is noted to have been turned laterally when the instrument is passed up what is thought to be the frontal recess, then it may have been channeled in this direction by a bulla frontalis or a supraorbital cell (Fig. 5.**61 a–c**).

The partition between the bulla frontalis and the frontal recess is best resected with through-cutting forceps as high as the instruments will allow. The same applies to supraorbital cells that encroach and extend up the posterior wall of the frontal sinus.

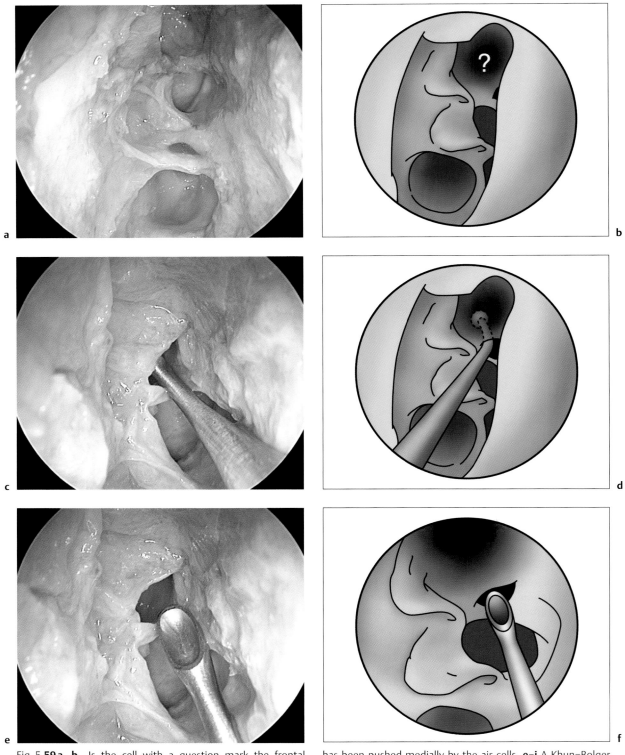

Fig. 5.**59a**, **b**  Is the cell with a question mark the frontal sinus? **c, d** A close-up view shows a sound locating a fine channel adjacent to the middle turbinate. It is as though the channel has been pushed medially by the air cells. **e–j** A Khun–Bolger curette is used to remove the roof of the second tier of cells, which then creates wide drainage for the frontal sinus.

Fig. 5.**59g–j**  ▷

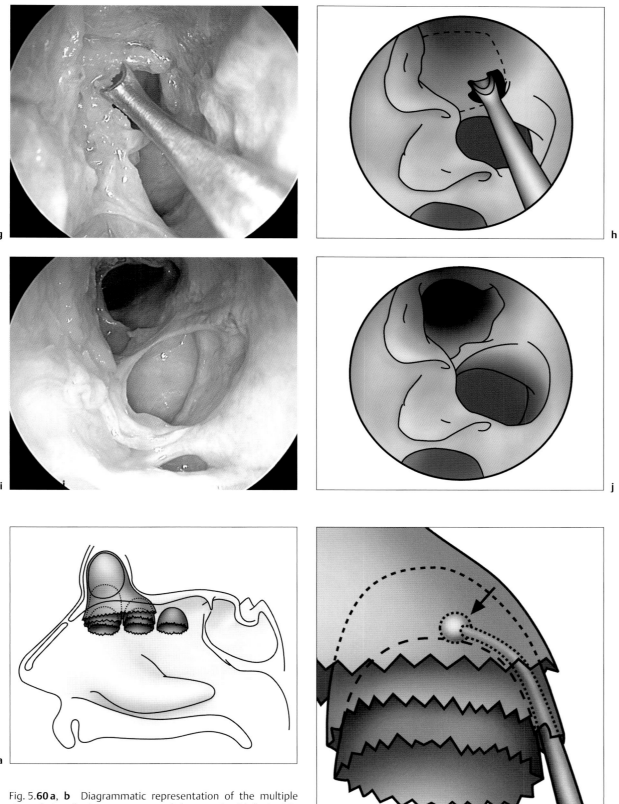

Fig. 5.**60 a**, **b**   Diagrammatic representation of the multiple tiers of air cells that can occur and that require "deflating" in order to drain the frontal recess.

If there is poor visibility because of bleeding or polyps, this is an area in which not to go blindly prodding around. Rather, it is best to use local vasoconstrictors and to return once visibility has improved.

When operating in the frontal recess, the following guidelines may be helpful:

- Work out the anatomy before you operate. Reconstruct a three-dimensional image in your mind of the anatomy and insertion of the uncinate process, the position of agger nasi air cells, whether there is a bulla frontalis or supraorbital cell, and the position and shape of air cells in and around the frontal recess. This is your map and you do not want to be lost in the wilderness! (Fig. 5.**62 a–f**).

- It is vital not to prod medially as you pass any instrument into the frontal recess, as the lateral lamella is usually the thinnest part of the skull base and it is easy to cause a CSF leak in this area.

- It is important not to palpate laterally in the frontal recess if there are small or no agger nasi air cells, as you can enter the orbit here. Check carefully on the CT image and ask the assistant to ballotte the eye while you are examining this area to make sure that you are not going to enter the orbit. Where there is doubt about where you are, it is safer to stay anterior, just behind the "beak" of the frontal bone. The bone is very thick anteriorly and if you approach the frontal recess staying just lateral to a sagittal plane, in line with the attachment of the middle turbinate to the skull base, you are less likely to traverse dura.

- The anterior wall of the ethmoid bulla is a good landmark in finding the frontal recess as its anterior wall will lead you up to the frontal recess. It also "guards" the anterior ethmoid artery if it is attached to the skull base, and when this happens the artery is often in the next undulation in the roof of the ethmoid bulla. *DVD* 6, 7, 8

You should not go searching for the anterior ethmoid artery as it is not a useful landmark and to do so is dangerous. It is important to be aware that it is partially dehiscent in 20% of patients. If the skull base is very well pneumatized, the artery can even be free like a tightrope, especially if there is a large supraorbital cell. (See Fig. 5.**63 a–g**.)

## Alternative Surgical Techniques

It is possible to approach the frontal recess anteriorly with a 0° scope if there is a large agger nasi air cell. A mucosal flap on the lateral nasal wall based anteriorly can be made so that the prominence in the lateral nasal wall created by the agger nasi air cell is uncovered. A Hajek–Kofler punch is then used to remove the "armpit" of this area where the middle turbinate

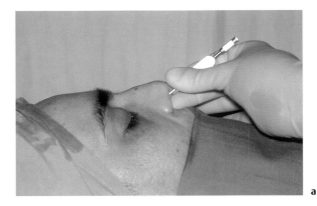

a

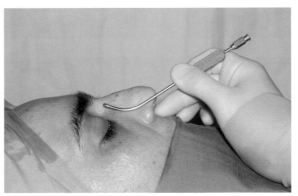

b

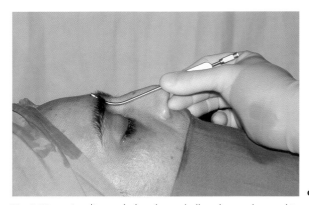

c

Fig. 5.**61**   **a** An olive ended sucker or ball probe can be used to help define whether you have located the frontal sinus. Place it within the "possible" frontal sinus and note its angle and pinch it with your fingers at the maxillary spine. **b** Then remove it and place it at the same angle and distance from the maxillary spine. If it is around the medial canthal area, you have not reached the frontal sinus. **c** If the probe is high above the supraorbital margin, it is probably in the frontal sinus. If it turns abruptly laterally, check that there is no bulla frontalis or supraorbital cell that can also extend this high up.

Fig. 5.**62 a–d**   Sequential coronal CT scans showing agger nasi  ▷ air cells, the drainage channel (arrow) of the frontal sinus: build up a 3D image of the cells in your mind. **e** View of right frontal recess from above with a track of blood going down to the infundibulum frontalis. **f** The same patient from below, showing that the frontal sinus drains medially (arrow).

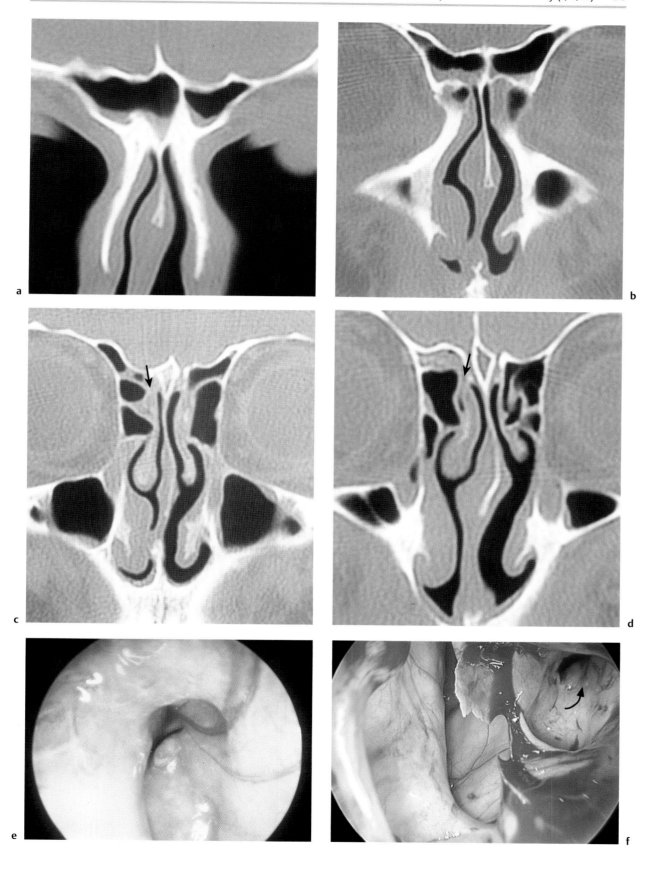

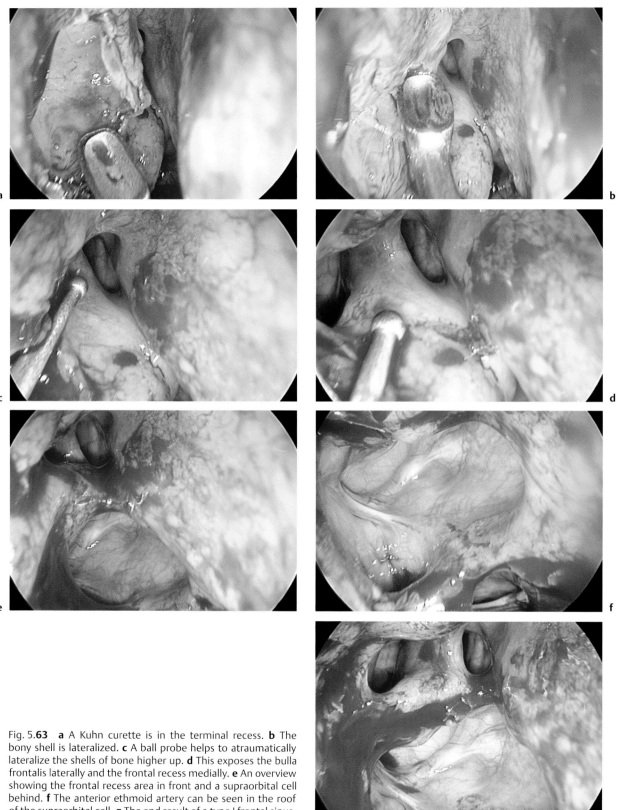

Fig. 5.**63**   **a** A Kuhn curette is in the terminal recess. **b** The bony shell is lateralized. **c** A ball probe helps to atraumatically lateralize the shells of bone higher up. **d** This exposes the bulla frontalis laterally and the frontal recess medially. **e** An overview showing the frontal recess area in front and a supraorbital cell behind. **f** The anterior ethmoid artery can be seen in the roof of the supraorbital cell. **g** The end result of a type I frontal sinusotomy.

attaches onto the lateral nasal wall and by doing this the anterior part of the agger nasi air cell is opened. The agger nasi cell can then be removed submucosally, the mucosa of the frontal recess lateralized, and the lateral flap placed over any raw bone to reduce the chance of any stenosis in this area. Surgery in the armpit area where the middle turbinate attaches to the lateral nasal wall often results in the middle turbinate becoming lateralized. We are not concerned about this as it helps to open the olfactory cleft.

If the middle turbinate has been resected in previous surgery or if the frontal sinus is very stenosed due to previous instrumentation in this area, this can make access to the frontal recess difficult. Extra care is needed as reported series have shown that complications are more common in this patient group. It is safest to palpate anteriorly where the bone is very thick, but you must not angle your probe medially (and risk a CSF leak) or laterally into the orbit. A "mini trephine" can help define the site of the frontal recess when the techniques mentioned have not worked.

A small incision is made within the eyebrow just medial to the notch on the supraorbital rim where the vessels and nerves come out. An incision of approximately 0.5 cm followed by soft-tissue dissection is needed before a small burr hole is made into the sinus. Fluorescein dye can then be placed into the frontal sinus and sought endoscopically within the nose to see where it comes out. Though it is often not necessary, but a blue filter can be used to define the site if there is only a small amount of fluorescein passing into the nose.

Where previous surgery has caused stenosis of the frontonasal duct, the main problem that needs to be overcome is the presence of all the scar tissue, and secondly the amount of prolapse of soft tissue that may have been caused by excessive removal of bone forming the lateral wall of the frontal recess. This is not uncommon after an external frontoethmoidectomy and is known to occur in approximately a one-third of patients who have had a Lynch–Howarth external ethmoidectomy approach. The alternative ways of overcoming this problem are discussed in Chapter 14.

## Useful Instruments

A 45° endoscope is invaluable and helps surgery in this area a great deal. Without the 45° endoscope it is extremely difficult to visualize whether the surgeon is looking at the roof of a bulla frontalis or has reached the frontal sinus.

An angled ball probe is helpful in the submucosal dissection and in mucosal preservation in this area. Mucosal preservation is essential to avoid frontal recess stenosis. Another technique is to dilate the frontal recess with the shaft of a ball probe or Kuhn curette

and fragment the shell of the agger nasi cells before carefully removing the bony fragments. The surgeon must avoid pulling on any loose mucosa as this runs the risk of stripping it off the frontal recess.

The Kuhn curette helps remove thicker bone in the frontal recess area and its shape and size can help deflate the cells intruding into this area.

The use of 45° through-cutting forceps helps in removing high fragments of bone or parts of partitions in this area and at the same time allows mucosal preservation.

Giraffe forceps (Kuhn–Bolger), designed with jaws that open in line with the instrument or at right angles to it, help to retrieve fragments of bone that ride up high into the frontal recess or sinus. This area can only be seen with a 45° endoscope.

## ■ Sphenoethmoidectomy ■ ■ ■ ± Sphenoid Sinusotomy (I, II, III) ■

Sphenoid sinusotomy is described on p. 100 as a separate entity. Sphenoid sinusotomy can be classified into types I, II, and III depending on its size. In a sphenoethmoidectomy it is usually only necessary to undertake a type II sphenoid sinusotomy. A sphenoid sinusotomy is usually only done to identify the level of the roof of the sphenoid sinus to obtain an idea of the level of the skull base.

### Terminology and Classification

**Sphenoethmoidectomy:** This is an extension of a partial anterior ethmoidectomy that involves surgery into the posterior ethmoid sinuses and the sphenoid sinus (Fig. 5.**64**).  *DVD* 7, 8

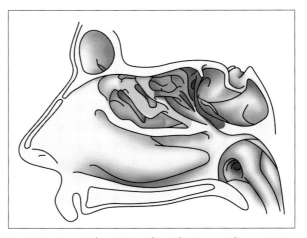

Fig. 5.**64**  A partial anterior ethmoidectomy with a posterior ethmoidectomy and sphenoid sinus surgery.

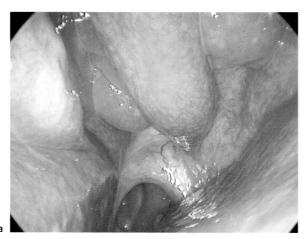
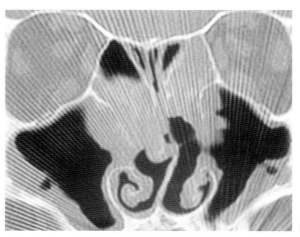

a                                                                                                                                      b

Fig. 5.**65**    **a** Endoscopic view and **b** CT scan of residual symptomatic polyps after oral and topical steroids.

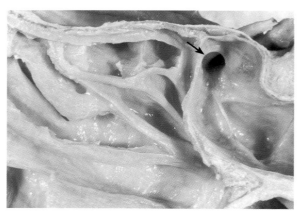

Fig. 5.**66**    This shows the right posterior ethmoid sinuses be-hind the basal lamella, and the optic nerve in the sphenoid sinus (arrow).

**Sphenoid sinusotomy:** A sphenoid sinusotomy is a transnasal approach to open the sphenoid sinus (see Fig. 5.**82**). For a classification, see p. 100.

## Indications

Surgery in this area is normally only warranted if there is polyposis after maximum medical treatment (Fig. 5.**65a**, **b**). Approximately 1 in 5 patients have a coexisting bacterial infection. In some countries, aspergillosis is more prevalent. In developed countries, polyposis associated with nonatopic asthma is common, and 1 in 6 will be sensitive to aspirin or non-steroidal anti-inflammatory drugs.

The procedure is also done for inverted papilloma, polyposis, and mucoceles involving these sinuses. If the ethmoid and sphenoid sinuses have been opened surgically, this does not necessarily mean that you need to

open the frontal recess, as mentioned in the section on anterior ethmoidectomy, as it greatly increases the risk of producing stenosis of the frontal recess.

## Anatomy

The posterior ethmoid sinuses lie behind the basal lamella and are few but often well pneumatized (Fig. 5.**66**). A sphenoethmoid (Onodi) cell has part of its extension lateral to the lateral wall of the sphenoid, which means that the optic nerve is likely to be exposed (Fig. 5.**67**). The degree of pneumatization of the sphenoid sinus varies, and knowledge of this is critical when instrumenting it. Its natural ostium lies high in the anterior wall of the sphenoid and can be hidden by the superior and middle turbinates. The bone of the sphenoid is thick from the ridge of the posterior choana up its anterior wall for about 1 cm, then it becomes thin (Fig. 5.**68**). The roof of the sphenoid sinus is a reliable landmark and the posterior ethmoid sinuses do not drop below this horizontal level of the skull base. The posterior ethmoid sinuses frequently do extend above the axial plane of the roof of the sphenoid sinus, but these will usually have been opened if the sphenoid sinus has been opened up to its roof. The vomer meets the sphenoid in the midline, but the sphenoid intersinus septum is asymmetric in over 75% of patients (Fig. 5.**69**). The lateral wall of the sphenoid contains the carotid artery, which is dehiscent in 30% of patients (Fig. 5.**70**). The superolateral aspect of the sphenoid sinus contains the optic nerve, which is visible in 20% of patients (Lang, 1989) (Fig. 5.**71**).

## Surgical Technique

The posterior ethmoidal cells are entered through the basal lamella and it is safest to enter these medially and inferiorly (Fig. 5.**72a–u**). Enlarge access to these

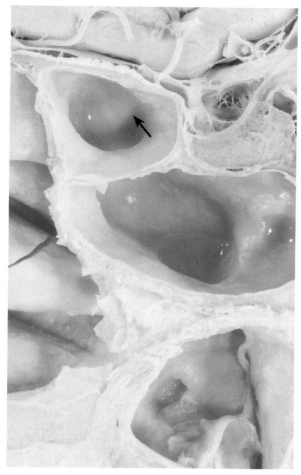

Fig. 5.**67**   A sphenoethmoid air cell above the sphenoid sinus—note the optic nerve in its lateral wall (arrow).

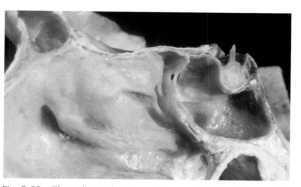

Fig. 5.**68**   The sphenoid ostia can be seen high on the anterior wall of the sphenoid—note that the bone becomes thin about 1 cm above the shoulder of the posterior choana.

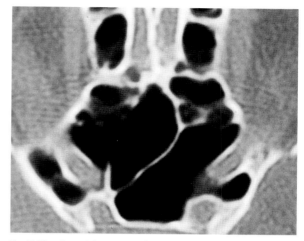

Fig. 5.**69**   An axial CT scan showing asymmetry of the sphenoid intersinus septum.

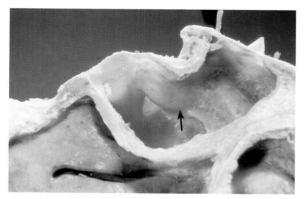

Fig. 5.**70**   Note the bulge of the carotid artery in the lateral wall of the sphenoid sinus (arrow).

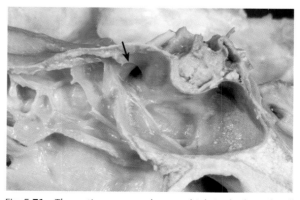

Fig. 5.**71**   The optic nerve can be seen high in the lateral wall of the sphenoid sinus (arrow).

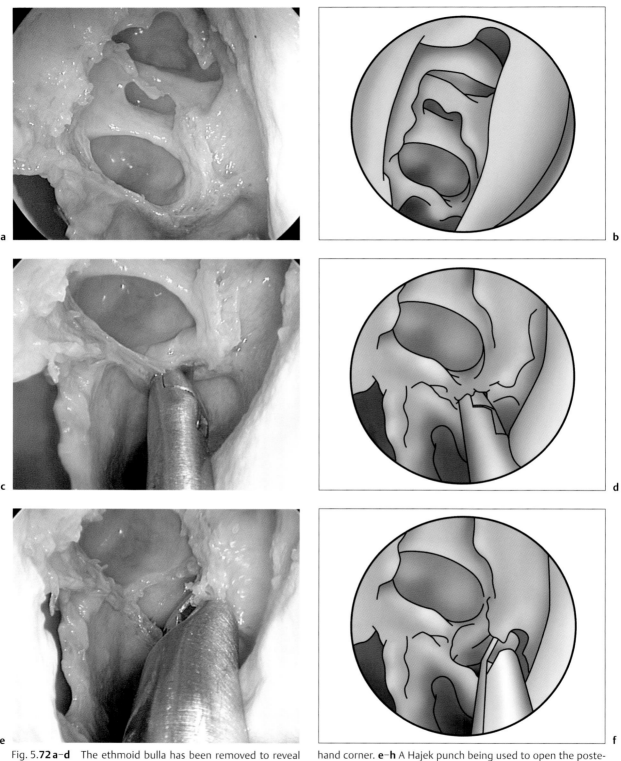

Fig. 5.**72 a–d**  The ethmoid bulla has been removed to reveal the basal lamella, which is punctured medially using straight Blakesley forceps. This is done medial to the medial wall of the maxillary sinus and above the horizontal inferior base of the ground lamella. Note the maxillary ostium in the bottom left-hand corner. **e–h** A Hajek punch being used to open the posterior ethmoid sinuses. Note preservation of the superior turbinate and its olfactory mucosa.

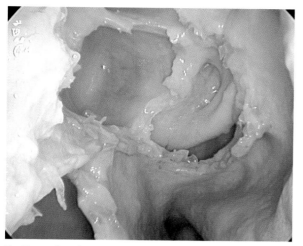
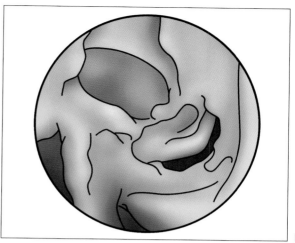

g

h

Fig. 5.**72 g, h** The superior turbinate can be seen through a "window" after some of the posterior ethmoid air cells have been removed.

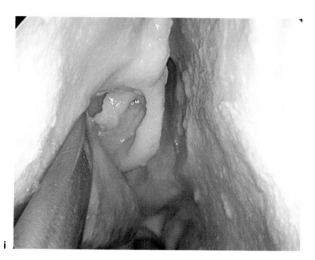
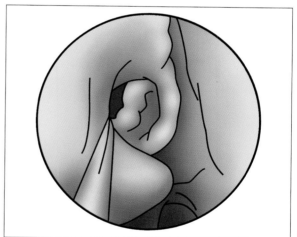

i

j

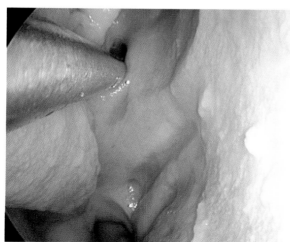
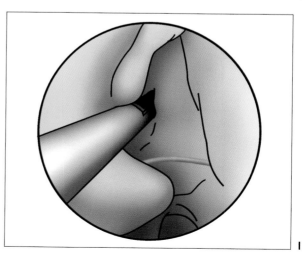

k

l

Fig. 5.**72 i, j** The middle turbinate is lateralized and the "window" between it and the inferior turbinate can be seen from the medial side. This allows the height of the roof of the sphenoid and posterior ethmoids to be compared. **k, l** The sphenoid sinus is located near the midline 1 cm above the posterior choana where the bone is thin.

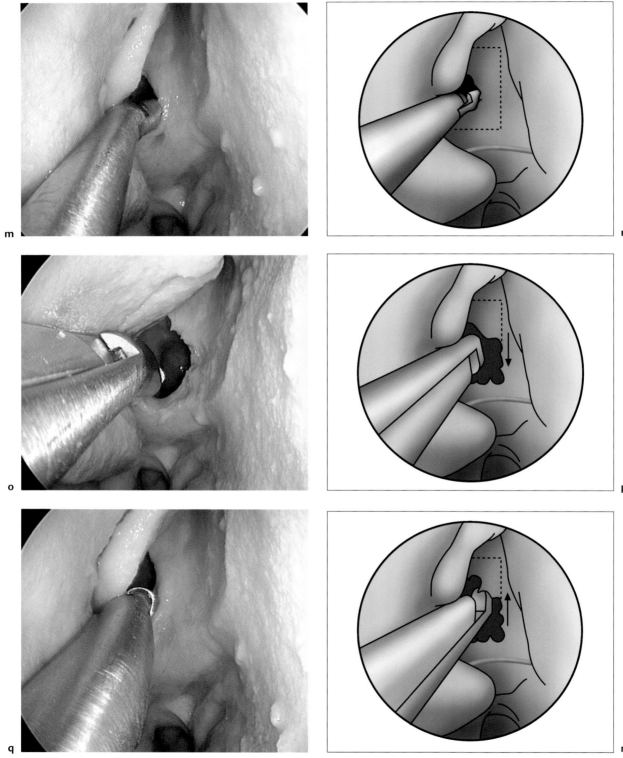

Fig. 5.**72 m**, **n**   The jaws of the Blakesley forceps are opened before it is withdrawn to help open the ostium. **o**, **p** The Hajek punch is used to take one downward bite in order to avoid the septal branch of the sphenopalatine artery. **q**, **r** A few upward bites enlarge the ostia up to the skull base.

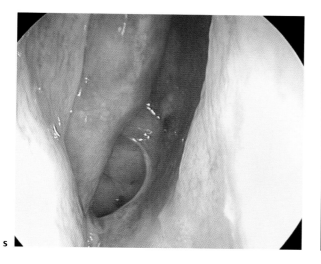

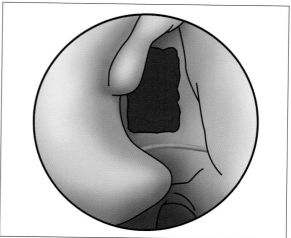

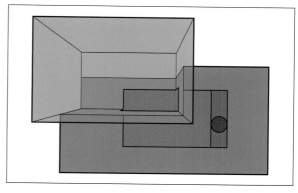

Fig. 5.**72**  **s** Sinusotomy, type I.  **t** Note the position of the septal branch of the sphenopalatine artery. **u** A line diagram to illustrate the size and position of a sphenoidotomy: type I, the dark circle; type II, the dark green vertical rectangle; type III, the dark green horizontal rectangle. The sphenoid and the pale green box that represents a posterior ethmoid air cell are joined. The sphenoid can be opened more extensively but requires ligation of the sphenopalatine artery and an exact knowledge of the position of the carotid and optic nerves.

cells and avoid making a tunnel. Beware that in some patients the next partition may be the skull base. If you are unhappy about visibility or the anatomy, it is best to find the sphenoid sinus first before venturing into uncharted waters. Even if you think you know where the sphenoid sinus is, do not be tempted to enter it through the posterior ethmoid complex as this is potentially dangerous. Always find the sphenoid sinus transnasally first if you intend opening up all the posterior ethmoid sinuses.

It is important to have landmarks by which to orientate yourself and to keep back with the endoscope so as to keep these in view. Our preferred strategy is to use the following landmarks to avoid traversing the boundaries of the paranasal sinuses:

- Check the CT scan to see that there is no Onodi cell as the optic nerve can sometimes be dehiscent in its lateral wall. Look at the posterior coronal CT slices of the maxillary sinus and look at the height from the roof of the maxillary sinus to the roof of the skull base. Sometimes this can be spacious but sometimes it is small and it will give the operator an idea of the extent of the posterior ethmoidal air cells.

- The roof of the sphenoid sinus is a useful landmark as the posterior ethmoid sinuses are not lower than it, so that if the operator stays in a plane that is lower than the roof of the sphenoid sinus, they are unlikely to traverse the skull base. Often the ethmoid sinuses will extend above this level, but when the posterior ethmoid sinuses have been opened to the level of the roof of the sphenoid sinus these are often apparent and can easily be palpated and opened.

- The posterior ethmoid sinuses that lie medial to the medial wall of the maxillary sinus in a sagittal plane can be removed without concern that the optic nerve or orbit will be damaged.

The sphenoid sinus can safely be found by staying adjacent to the vomer. It lies approximately 1.0–1.5 cm above the bridge or "shoulder" of the posterior choana. Often the bulk of the middle turbinate restricts access to this area and it may be necessary to gently displace the middle turbinate with the side of a Freer's elevator in order to be able to visualize the sphenoethmoid recess. This is easier after an anterior ethmoidectomy

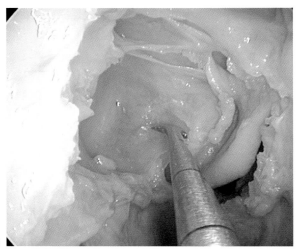

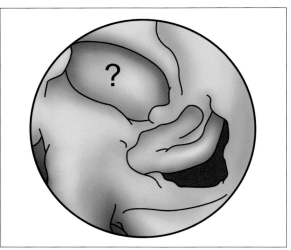

Fig. 5.**73**   **a** After completion of the transnasal sphenoid sinusotomy, the cavity of the posterior ethmoids is inspected. **b** How do you know whether it is safe to go further back to open the sphenoid sinus more? (See Fig. 5.**74a**, **b** and Fig. 5.**75a–j** for the answer.)

and when the basal lamella has been entered just above its inferior horizontal connection to the posteroinferior edge of the middle turbinate. Occasionally a bubble of air will be seen coming from the sphenoid ostium that is positioned much higher in the sphenoethmoid recess. The anterior wall of the sphenoid sinus is so thin that if a straight sucker (diameter 2–3 mm) is walked up the anterior wall of the sphenoid bone from the posterior choana then at 1.0–1.2 cm the sucker will enter the sinus with moderate pressure. It is wise to stay next to the vomer as to go more laterally runs the risk of damaging the structures in the lateral wall of the sphenoid sinus.

Once you have identified the sphenoid sinus, its anterior wall can be removed up to the skull base. It is wise not to open more than one bite inferiorly unless there is a good reason because of the septal branch of the sphenopalatine artery. Having established the level of the skull base below which it is safe to operate, you can then easily make a window between the superior and middle turbinates that will allow you to check where you are when you return to the posterior sinuses.

Now you can return to the posterior ethmoid sinuses, and after checking that there is a connection through the superior meatus, you can remove more cells that are medial and inferior toward the sphenoid sinus (Fig. 5.**73a**, **b**). Doing this creates more space in the posterior complex. The next step is to join the posterior ethmoid sinuses to the sphenoid sinus (Fig. 5.**74a**, **b**). This can safely be done by placing an instrument at the most posterosuperior aspect and then moving it vertically downward and then medially, pointing it toward the sphenoid sinus. With this maneuver the posterior ethmoid and sphenoid sinuses

can be joined safely (Fig. 5.**75a–j**). It is important to identify the level of the roof of the sphenoid sinus before opening any ethmoidal air cells superiorly, in order to avoid traversing the skull base (Fig. 5.**76a–d**). It is vital to preserve the superior turbinate at all costs because it is valuable olfactory epithelium. The remaining posterior ethmoid sinuses can be cleaned; a curved sucker is useful to palpate for space behind any partitions to help define the extent of the remaining air cells. A Hajek–Kofler punch is excellent for removing these bony remnants.

If the CT scan shows a "black halo" of air at the periphery of the posterior ethmoidal air cells, this will be helpful because when they are opened the clear mucosa lining the skull base will be seen. If there is a "white out" then care will be needed to ensure that you stay below the level of the roof of the sphenoid sinus. Very rarely, the anterior wall of the sinus is thicker, with hyperostosis secondary to chronic infection, or the sinus is hypoplastic and it will not be possible to enter it. This should be visible on the CT scan preoperatively.

It is best to limit the use of powered instrumentation in the sphenoid sinus unless visibility is good. If such an instrument is used, then the mouth of it should be pointed medially to avoid the risk of damaging any lateral structure.   **DVD** 7, 8

### Alternative Surgical Techniques

Some workers have advocated finding the sphenoid sinus from a lateral to medial approach by going through the posterior end of the superior turbinate. This can be done, but it runs the potential risk of going through the skull base or damaging the optic nerve if

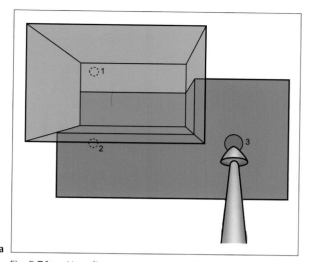

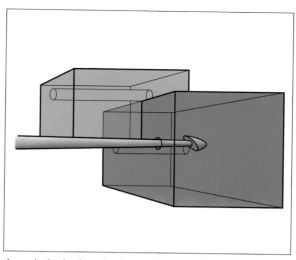

Fig. 5.**74 a**    Line diagram to represent the anterior aspect of the right sphenoid and posterior ethmoid sinuses. (1) Define the most posterior-superior-lateral part of the posterior ethmoid sinuses. (2) Move vertically downward and do not push through the back wall. (3) Move horizontally medially; it is at this point that the sphenoid sinus can safely be identified. **b** Antero-medial view of the right sphenoid and posterior ethmoid sinuses.

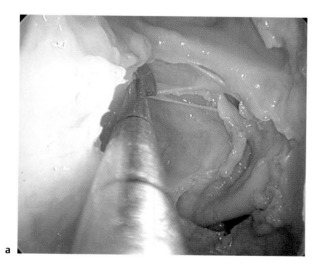

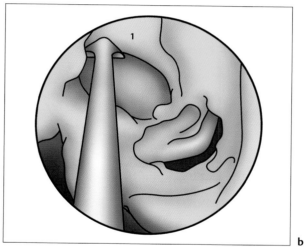

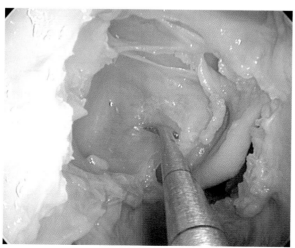

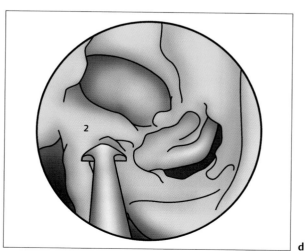

Fig. 5.**75 a**, **b**    The most superior-lateral-posterior aspect of the posterior ethmoid sinuses. **c**, **d** Move vertically downwards.

Fig. 5.**75 e–j**  ▷

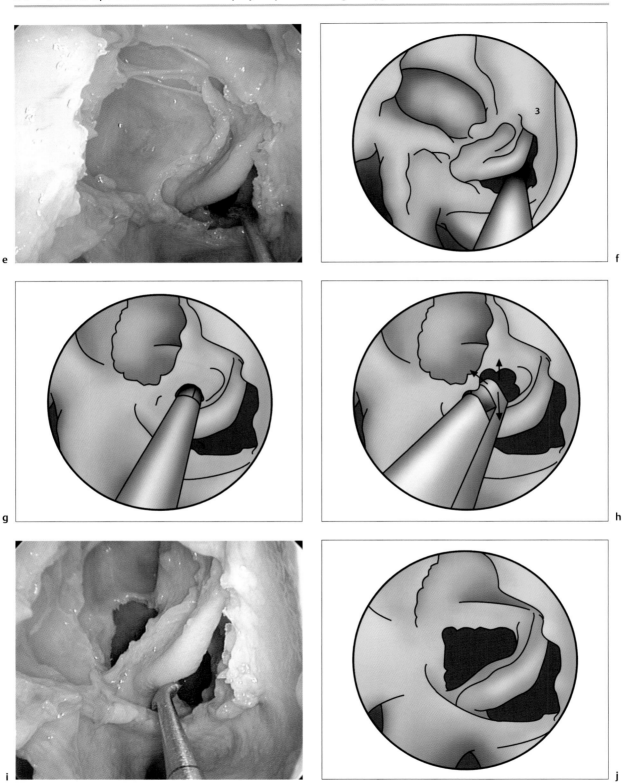

Fig. 5.**75 e, f** Then move horizontally-medially where the sphenoid can safely be found and the sphenoid ostium opened as necessary. The instrument may fall into the sinus or gentle pressure may be needed. **g–j** The medial aspect of the poste-rior wall of the posterior ethmoid sinuses can then be traversed safely and enlarged. It is important to preserve the superior turbinate.

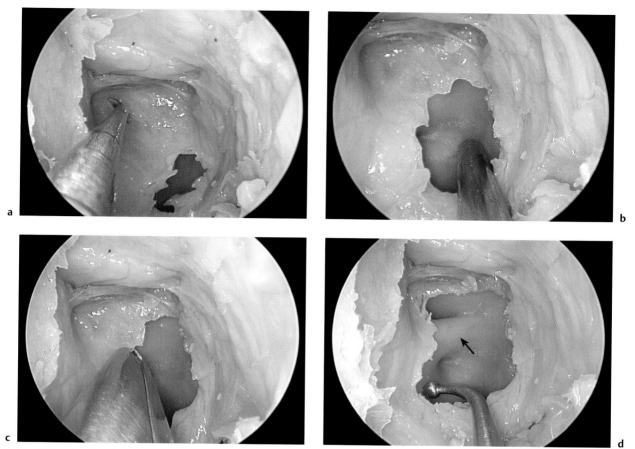

Fig. 5.**76 a–d**   This shows how dangerous it is to puncture a posterior ethmoid cell laterally. The optic nerve (arrow) can be exposed laterally. Note that it is safer to enter the sphenoid sinus from the posterior ethmoids at their most medial point.

there is an unrecognized posterior ethmoid air cell that rides above the sphenoid sinus or around the optic nerve (Fig. 5.77). It also removes valuable olfactory mucosa that should be preserved wherever possible.

## Useful Instruments

The shaver helps to remove polyps without avulsing them. It works best in the oscillating mode, but it is important not to use it to remove any polyps that are based on the turbinates or septum because this removes olfactory epithelium. It is important to send tissue for histological examination in every case. A Kerrison punch is a useful addition to allow the removal of fine partitions of bone.

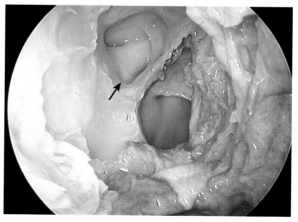

Fig. 5.**77**   The optic nerve in a sphenoethmoid air cell (arrow) above and lateral to the sphenoid sinus.

## ■ Frontosphenoethmoidectomy ■ ■ ■ ■
### ± Frontal Sinusotomy (I, II, III) ■
### ± Maxillary Sinusotomy (I, II, III) ■
### ± Sphenoid Sinusotomy (I, II, III) ■

### Terminology and Classification

This includes an anterior ethmoidectomy, posterior ethmoidectomy, sphenoid sinusotomy (see section on sphenoid sinusotomy, p. 100) along with opening the frontal recess. It is a combination of all these sections already described (Fig. 5.78). **DVD** 7, 8

### Indications

This is mainly reserved for those with persistent symptoms after anterior ethmoid surgery. In patients with severe recurrent polyposis, the best way to provide the patient with a longer symptom-free interval is to open up all the cells including the frontal recess (Fig. 5.79 a–c). A small proportion of patients with polyposis have frontal symptoms and in these patients we would open the frontal recess.

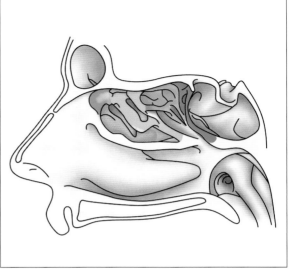

Fig. 5.**78**   A frontosphenoethmoidectomy. In addition to a sphenoethmoidectomy, the frontal recess is opened.

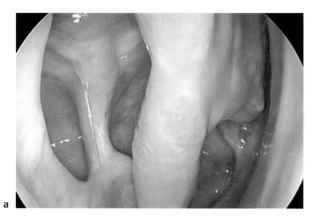

a

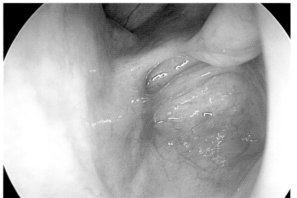

b

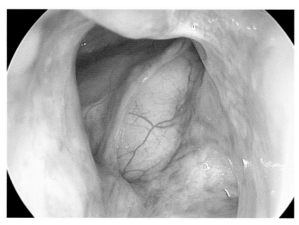

c

Fig. 5.**79 a, b**   Postoperative appearance after a frontosphenoethmoidectomy for severe polyposis. **c** A frontal sinusotomy type II in the same patient as in **a** and **b**. Note that there is residual mucosal inflammation that requires regular douching and topical nasal steroids to control it.

Patients with postoperative stenosis of the frontal recess and with symptoms require opening of the frontal recess (Fig. 5.**80**). Patients with pathology involving the frontal recess such as fungal disease and mucoceles need wide opening of the frontal recess area. (Fig. 5.**81 a–c**). Osteomas rarely cause symptoms except when they are large enough to cause a cosmetic deformity or a mucocele (Hehar and Jones, 1997). Beware if a patient has other symptoms, e.g., pain, as an osteoma rarely causes these symptoms and they are so common that they are likely to be a coincidental finding.

**Be careful to review the patient's symptoms and endoscopic signs to make sure that you are addressing genuine frontal sinus pathology.**

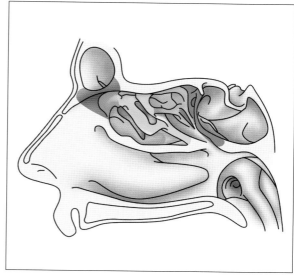

Fig. 5.**80**   Frontosphenoethmoidectomy and median drainage procedure.

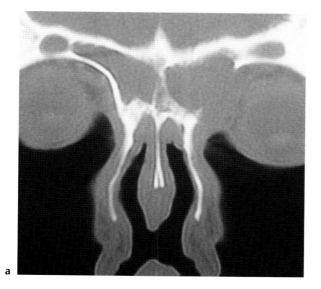

a

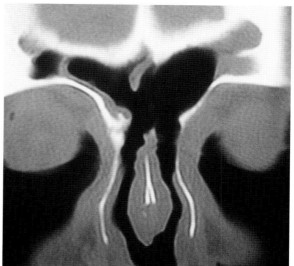

b

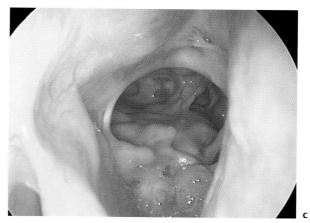

c

Fig. 5.**81 a–c**   The pre- and postoperative appearance after a frontosphenoethmoidectomy and median drainage procedure for severe polyposis and a left mucocele.

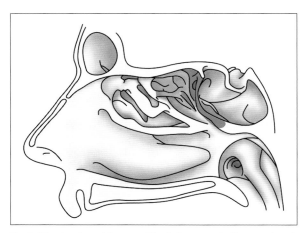

Fig. 5.**82**  A sphenoidotomy. The light green indicates when it is necessary to enlarge it into the posterior ethmoid sinuses.

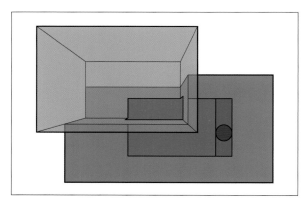

Fig. 5.**83**  Line diagram to represent the anterior aspect of the right sphenoid and posterior ethmoid sinuses. A type I sphenoidotomy defines the ostium—here a shaded round circle. A type II sphenoidotomy enlarges the ostium superiorly and inferiorly—here the vertical rectangle. A type III sphenoidotomy amalgamates the sphenoid with the posterior ethmoid sinuses—represented here by joining the light and dark green boxes.

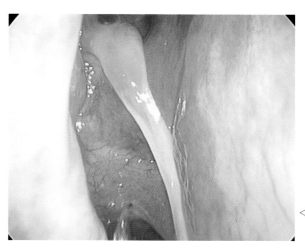

## ■ Sphenoid Sinusotomy (I, II, III) ■

### Terminology and Classification

This is a transnasal approach to open the sphenoid sinus (Fig. 5.**82**).

**Sphenoid sinusotomy I:** Identifying the sphenoid ostium without further instrumentation.

**Sphenoid sinusotomy II:** Opening the sphenoid inferiorly to half its height and upward to the skull base.

**Sphenoid sinusotomy III:** The sphenoid sinusotomy is extended to the floor of the sinus and laterally to the vital structures (Fig. 5.**83**).  **DVD**  7, 8

### Indications

Isolated sphenoid sinus disease, e.g., aspergillosis, purulent bacterial infection, inverted papilloma, mucocele, and biopsy of skull base lesions.

### Anatomy

The only point we wish to add to those already mentioned earlier is that the course of the septal branch of the sphenopalatine artery runs horizontally across the anterior wall of the sphenoid bone. In a type III sphenoid sinusotomy it is inevitable that this artery will be cut and require diathermy close to the sphenopalatine foramen.

### Surgical Technique

The sphenoid ostium can be found at the level of the superior turbinate. It is often necessary to lateralize the middle and superior turbinate in order to visualize it (see Fig. 5.**72k**). The ostium can then be enlarged as necessary.

If visibility is poor because of polyps or bleeding, the sphenoid sinus can safely be approached by staying close to the septum in the midline and palpating with the straight sucker up the posterior wall of the sphenoid (Fig. 5.**84**). At 1–1.5 cm above the posterior choana, the bone of the anterior wall of the sphenoid sinus is thin and it can be punctured by applying moderate pressure with a straight sucker (2–3 mm diameter). It may be necessary to gently lateralize the middle turbinate in order to obtain access to the sphenoethmoid recess. Once the sphenoid sinus is located, it can be enlarged with a small 45° forceps while a Hajek–Kofler punch or a Stammberger circular cutting punch or "mushroom" punch is used to enlarge it. It is best to

◁ Fig. 5.**84**  The sphenoid ostium with mucus coming out of it. This is a type I sphenoidotomy where suction and inspection were done, but it was not enlarged.

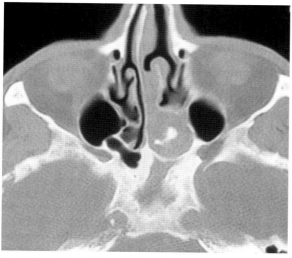

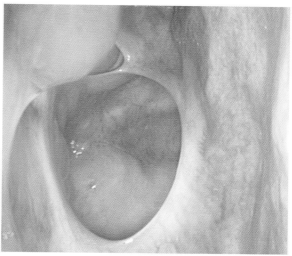

a    b

Fig. 5.**85**    **a** Aspergillosis of the sphenoid sinus. **b** The endoscopic appearance after a type II sphenoidotomy.

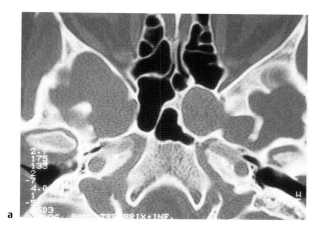

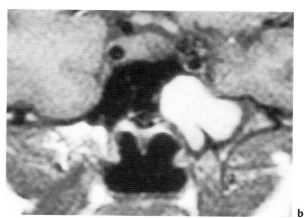

a    b

stay near the midline in order to avoid damaging a dehiscent carotid or optic nerve that may not be readily discernible on a CT scan if it is opaque with mucus retention or polyps.

It is advisable not to open the sphenoid ostium downward to a level lower than half the total height of the sinus, as a branch of the sphenopalatine artery runs along its anterior wall and if cut this can bleed briskly (see Fig. 5.72 k–t). Occasionally, the intersinus septum of the sphenoid is so oblique that one side can be very small. Care needs to be taken when removing the intersinus septum as it is oblique in over 75% of patients and can be based on the bone over the internal carotid artery. If the sphenoid is rudimentary or the bone around it is hyperostotic, then careful consideration needs to be given as to whether opening it serves any purpose. This is rarely the case (Fig. 5.85 a, 5.86 a–c).

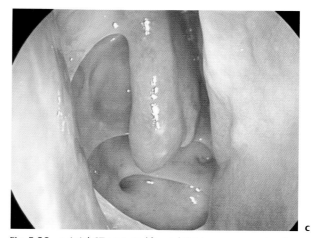

c

Fig. 5.**86**    **a** Axial CT scan and **b** axial MR image scans showing a dermoid in the sphenoid sinus extending laterally. **c** Postoperative appearance after a type III sphenoidotomy.

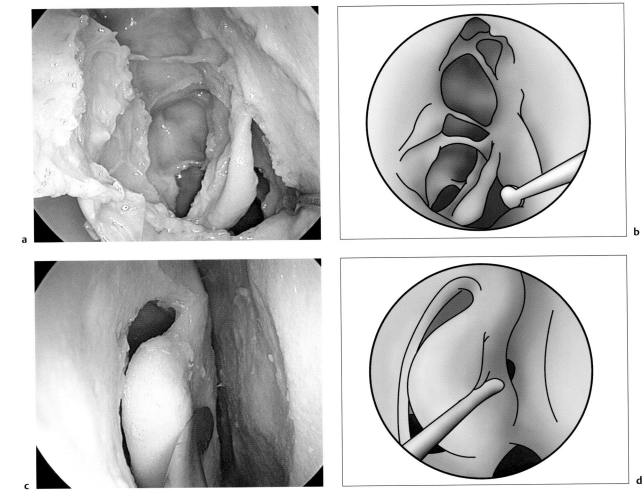

Fig. 5.**87**  **a**, **b** Appearance after a sphenoethmoidectomy. **c**, **d** Gentle lateralization of the middle turbinate to open up the olfactory cleft.

## ■ A Comment on the Management of the Middle and Superior Turbinates

One of the main differences between this and other texts is our concern for the sense of smell and our respect for the turbinate and therefore olfactory tissue. Some authors have advocated resection of the middle turbinate to help access and with the aim of reducing the incidence of adhesions. We do not do this as we try to preserve all the olfactory mucosa on the medial surface of the ethmoturbinals and the septum.

The patient who has had anosmia or severe hyposmia might not "miss" their sense of smell after surgery as it was poor in the first place. This has led surgeons to become complacent about the sense of smell, particularly in those with late-onset asthma and polyps medial to the middle turbinate, where the results of surgery have been mixed (70% with hy-

posmia are improved but this rarely lasts for longer than 6 months even in the presence of continued medical treatment). However, if you do restore patients' sense of smell their quality of life is much improved and they are extremely grateful. By preserving "all" the mucosa in the olfactory area on the septum and the turbinates, as well as opening the olfactory cleft, this can be done.

### Surgical Technique

The middle and superior turbinates should gently be lateralized after a complete frontosphenoethmoidectomy to open up the olfactory cleft. Atraumatic lateralization of the turbinates is only possible after making space for them (Fig. 5.**87 a–d**). This reduces the mucosa-mucosa contact in this area and allows better access for topical nasal steroids.

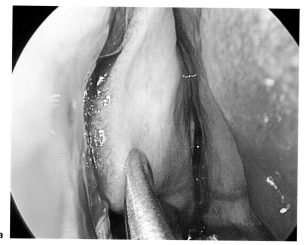

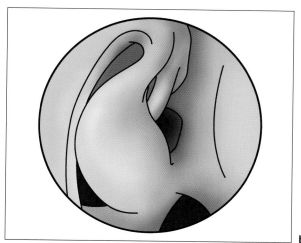

Fig. 5.**88 a, b**   The maxillary sinusotomy can be seen to extend below the inferior edge of the middle turbinate.

It is difficult to resist the temptation to remove or debulk polyps medial to the middle turbinate, but it is best to preserve this mucosa. A course of preoperative steroids will help reduce the size of the polyps. Only remove polyps that come from the posterior ethmoid cells under the superior turbinate and not polyps that are based on the septum or the middle turbinate.

If the surgeon displaces the middle turbinate in this way, the surgeon should ensure that the middle meatal antrostomy is undertaken such that it lies at a level below the inferior edge of the middle turbinate, so that if the middle turbinate lateralizes, the maxillary ostium can still drain (Fig. 5.**88 a, b**) and it is possible to visualize the maxillary sinusotomy and the frontal recess as well as the ethmoids with a 45° endoscope. The middle turbinate should remain relatively stable as long as it is only gently lateralized and the base or inferior horizontal component of the ground lamella is preserved. Even when it is very mobile we would prefer for it to lateralize rather than for it to adhere to the septum and run the risk of making olfaction worse.

When the olfactory cleft is opened, even large polyps medial to the middle turbinate resolve, so do not be worried about leaving them behind (Fig. 5.**89 a–c**). Note that no polyps were removed from the middle turbinate in order to preserve olfactory mucosa. It is easy to remove them, but not easy to put back the olfactory epithelium that is removed with them!   *DVD* 7, 8

## Alternative Surgical Techniques

If there is a concha bullosa, the lateral half of the turbinate can be resected. This can be done by incising the anterior surface with a sickle knife and then removing the lateral portion by cutting it free with microscissors or with straight through-cutting forceps (Fig. 5.**90 a–c**).

Occasionally a concha bullosa restricts access when only an infundibulotomy is required. A minimally traumatic technique is to gently crush the turbinate; this preserves the olfactory mucosa and there is no bleeding, so patients can go home the same day.

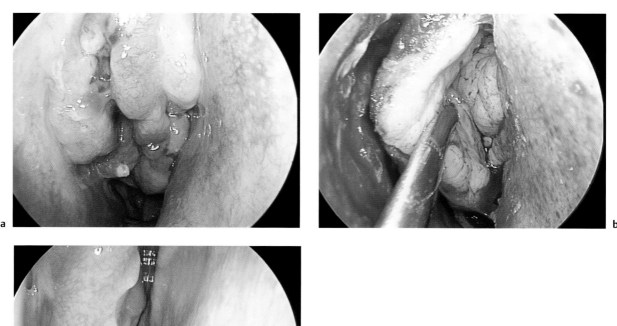

Fig. 5.**89**   **a** Preoperative polyps in the olfactory cleft. **b** Peroperative gentle lateralization of the middle turbinate after a sphenoethmoidectomy. **c** The appearance one year later—the patient complied with topical nasal steroids.

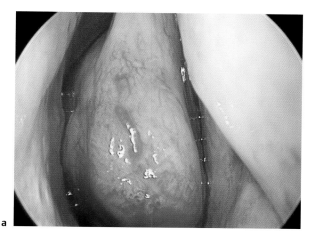

a

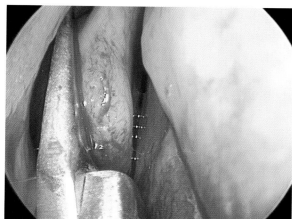

b

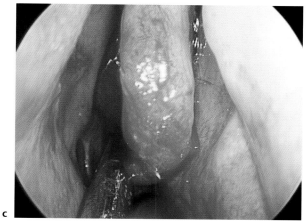

c

Fig. 5.**90 a–c**  The lateral half of a concha bullosa is removed using the Zurich microscissors.

# 6 An Endoscopic Tour:
## Endoscopic Examination, Anatomical Variations, and Specific Conditions

We need to be able to recognize the wide range of structural variations in the bony architecture of the paranasal sinuses and to distinguish normal from diseased mucosa. It helps to have a system for looking for these in order to build up as complete a picture of the patient's situation as possible (Fig. 6.1). In this section we will discuss various techniques, devices, and particular problems.

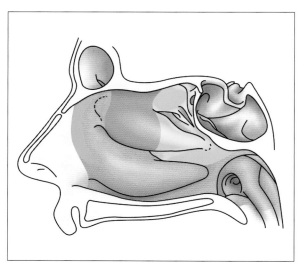

Fig. 6.1 Three steps to examine the nasal airway and conduits of the paranasal sinuses.

## ■ Outpatient Examination

It is best to examine the nose initially without any anesthetic as the solution can irritate the mucosa, producing a reactive rhinorrhea and edema, which makes it difficult to know whether there is any underlying mucosal disease or not. A rigid 30°, 2.7 mm endoscope is good for outpatient examination (Fig. 6.2 a, b). It provides good access and control and is also a durable instrument. Its only drawback is that it does not provide enough light or a wide enough view to record a good image. For this, a 4 mm rigid endoscope is needed.

It is important not to produce any discomfort, so the endoscope should be advanced slowly, avoiding any contact with the septum or lateral nasal wall. The middle meatus is often the most spacious area to examine, and this is often the best area to examine first so as to give patients confidence that they will not feel much discomfort during this procedure. It is possible to advance the endoscope to visualize the postnasal space and to see whether there is any mucopus tracking back from the middle meatus, the posterior ethmoid sinuses, or the sphenoethmoid recess (Fig. 6.3). The anterior aspect of the olfactory cleft can be seen by angling the endoscope upward as soon as it is introduced past the nasal vestibule. However, it is important not to touch the anterior end of the middle turbinate when you do this, as it is very sensitive. One key aspect of using the endoscope is to make every move-

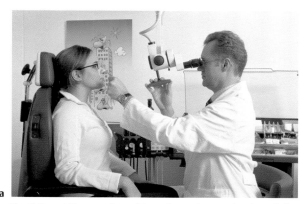
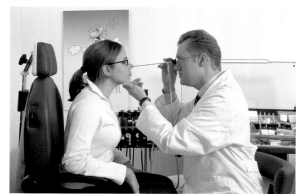

Fig. 6.2 **a** Microscopic and **b** endoscopic examination of the nose.

ment slowly and gently. Patients can tolerate some pressure on the mucosa as long as it is applied very slowly; sudden movements cause more discomfort. We tell the patient to let us know by grunting if they are going to sneeze in order to warn us to withdraw the endoscope.

After the overview, you may think that local anesthetic should be applied for a more thorough examination, for example, when the nose is crowded or the initial inspection has produced discomfort. We use cotton wool soaked in a local anesthetic and a decongestant, placing it in the middle meatus or where we need to examine.

## ■ The Endoscopic Tour

The lateral nasal wall and cavity are inspected in three steps.

1  Step 1 involves advancing the endoscope along the inferior meatus. If there is no room because of a septal spur, advance the endoscope between the middle and inferior turbinate toward the nasopharynx (Fig. 6.**4**). The posterior aspect of the nasal cavity is inspected before coming forward to inspect the front.

   The following structures should be examined: the back of the inferior turbinate (Fig. 6.**5**), the tubal orifice, and the fossa of Rosenmüller (Fig. 6.**6**), as well as the posterior wall of the nasopharynx. It is important to look for mucopus tracking down from the lateral nasal wall over the tubal orifice.

2  Step 2 involves coming forward a little and angling the endoscope upward to see the sphenoethmoid recess area (only a limited view of the sphenoid

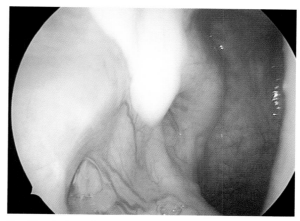

Fig. 6.**3**   A view of mucopus tracking down the nasopharynx from the middle meatus.

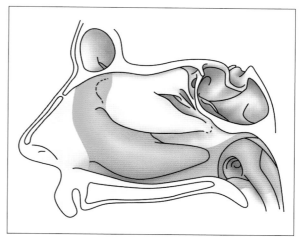

Fig. 6.**4**   Step 1 examines these areas.

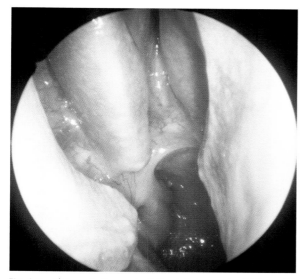

Fig. 6.**5**   The posterior end of the inferior and middle turbinate.

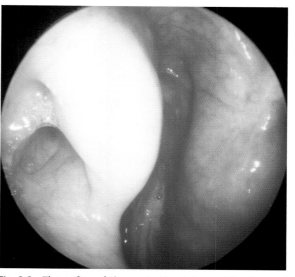

Fig. 6.**6**   The orifice of the eustachian tube and the fossa of Rosenmüller behind and medial.

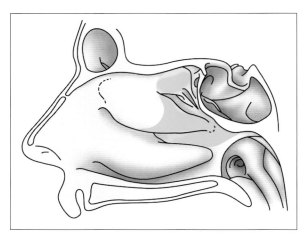

Fig. 6.**7**   Step 2 examines the sphenoethmoid recess and the anterior wall of the sphenoid.

ostium and the higher part of the anterior wall of the sphenoid is possible because the superior turbinate gets in the way) (Fig. 6.7). Look for mucopus tracking down from the sphenoid ostia as you try, if possible, to maneuver the endoscope to visualize the superior turbinate, the sphenoid ostium, and the posterior olfactory cleft (Fig. 6.**8 a**, **b**). Look out for polyps coming out of the superior meatus under the superior turbinate as these indicate disease in the posterior ethmoid sinuses (Fig. 6.**9**). Mucopus may be seen draining from the posterior ethmoid sinuses above the root of the middle turbinate.

3   Step 3 is accomplished by gently rolling the endoscope under the middle turbinate to see whether mucopus is tracking under the ethmoid bulla from the maxillary sinus (Fig. 6.**10**). The accessory ostium (Fig. 6.**11**), the posterior edge of the uncinate process, and the bulla ethmoidalis (Fig. 6.**12**), as well as the outflow area of the frontal recess are then visible (Fig. 6.**13**). You then come forward to obtain an overview of the middle meatus (Fig. 6.**14 a**, **b**). If you can see a maxillary ostium, it is always an accessory ostium, as the natural one is hidden by the uncinate process.

It is less stimulating to the middle turbinate to inspect the hiatus semilunaris while withdrawing the endoscope than to try to enter this area from the front, where the slightest touch to the anterior end of the middle turbinate causes pain. It is possible to use a flexible endoscope, but it is more difficult to maintain fine control and the visibility is not as good because of the optical properties of the endoscope. A 45° endoscope can help visualize the sphenoid ostium or Hasner's valve under the inferior turbinate. Hasner's valve is found approximately 1 cm be-

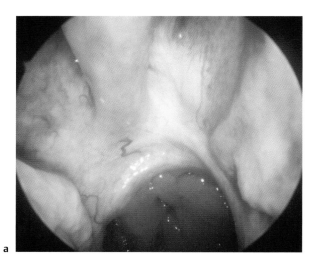

a

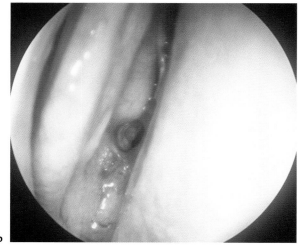

b

Fig. 6.**8**   **a** The initial view of the sphenoethmoid recess and **b** A view of the upper part of the sphenoethmoid recess showing the sphenoid ostium that is sometimes possible.

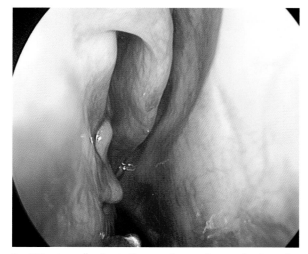

Fig. 6.**9**   A small polyp in the superior meatus coming from the posterior ethmoid sinuses under the superior turbinate.

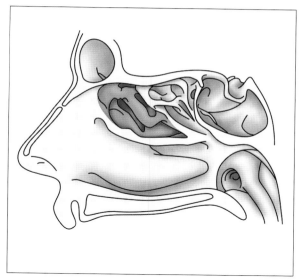

Fig. 6.**10**   The areas examined in step 3: the middle meatus, the ethmoid bulla, the hiatus semilunaris, and the uncinate process.

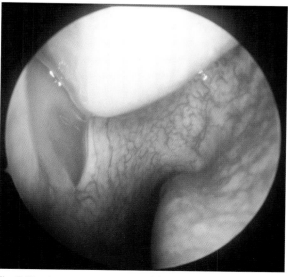

Fig. 6.**11**   An accessory ostium of the right maxillary sinus with clear mucus filling it.

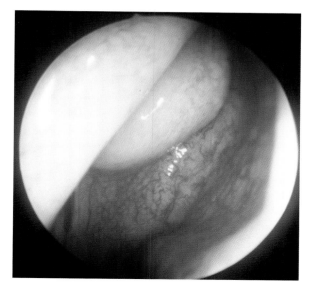

Fig. 6.**12**   The posterior edge of the uncinate process and the bulla ethmoidalis with an accessory ostium in the posterior fontanelle.

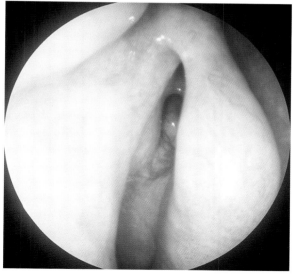

Fig. 6.**13**   The outflow area of the frontal recess.

hind the anterior end of the inferior turbinate high in the lateral wall of the inferior meatus (Fig. 6.**15**).

## ■ Endoscopic Evidence of Mucosal Disease

Endoscopic findings must be interpreted in the light of patients' symptoms and response to medical treatment. You will be caught out if you intervene on the basis of an abnormal endoscopic examination alone.

However, endoscopy is far more reliable than CT—we cannot emphasize this point enough (Fig. 6.**16**). Endoscopy is particularly helpful in patients who have had radiology that has shown changes, and when the history and examination indicate that the problem is not due to their sinuses. These patients can be told or shown via a camera their endoscopic appearance. For most patients an intranasal view of their disease with an image on a monitor is particularly helpful in supporting the surgeon's opinion and may help

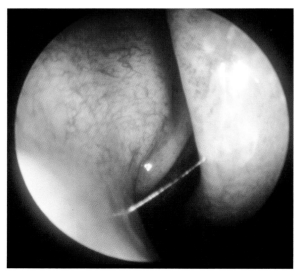

a

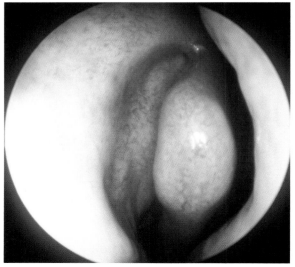

b

Fig. 6.**14 a, b**   When the endoscope is withdrawn, you obtain an overview of the anterior part of the middle meatus.

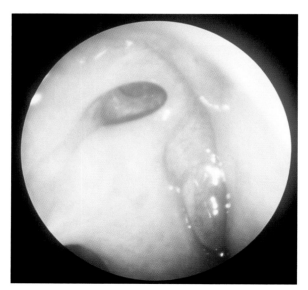

Fig. 6.**15**   Hasner's valve lies 1 cm behind the anterior end of the inferior turbinate.

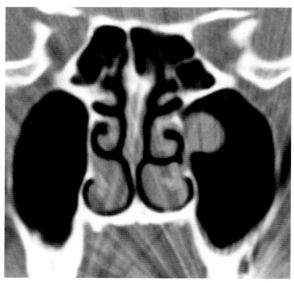

Fig. 6.**16**   An incidental mucus retention cyst found in 1 in 30 asymptomatic people.

counteract any information they have gleaned from their radiology report that may have insinuated that they have significant paranasal sinus pathology when these changes are often incidental (Bolger and Kennedy, 1992; Benninger, 1997; Hughes and Jones, 1998).

One of the key aspects of the examination is to establish whether the lining of the nose and the outlet areas of the sinuses have normal mucosa. Nineteen percent of most populations have allergic rhinitis. Of these, many will have marked hypertrophy of the inferior turbinates, but on inspection of the middle meatus that area of mucosa will look normal. A minority, particularly those with intermittent (seasonal) rhini-

tis, will have some edema of the mucosa throughout the nasal airway. They will often have "wet" mucosa with clear mucus, although occasionally this will have a light yellow stain because of the presence of eosinophils. The same can be found in patients with late-onset asthma who have rhinitis. Patients with late-onset asthma or allergic rhinitis pose a diagnostic problem, as it is not possible to be sure whether there is any coexisting paranasal sinus disease on the basis of endoscopy (and often on history). A trial of medical treatment is often a useful indicator, but it is best to focus on the patient's main symptoms and response to medical treatment in the light of the endoscopic signs rather than the other way around. You may make use of a diary of symptoms kept by the patient, see the patient on more than one occasion or, best of all, see them when they are symptomatic in order to help ascertain whether there is any infective component contributing to their symptoms.

In the majority of patients, with a clear middle meatus and a normal lining, the normal appearance is of particular value as it means that symptoms of pain and pressure are extremely unlikely to be attributable to sinus disease. It is worth asking a patient who has recurrent acute episodes of pain to attend when they are symptomatic—you may be surprised to find out how infrequently these patients have an abnormal endoscopic examination when they are examined. In patients who have had previous surgery, endoscopy is also far more useful than CT. When a patient returns after previous sinus surgery and has some residual symptoms, it is tempting to arrange for a CT scan. Resist the temptation. You will serve your patients better by retaking the history and doing a thorough endoscopic examination (Fig. 6.**17**). A CT scan will often show some mucosal thickening, which is often an incidental finding (Maclennan and MacGarry, 1995).

## ■ Anatomical Variations

The prevalence of anatomical variations is well documented, and it appears that they are not consistently different between asymptomatic groups and those with proven rhinosinusitis. This is contrary to early reports that labeled them as anatomical "abnormalities," for they now appear to be normal variations. This implies that anatomical variations play a minor role, if any at all, in initiating rhinosinusitis or causing it to persist. Perhaps the primary concern of anatomical variations is their tendency to lead the surgeon astray during an operation. For example, a septal deviation is often found with a compensatory concha bullosa on the contralateral side. These findings are as common in an asymptomatic population as in a population with rhinosinusitis (Havas et al., 1988; Lloyd, 1990; Lloyd et al., 1991; Bolger et al., 1991; Jones et al., 1997a).

### Agger Nasi Air Cells

Endoscopically, it is possible to get an idea whether there is a sizable agger nasi cell from the prominence in the lateral nasal wall where it meets the middle turbinate (Fig. 6.**18**a, b).

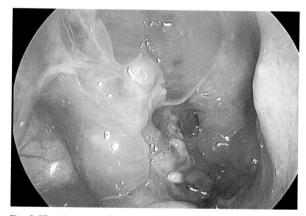

Fig. 6.**17** History and endoscopy are more reliable in assessment than CT after previous surgery. Endoscopic signs supported by a history suggestive of sinus pathology.

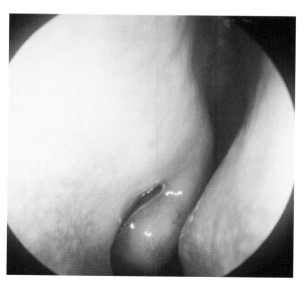

a

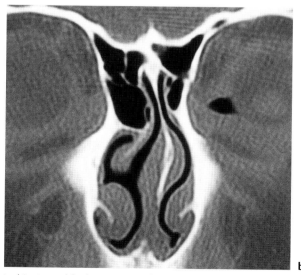

b

Fig. 6.**18** **a** A well-pneumatized agger nasi cell producing a bulge in the lateral nasal wall near the origin of the middle turbinate and **b** the corresponding CT image from the same patient.

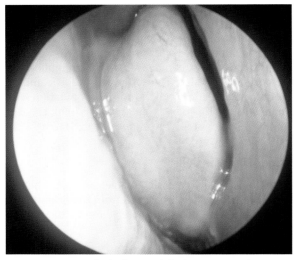
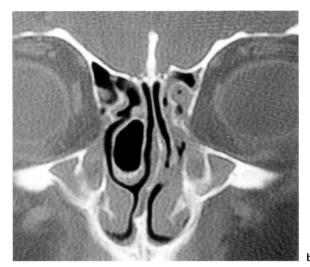

a                                                          b

Fig. 6.**19**    **a** A concha bullosa with **b** the corresponding CT image.

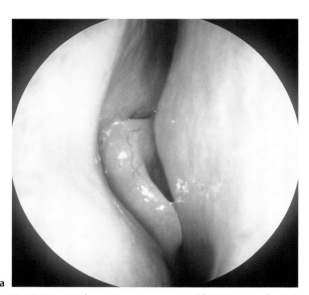
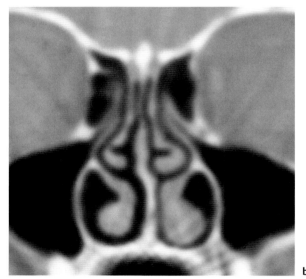

a                                                          b

Fig. 6.**20**    **a** Endoscopic appearance and **b** CT image of a right paradoxical middle turbinate.

## Concha Bullosa

Endoscopically, a concha bullosa has the appearance of an inflated anterior end of the middle turbinate, and that is essentially what it is. It is found in about one-third of normal individuals. It often restricts access to the middle meatus and the posterior nasal cavity (Fig. 6.**19**a, **b**). On CT, as the anterior end of the middle turbinate is followed backward, its base starts to lateralize with ethmoid air cells forming much of its midsection and base until more posteriorly it comes off the lateral nasal wall in a near coronal plane. The posterior half has a condensation that forms the basal lamella or the partition between the anterior and posterior ethmoid air cells. In the coronal section, most middle turbinates have one or more air cells within the posterior half, but this does not mean that this is abnormal or in itself will predispose them to harm.

## A Paradoxical Middle Turbinate

This is a middle turbinate that has a concave medial surface facing the septum. This occurs in approximately 11 % of normal people and is a normal variation (Fig. 6.**20**a, **b**). The middle turbinate is often thin and frail and should be gently mobilized by pressing it medially with a Freer's elevator to help access to the middle meatus.

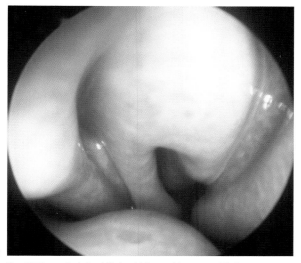
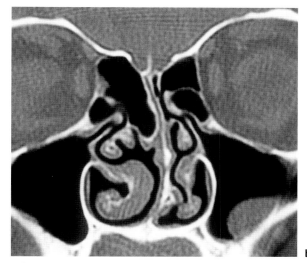

Fig. 6.**21**   **a** A right bifid middle turbinate and **b** its appearance on CT.

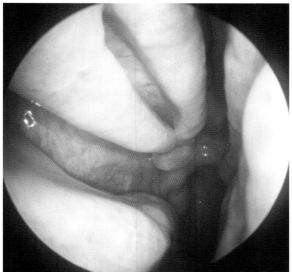
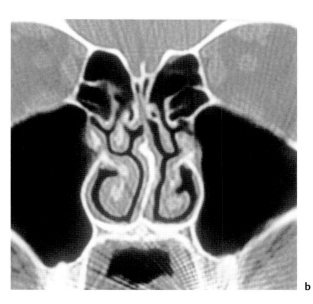

Fig. 6.**22 a**, **b**   Posterior bifidity of the middle turbinate.

## A Bifid Middle Turbinate

The degree of bifidity of the middle turbinate can vary from a shallow groove on its medial aspect to a deep one that almost divides it in two (Fig. 6.**21 a**, **b**). A bifid middle turbinate will often only be seen if you examine the medial surface, and its bifidity can be confirmed on CT (Fig. 6.**22 a**, **b**). When the groove almost splits a bifid middle turbinate into two, the bifidity can make it look like two turbinates or a paradoxical uncinate process and a middle turbinate. Whether it is a bifid middle turbinate or a paradoxical uncinate process can be found by following the lateral surface of the lateral bulge to define whether the groove has a blind end or one that continues upward out of reach into the middle meatus.

## A Polypoidal Anterior End of the Middle Turbinate

It can sometimes be relatively difficult to differentiate middle meatal polyps from sessile polypoidal mucosa based on the middle turbinate as they can look the same (Fig. 6.**23 a**, **b**). It is wise to gently palpate any polyp in this area to help define whether it is based on the middle turbinate. The middle turbinate is a useful landmark and, as it is attached to the skull base, it is important not to avulse it. Polyps on the medial surface of the middle turbinate that do not come from the superior meatus or sphenoid should be left alone as they contain valuable olfactory sensory neurons.

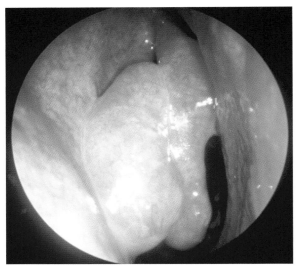
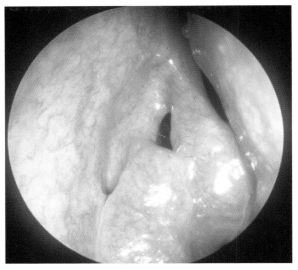

Fig. 6.**23**   A sessile polyp based on the anterior end of the middle turbinate—**a** initial and **b** close-up view.

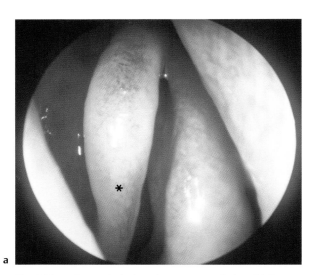
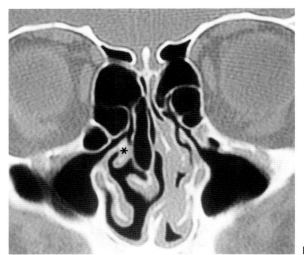

Fig. 6.**24**   **a** A paradoxical uncinate process (∗) and **b** its appearance on CT.

### A Paradoxical Uncinate Process

A true paradoxical uncinate is one that curves back on itself. In this case, the uncinate process can give a strange appearance to the middle meatus and look like an extra turbinate (Fig. 6.24 a, b). Be careful not to go through it in the belief that its end is the ethmoid bulla, as you may inadvertently enter the orbit. Nasal polyps in the infundibulum often push the uncinate process forward, even to the extent that it can turn back on itself.

### Pneumatized Uncinate Process

This can look like an extra turbinate and can lead the unwary surgeon astray (Fig. 6.25 a, b). If it is recog-

nized, with the help of a CT scan, then it should be opened and removed with the help of through-cutting forceps and back-biters.

### Accessory Ostia of the Maxillary Sinus Anterior to the Uncinate Process

If an ostium to the maxillary sinus can readily be seen by endoscopy in outpatients, it is probably an accessory ostia. The accessory ostium that is most readily seen lies anterior to the edge of the uncinate process (Fig. 6.26 a–d). Such ostia are said to be the result of recurrent acute maxillary infections, but this is conjectural.

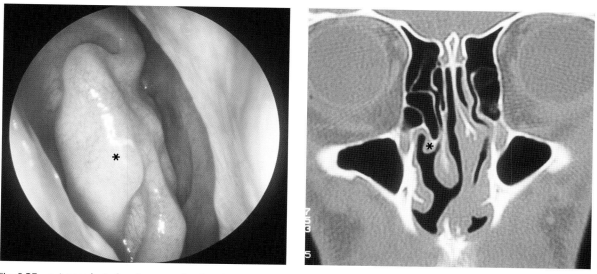

Fig. 6.**25**    **a** A paradoxical and pneumatized uncinate process (∗) and **b** its appearance on CT.

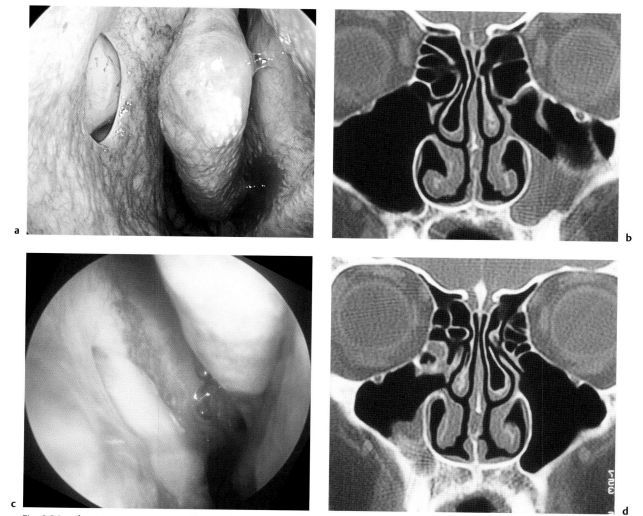

Fig. 6.**26 a–d**    Anterior accessory ostium and its appearance on CT.

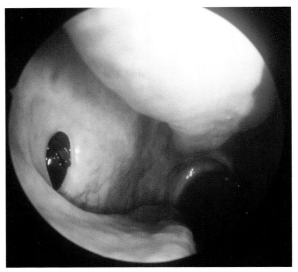

a

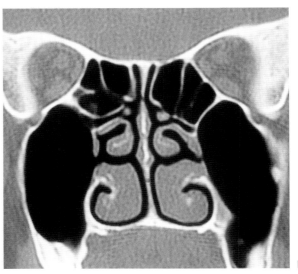

b

Fig. 6.**27**    **a** An endoscopic view of a right posterior accessory ostium and **b** its appearance on CT. Note the left posterior accessory ostium on CT.

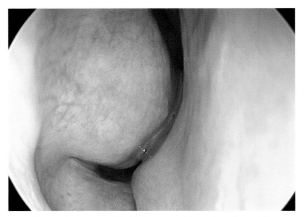

Fig. 6.**28**    A hypertrophied inferior turbinate in idiopathic rhinitis.

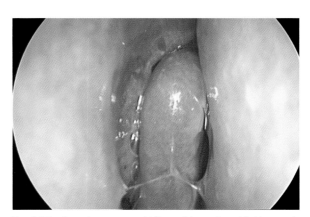

Fig. 6.**29**    An edematous middle turbinate in a highly atopic patient. Allergic secretions can look like pus when they are lightly stained yellow by eosinophils.

## Accessory Ostium of the Maxillary Sinus in the Posterior Fontanelle

This is found behind the posterior edge of the uncinate process between the inferior and middle turbinate and is a fistula into the maxillary antrum (Fig. 6.**27** a, **b**).

## ■ An Atlas of Specific Conditions To Help Recognize Variations in Anatomy and Different Pathological Conditions

### Allergy

1  Hypertrophied inferior turbinate (Fig. 6.**28**).
2  Edematous middle turbinate (Fig. 6.**29**).

### Infection

1  Bacterial rhinosinusitis:
   ● Pus in the middle meatus (Fig. 6.**30**).
   ● Pus down the posterior lateral wall (Fig. 6.**31**).
2  Aspergillosis (Fig. 6.**32**).

### Inflammatory Diseases

1  Pyogenic granuloma (Fig. 6.**33**).
2  Wegener granulomatosis (Fig. 6.**34** a, **b**).
3  Sarcoidosis (Fig. 6.**35** a, **b**).

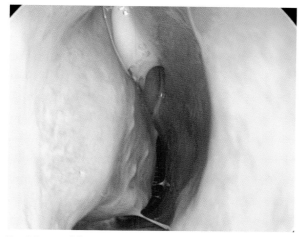

Fig. 6.**30** Middle meatal pus in acute maxillary sinusitis.

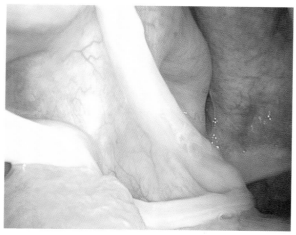

Fig. 6.**31** Pus tracking over the eustachian tube orifice.

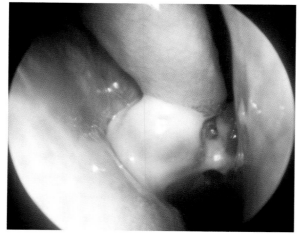

Fig. 6.**32** The thick green plug of mucus sometimes seen in aspergillosis.

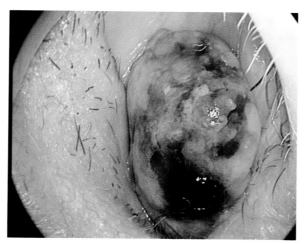

Fig. 6.**33** A pyogenic granuloma, which often bleeds spontaneously.

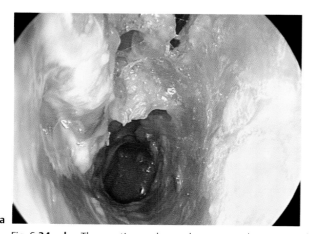

a

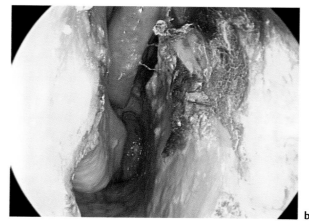

b

Fig. 6.**34 a**, **b** The crusting and granular mucosa show some of the spectrum of Wegener granulomatosis.

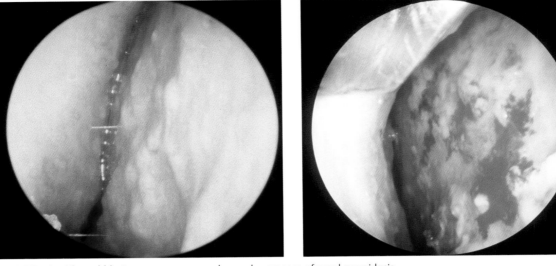

Fig. 6.**35 a**, **b**   The cobblestone appearance and granular mucosa of nasal sarcoidosis.

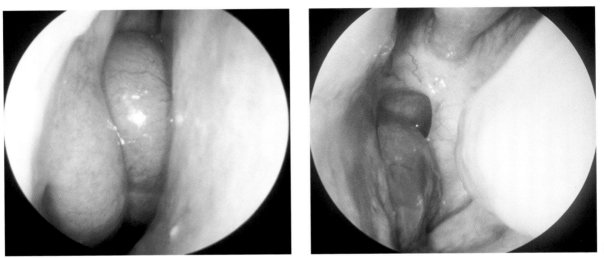

Fig. 6.**36 a**, **b**   Right antrochoanal polyp also visible in the posterior choana from the left side.

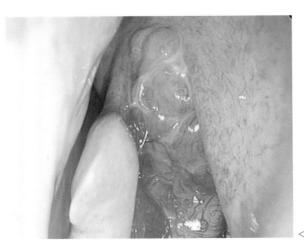

## Benign Tumors

1   Antrochoanal polyp (Fig. 6.**36 a**, **b**).
2   Inverted papilloma (Fig. 6.**37**).
3   Chondroma (Fig. 6.**38**).
4   Angiofibroma (Fig. 6.**39**).

## Malignant Tumors

1   Olfactory neuroblastoma (Fig. 6.**40**).
2   Postnasal space tumor (Fig. 6.**41**).
3   Malignant melanoma (Fig. 6.**42**).
4   Adenocarcinoma (Fig. 6.**43**).

◁ Fig. 6.**37**   Inverted papilloma in the left frontal recess.

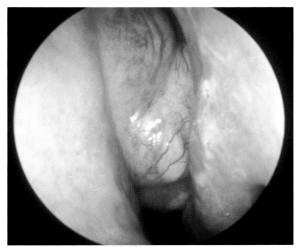

Fig. 6.**38**   Chondroma of the septum.

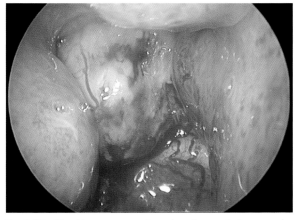

Fig. 6.**39**   The blue or magenta color of a posterior vascular mass in an adolescent—an angiofibroma.

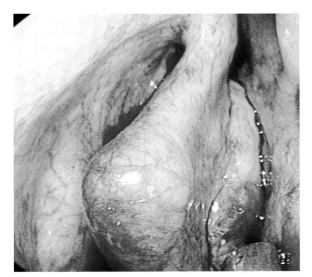

Fig. 6.**40**   A solitary hemorrhagic polyp medial to the turbinate—an olfactory neuroblastoma.

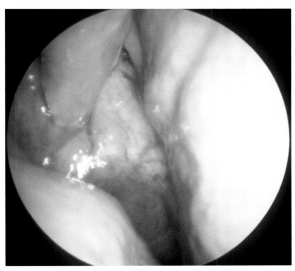

Fig. 6.**41**   A mass in the nasopharynx due to a lymphoma.

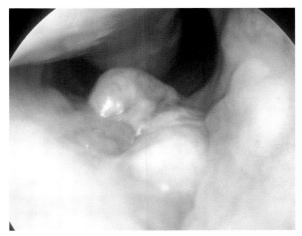

Fig. 6.**42**   Amelanotic melanoma on the floor of the nose.

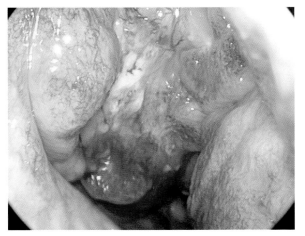

Fig. 6.**43**   Adenocarcinoma of the lateral nasal wall.

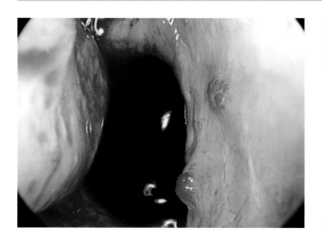

## Miscellaneous

Hereditary hemorrhagic telangiectasia (HHT) (Fig. 6.**44**).

Fig. 6.**44**  Telangiectasia in HHT.

# 7 The Place of Radiology

## ■ The Role of Conventional Radiology

Plain radiographs have a limited role in the modern management of paranasal sinus disease because they have so many false-positive and false-negative findings. In acute maxillary or frontal sinusitis, they can help confirm the diagnosis, but otherwise they have been superseded by CT (Fig. 7.1 a–c).

## ■ The Role of Computed Tomography

CT shows the bony anatomy very well; this provides a map for endoscopic sinus surgery. However, the mucosal changes that it can show rarely tell us about the pathology in the sinuses (Goldwyn et al., 1995; Cousin et al., 2000).

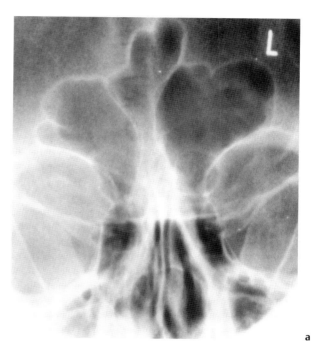

Fig. 7.**1 a–c**   The plain radiograph (**a**) does not show that the frontal sinus that is diseased drains into the left frontonasal infundibulum, as is shown on CT (**b** and **c**).

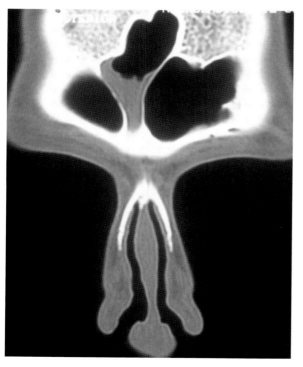

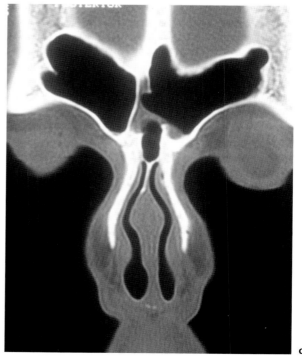

b

c

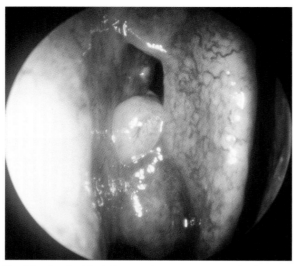
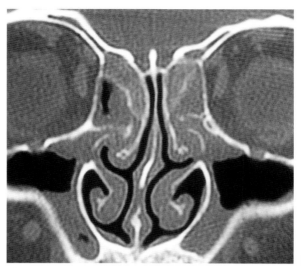

a

b

Fig. 7.2a, b   Residual disease after maximum medical treatment. *Then* CT shows more detail of the extent of sinus disease.

It is easy to fill out a CT request form, but this may be a mistake—although CT has good sensitivity for diagnosing paranasal sinus disease, it has poor specificity; for example, there are many false-positive changes. Before you request a CT scan, think why you are doing it and what information it will provide. Without a clinical picture based on the history, examination, and a trial of medical treatment, it is impossible to give any specific meaning to a finding of "mucosal changes" on a CT scan (Jianetto and Pratt, 1995).

Unfortunately, one in three asymptomatic people have an abnormal CT scan, which makes CT a poor diagnostic tool for rhinosinusitis. It is, therefore, important not to request a CT scan in the initial management of patients unless there are specific reasons to do so. These include:

- Suspected intracranial or intraorbital involvement as a complication of rhinosinusitis
- Suspected atypical infection or malignancy
- Specific pathology, e.g., mucoceles, benign tumors of the paranasal sinuses, where the extent of the lesion needs to be defined
- Prior to orbital or optic nerve decompression

### ■ When to Request CT in the Management of Rhinosinusitis

CT for rhinosinusitis is best reserved for patients who have not responded to maximum medical treatment. After maximum medical treatment, CT can help confirm that there is paranasal sinus disease and give an indication of the extent of residual disease (Fig. 7.2 a, b). It can also provide a map for the surgeon to use for in-

traoperative navigation and help to stage the extent of the disease.

If the CT scan shows no signs of any mucosal disease, this should prompt the surgeon to reconsider whether the patient's symptoms are due to rhinosinusitis, especially if the primary symptom is pain. In a minority of patients it can be unclear, despite repeated consultations, endoscopic examination, trials of medical treatment, and a patient's diary, whether their symptoms are due to paranasal sinus disease. CT or MRI is indicated if there are progressive symptoms of pain or any neurological signs in order to exclude malignancy or central pathology (Jones, 2002; Marshall and Jones, 2003).

It is important for the surgeon to look at the CT scan preoperatively to get an idea of the anatomy and to relate the changes revealed on the CT scan to the patient's clinical condition (Simmen and Schuknecht, 1997). It is very helpful to show the CT scan to the patient when trying to explain their disease, the planned surgery, and the possible complications (Fig. 7.3).

### ■ CT Parameters

Spiral CT performed with axial 1 mm sections is the current ideal for CT imaging of the paranasal sinuses (see Table 7.1). Coronal reconstructions with 2–3 mm sections are sufficient for most endoscopic sinus surgery, but finer cuts are required to answer specific questions about the site and extent of a CSF leak.

Axial sections with coronal reconstruction will remove any dental artifacts; these can be excluded be-

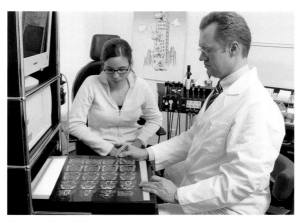

Fig. 7.**3**   The CT images help to communicate what the problem is to the patient.

Table 7.**1**   Zurich Protocol for CT of the paranasal sinuses

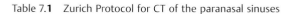

- Scan plane axial:
  alveolar recess of maxillary sinus to roof of frontal sinus
- Slice collimation:
  1 mm (e.g. 4 × 1 mm), table feed 3.5, rotation time
  0.75 s
- Slice reconstruction:
  1.2/0.7 mm overlap ultrahigh bone algorithm
  1.2/0.7 soft-tissue algorithm
- Multiplanar reconstructions:
  Axial/sagittal 2.0/2.0 mm ultrahigh and soft tissue
  Coronal 1.5–2.0 mm
- Filming (window/level):
  Ultrahigh-resolution bone algorithm 3200/700
  Soft-tissue algorithm 270–300/100

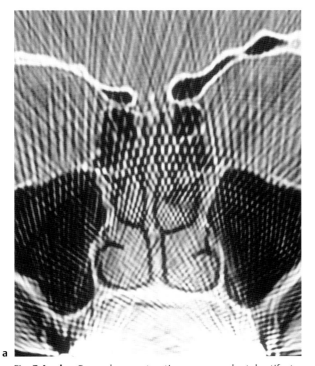

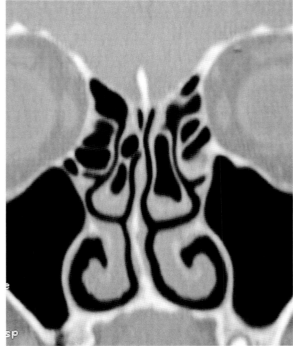

a                                                                                                 b

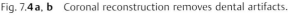

Fig. 7.**4 a**, **b**   Coronal reconstruction removes dental artifacts.

cause they lie in the axial plane, and this produces better images with less artifact (Fig. 7.**4 a**, **b**). The axial plane is also more comfortable for the patient. It is also possible to alter the angle of the coronal reconstruction from the axial data. Sagittal reconstructions in conjunction with axial images are helpful for frontal surgery, giving the surgeon a better understanding of the complex relationship between the anterior ethmoid sinuses and the frontal recess (Fig. 7.**5**). It is now possible to reconstruct the images in any plane (Fig. 7.**6**).

Thin CT sections help to distinguish true osseous defects from partial volume effects that result from inadequate slice thickness. Thinner slices, in general, provide a better anatomical resolution in critical areas such as the frontal recess, optic canal, sphenopalatine foramen, and nasolacrimal duct. If thin sections are used, it is easier to see a small lesion such as a circumscribed osseous erosion produced by a carcinoma, which might be missed on thicker sections. High spatial resolution may also provide additional information about the lesion's intrinsic composition, e.g., the

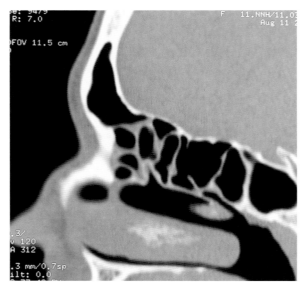

Fig. 7.**5**   A sagittal reconstruction showing the air cells around the frontal recess.

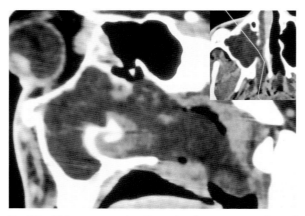

Fig. 7.**6**   Oblique reconstruction showing an antrochoanal polyp as it extends down the posterior choana.

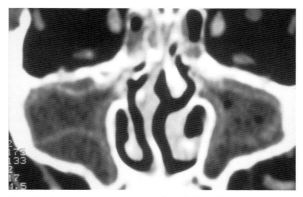

Fig. 7.**7**   Intravenous contrast helps distinguish mucosa from secretions or tumors. The dense line indicates the contrast enhancing mucosal surface, which thus can be distinguished from edema within the mucosa in the periphery of the sinus and the central intraluminal fluid.

presence of calcification in inverted papilloma or hyperdense areas in mycetomas. Intravenous contrast is only required for tumors, vascular lesions, and the orbital and intracranial complications of infection (Schuknecht and Simmen, 2002) (Fig. 7.**7**).

If a spiral CT is not available to allow reconstruction, then axial cuts are indicated if there is specific pathology in the sphenoid sinus or if surgery in this area is planned, e.g., orbital decompression.

## ■ Radiation Exposure

CT utilizes X-rays to obtain diagnostic information. While the radiation exposure should be limited as much as possible, a certain quantum of X-rays is required to achieve an acceptable image quality. The X-rays emitted by the CT scanner interact with the body tissue by depositing energy, called "dose." Rather than the "ion dose" (unit Roentgen, R), the absorbed dose (unit Gray, Gy) is most frequently considered.

The absorbed dose is determined by a number of technical parameters dependent on the type of CT scanner and its dose specification. There are no significant differences between comparable CT scanners.

However, a number of parameters such as tube voltage (referred to as "kV"), current (referred to as "mA"), scan mode, slice collimation, and rotation time are subject to modification. Decreasing the kV, using a thicker slice collimation, and increasing the table feed per rotation will reduce the amount of dose applied. The trade-off obtained by modifying the parameters in this way will lead to a decrease in image quality. It has been shown, however, that in a given setting of parameters, decreasing the tube current/scan time product (mA s) effectively reduces the dose to the eye lens by as much as 77 % (Sohaib et al., 2001) while still providing adequate image quality. In two studies, the dose applied to the eye lens was measured between 3.1 and 13.5 mGy at 50 and 200 mA s, respectively (Sohaib et al., 2001), and ranged between 1.88 and 31 mGy (Dammann et al., 2000) at corresponding values of mA s. A single-dose irradiation of 2 Gy may cause cataract of the eye lens; repetitive fractionated-dose applications are tolerated to a significantly higher degree.

Compared with conventional nonspiral CT machines, the dose may be reduced by using a spiral CT scanner to reconstruct coronal and sagittal planes from the original data set. An extra examination in an additional plane can thus be avoided.

Overall, the best way of reducing radiation exposure is to avoid unnecessary examinations and to use the correct settings to minimize dose.

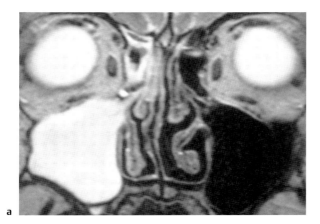

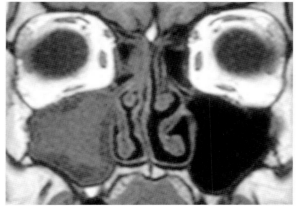

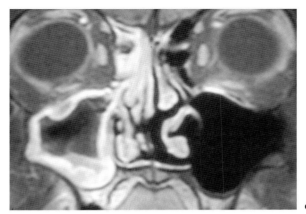

Fig. 7.**8**  **a** Coronal MR image with T2 weighting shows fluid and the edematous mucosa with a high signal (bright). **b** The corresponding T1-weighted image without contrast depicts fluid with a low signal (dark). Following intravenous contrast enhancement, a signal increase on the mucosal surface (**c**) is noted, while the centrally located fluid does not take up contrast.

## ■ Indications for MRI

The prevalence of incidental changes on MRI is so great that the technique is of little use in the diagnosis of rhinosinusitis (Cooke and Hadley, 1991). A comparison between a T2-weighted image (fluid bright), a T1-weighted image (fluid dark), and a T1-weighted image with nonionic contrast provides useful information about soft-tissue lesions (Fig. 7.**8 a–c**). This is particularly helpful in defining the boundary of pathology in relation to the dura, orbital apex, or optic nerve.

MRI is unable to delineate the fine osseous details required for endoscopic paranasal sinus surgery. On its own, MRI provides information about the extent of a tumor confined to bone, but it rarely allows the lesion to be characterized. This usually requires a CT scan.

MRI is complementary to CT in the following circumstances:
- Where malignancy has reached the dura of the anterior skull base, the orbital apex, and the optic nerve (Fig. 7.**9 a**, **b**).
- If there is intracranial or intraorbital involvement from an atypical infection or inflammatory process (Fig. 7.**10 a**, **b**).

- In vascular tumors like a juvenile angiofibroma. Imaging is particularly important in angiofibroma because it is one of the few instances where a diagnosis can be based on radiology. A biopsy, which is to be avoided in angiofibroma, can therefore be obviated (Fig. 7.**11 a**, **b**).
- If you suspect an intrasphenoid extension from an internal carotid artery aneurysm (Fig. 7.**12 a–c**).
- In congenital midline lesions such as meningocele, meningoencephalocele, or sinonasal glioma (Fig. 7.**13 a**, **b**).
- When a high-resolution CT scan has shown the skull base defect, MRI can help define any pathology associated with a CSF leak, e.g., brain, hematoma, CSF.
- MRI can complement CT in determining how extensive an inverted papilloma is. It defines how much of the opacification shown on CT is due to secretions and how much is due to the tumor. This is important in planning surgery if it involves the frontal or maxillary sinus.

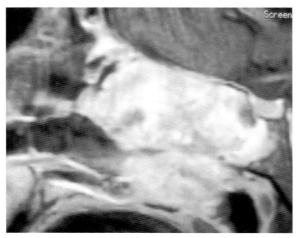
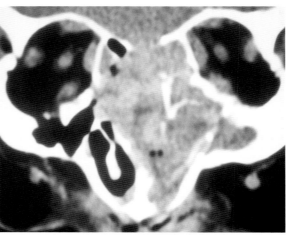

Fig. 7.**9**  A 64-year-old patient with squamous cell carcinoma of the nasal cavity. **a** On the sagittal T1-weighted MR image with intravenous contrast enhancement, the extension of the tumor is delineated, reaching from the frontal recess anteriorly and into the sphenoid sinus posteriorly as well as into the inferior meatus. The dura is visualized as a linear hyperintense structure in direct contact with the tumor along the cribriform plate where infiltration starts and extends along the sphenoid roof to the tuberculum sellae posteriorly. **b** The coronal contrast-enhanced CT shows a lesion that has eroded the ethmoid, part of the cribriform plate, and the nasal septum.

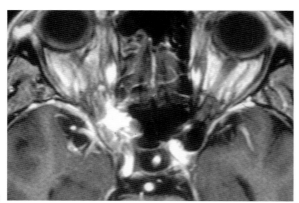
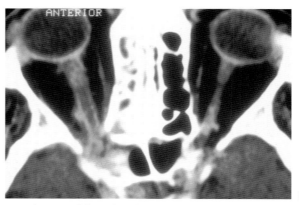

Fig. 7.**10**  **a** Axial contrast-enhanced T1-weighted MR image depicts infiltration of the optic nerve within the optic canal and orbital apex. **b** An axial CT 1.5 mm slice with intravenous contrast shows contrast-enhancing tissue arising from the optic-carotid recess of the right sphenoid sinus. The lateral sinus wall is eroded; the orbital apex and the optic nerve sheet are infiltrated. Note marked thickening of the optic nerve compared to the opposite side. Diagnosis: Invasive apergillosis.

## ■ MR Angiography

MR angiography (MRA) delineates flow within vessels by suppressing the signal from stationary tissue. It is performed as part of an MR examination and does not necessarily require contrast injection. MRA provides information with respect to the principal feeding arteries in vascular tumors (such as angiofibromas, hemangiopericytomas, or paragangliomas, and certain metastases) and in vascular lesions (such as angiomas or aneurysms located at the skull base). Delineation of increased flow by MRA is an indication to proceed to additional digital subtraction angiography—not for diagnostic purposes but to perform preoperative embolization.

A negative result on MRA does not definitively rule out a vascular lesion. A minor amount of flow or the presence of slow flow such as in a capillary hemangioma, esthesioneuroblastoma, and even in an angiofibroma may be invisible to MRA.

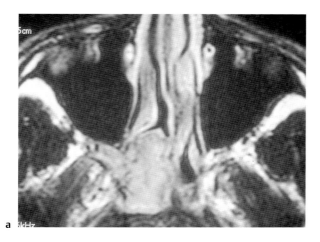

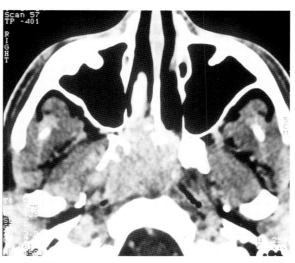

Fig. 7.**11**  **a** Axial T2-weighted MR image and **b** contrast-enhanced CT image in a 17-year-old patient with a juvenile angiofibroma. The typical appearance consists of a markedly contrast-enhancing lesion (**b**) that displays multiple intralesional vessels with punctate signal loss on MRI and high density on CT. The typical location is within and adjacent to the sphenopalatine foramen. Tumor extension into the foramen and pterygopalatine fossa is particularly well seen on the MR image.

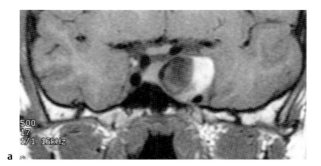

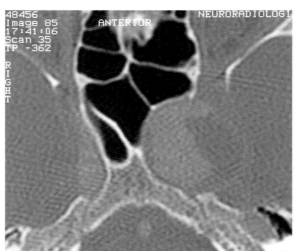

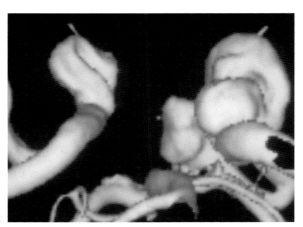

Fig. 7.**12**  A 59-year-old woman with retro-orbital pain and a single episode of epistaxis 9 weeks previously. **a** Coronal T1-weighted image delineates the aneurysm with a thrombosed, signal-intense component within the cavernous sinus and signal loss due to flow within the "open" part. Note the displacement and close contact of the aneurysm to the mucosal lining of the sinus. **b** Pressure erosion of the osseous wall is shown by high-resolution CT. **c** MR angiography giving an impression of the three-dimensional bilobulated configuration and the medial intrasphenoid projection of the aneurysm.

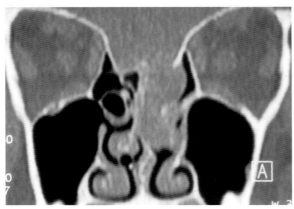

a

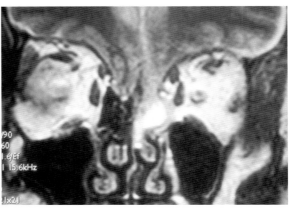

b

Fig. 7.**13   a** Coronal high-resolution CT scan depicts an os-seous defect within the cribriform plate and the ethmoid roof and soft-tissue obliteration of the olfactory rim and the frontal recess. Even on soft-tissue images, CT is not able to reliably dis-tinguish a pseudomeningocele, a meningoencephalocele, or a tumor such as an esthesioneuroblastoma in this location. **b** This is achieved by the T2-weighted MR image showing herniation of the frontal lobe through the defect and a concomitant pseu-domeningocele with a bright signal of CSF in the middle mea-tus.

## ■ Digital Subtraction Angiography

Digital subtraction angiography (DSA) is the best method to delineate the vascular supply of a specific anatomical area or lesion. Intra-arterial contrast injec-tion is required in order to delineate the vascularity. This may be performed by a catheter inserted via a transfemoral approach into the territory of the exter-nal carotid artery or via a microcatheter, which allows superselective evaluation of a specific artery or arterial branch.

Only in very rare circumstances is DSA required as a diagnostic tool:

- In a lesion (e.g., chordoma or neoplasm) that abuts the internal carotid artery at the foramen lacerum or within the cavernous sinus. In these cases, per-manent occlusion of the internal carotid artery may be necessary in order to achieve radical resection. A test occlusion with a balloon is mandatory to assess the quality of the collateral circulation.
- In recurrent epistaxis, DSA may be required as a means to verify the source of repeated hemorrhage.

DSA is performed with both diagnostic and therapeu-tic intention when a lesion is demonstrated that is amenable to endovascular treatment (e.g., a pseudo-aneurysm or telangiectasis in Osler disease). Super-selective treatment may consist of intralesional deposition of microparticles or tissue adhesives (glue) to occlude the blood supply. In case of an aneurysm, this may be achieved by deploying small platinum coils.

Embolization of epistaxis and nasal cavity tumors with microparticles close to the nasal septum carries a small risk of occluding collaterals to the ophthalmic artery via septal branches of the sphenopalatine and ethmoid arteries. If unrecognized, loss of vision may ensue. The same risk from particle embolization ap-plies to the anterior ethmoid artery.

## ■ Interdisciplinary Cooperation

The surgeon and the radiologist can get the most out of imaging techniques by working together. Each needs to learn from the other. Radiologists need to under-stand the pathology of rhinosinusitis, otherwise they are in danger of writing misleading statements like "mucosal thickening showing rhinosinusitis" when a better interpretation would be "mucosal thickening consistent with rhinosinusitis." On the other hand, the surgeon needs to know the CT parameters for window settings and how these affect the images. It is impor-tant that the surgeon knows how to interpret CT films and does not rely on a written report, because words cannot adequately describe patterns of changes or the complexity of anatomy.

**Hold regular meetings together, which will pro-vide the basis for a mutually productive learning ex-perience that in the end will benefit both you and your patients.**

# ■ Points to Mention on a CT Request

The radiologist and radiographer will provide you with much better images and a much better report if they have information that will help them choose the optimum scan settings and interpret the images in the light of the clinical picture.

1   Write down the provisional diagnosis, e.g., "severe polyposis unresponsive to medical treatment."

2   Say why you want the scan, e.g., to define the anatomy before surgery.
3   Detail what surgery has been done.
4   Ask for fine cuts if indicated, e.g., in case of a CSF leak or when sagittal reconstruction is needed.
5   Name the area you want examined, e.g., the frontal recess.
6   If you suspect a tumor, say so and ask for a contrast study.

# 8 Preoperative Checklist

Imagine that you have decided that the patient will need surgery as part of their treatment. This decision is rarely made after the first consultation but rather after a trial of medical treatment. Having made the decision to operate, what should you do before operating? See the preoperative checklist below.

It is important to prepare your patient in order to:

- Minimize the amount of surgical manipulation required.
- Preserve as much olfactory mucosa as possible.
- Reduce peroperative bleeding to reduce the likelihood of complications.
- Work out the surgical anatomy in order to minimize the chance of entering the orbit or skull base.
- Set clear goals for yourself and your patient: A disciplined approach to surgery will mean that you will be less likely to embark on an "endoscopic safari", which could result in excessive surgery, increased recovery time for your patient, and the risk of complications.

*The Preoperative Checklist*
1  Confirm the diagnosis.
2  Review previous medical treatment.
3  Optimize the immediate preoperative condition.
4  Check that relevant investigations have been done:
    - Allergy tests
    - Immune status
    - Hematological parameters
    - Olfaction
    - Vision
5  Review the relevant medical history, e.g., drug allergies, medication.
6  Preoperative CT checklist.
7  Planning and staging the procedure.
8  Informed consent.

It is good practice to see the patient 10–14 days before surgery in order to maximize the appropriate preoperative medical treatment and to go over advice and consent. It is not best practice to obtain consent on the day of surgery as the patient may feel pressurized.

## ■ Confirm the Diagnosis

Patients with genuine chronic bacterial rhinosinusitis who do not respond to medical treatment are often helped by surgery, unless they are immunosuppressed, when caution is needed (Fig. 8.1). It is important to make sure as far as possible that your patient has a diagnosis that is likely to respond, at least in part, to surgical intervention. Operating on a patient who has only allergic rhinitis is very unlikely to help them (Fig. 8.2). If their CT is normal or shows turbinate hypertrophy without evidence of sinus disease, retake

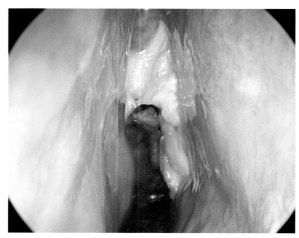

Fig. 8.**1**   A patient who has not responded to multiple courses of antibiotics—consider their immunity before operating.

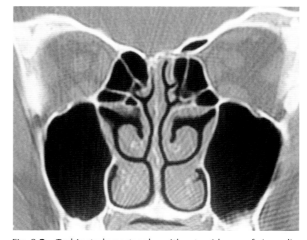

Fig. 8.**2**   Turbinate hypertrophy without evidence of sinus disease—think twice before operating on these patients.

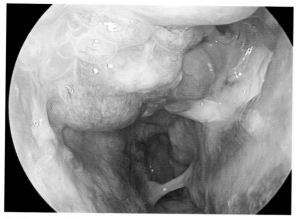
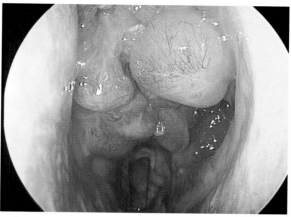

a

b

Fig. 8.**3** **a** Endoscopic view at presentation. **b** Endoscopic view after maximum medical treatment. Give a cautious prognosis in the patient who fails to respond symptomatically and whose polyps remain large after steroids and antibiotics.

the history, try more medical management, ask the patient to keep a diary of their symptoms, and wait for a pattern of their symptoms or exacerbating or relieving factors to become clearer. If the problem is tension-type headache, then surgery will not help (although it is interesting to note that in about one-third the alteration in central neuroplasticity that results from surgery leads to an improvement for a few months). One-third of patients with tension-type headache who inadvertently had surgery have an increase in their symptoms and, this is why it is important to make the correct diagnosis and avoid surgery (Jones and Cooney, 2003; Jones, 2004).

### ▪ Reviewing the Effect of Maximum Medical Treatment Helps in Determining Prognosis

After a trial of maximum medical treatment, you should be able to predict how reversible the patient's mucosal disease is and offer more accurate information about their prognosis after surgery. The extent of any response to maximal medical treatment, and how long it lasts, will indicate the extent and likelihood that postoperative medical treatment will be needed (Fig. 8.3 a, b). A short-lived improvement in the nasal airway with only a minimum and transient improvement in the sense of smell after a course of oral steroids will lead the surgeon to give a more guarded prognosis about the benefits of surgery. A short-lived response to maximal medical treatment would also indicate that long-term medical treatment after surgery may be required.

### ▪ Optimize the Immediate Preoperative Condition

Check that the patient has had maximum preoperative medical treatment. It is surprising how often this is overlooked. Reducing the amount of inflammation at the time of surgery will make the operative field easier work in and will enable the surgeon do a safer and better job. The patient with infective rhinosinusitis should have had at least a minimum of 2 weeks of a broad-spectrum antibiotic with anaerobic cover: for example, coamoxiclav or cefuroxime and metronidazole (Fig. 8.4). For allergic rhinitis, the current ARIA guidelines summarize the best medical treatment (see Chapter 3, Table 3.1). It is particularly important to

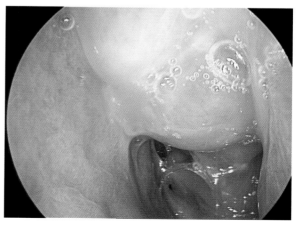

Fig. 8.**4** A patient with polyps and purulent secretions who says they have had antibiotics. Patients often say they have had "lots" of courses of antibiotics—but check that they had ones with the right bacterial spectrum and for long enough.

check compliance with topical nasal steroids. In severe nasal polyposis, and in particular when polyps lie medial to the middle turbinate and there is a reduction or absence of sense of smell, a course of oral steroids in the week before surgery should help reduce surgical damage to the olfactory mucosa. Oral steroids should be given as long as there are no contraindications and their side effects are explained to the patient. A dose of 40–70 mg of prednisolone (depending on body mass) with breakfast for 4–7 days is recommended as long the patient does not have diabetes, cardiac disease, gastric or duodenal ulcers, or osteoporosis. Patients with allergic rhinitis, especially in the hay fever season, should have a prophylactic nonsedative antihistamine preoperatively as this will reduce hyperreactivity and the amount of exudate that occurs with surgery.

### ■ Check That Relevant Investigations Have Been Done

#### Allergy Tests

Skin-prick tests have good sensitivity and relatively good specificity. They not only define the allergens whose avoidance may help the patient, they also demonstrate to the patient that part of their problem is their own reaction to the environment and that surgery on its own may not be the whole solution.

Total IgE is not very specific or sensitive, being positive in only approximately 60 % of patients with allergic rhinitis. It has a role as an adjunct to history, clini-

cal findings, and skin-prick tests. However, it is of particular use in a patient who is taking antihistamines or who has dermatographism. It can happen that a total IgE is normal yet the specific IgE can be raised.

As the upper and lower respiratory tract are in continuity, it is worth having a peak flow meter (and in children a height–peak flow chart) to check for possible asthma. It is pertinent to remember that 16 % of those with rhinosinusitis have asthma and that 80 % of asthmatics have rhinosinusitis. Cytology of the nasal mucosa has not been standardized, and what is termed eosinophilia varies from study to study. It is said that those with eosinophils will respond better to topical nasal steroids, but it is simpler to do a trial of medical treatment than do nasal cytology, particularly as this is the clinical strategy that will be used whatever the result of cytology. Cytology does not differentiate reliably between "eosinophilic" and "noneosinophilic" rhinitis, if there is indeed such a distinction to be made. Rhinomanometry and acoustic rhinometry are mainly used as research tools, although they can be used to provide objective data after a nasal challenge.

#### Immune Status

If ciliary dysmotility is suspected because of coexisting bronchiectasis or a failure to respond to medical treatment, the saccharin clearance test is a useful and easy screening test (Fig. 8.5). However, it is only of use when the patient's infection is under control as infection on its own will lead to an abnormal result (Lale et al., 1998). Similarly, if specimens are taken for cytology or histology to look for ciliary activity or morphology, they should be taken from an area of healthy-looking mucosa. A sweat test remains the investigation of choice if cystic fibrosis is suspected, although genetic testing will pick up over 80 % of those with the most common alleles.

In testing for immunity, if a patient has had two or more serious sinus infections within a year or has had two or more courses of antibiotics with little effect, then their immunity should be investigated (Jeffery Modell Foundation). The first-line investigations for immune deficiency include microbial samples for cultures; a full blood count with differential white cell count; immunoglobulins IgG, IgA, IgM; vaccine specific IgG responses to tetanus, Hib, and pneumococcus; electrolytes and urea; liver function tests and a fasting blood glucose; and an HIV test. Second-line investigations include a nitroblue tetrazolium reduction test; IgG subclasses; functional complement assays; and tests for cell-mediated immunity, which include lymphocyte subset analysis, lymphocyte stimulation with antigens and mitogens, and delayed hypersensitivity skin tests (Cooney and Jones, 2001). There are

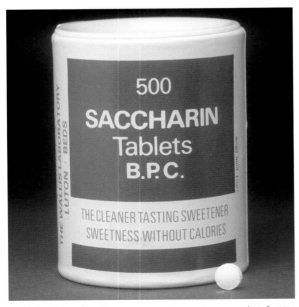

Fig. 8.**5**   If a patient has nonresponsive or temporarily infective rhinosinusitis and bronchiectasis, perform a saccharin test while their mucosa is as healthy as you can get it.

numerous tests for different aspects of cell-mediated immunity both in vitro and in vivo, and it is worth liaising with an immunologist to choose the correct tests. Abnormal test results or a strong suspicion justify referral to an immunologist.

## Hematological Parameters

Where it is clinically indicated, the patient's hemoglobin, differential white cell count, clotting studies, electrolytes, and liver function test may be requested.

## Olfaction

The patient and surgeon often overlook the importance of sense of smell (Simmen et al., 1999). There are few reports on the incidence of the loss of sense of smell following endonasal surgery, but it may be as much as 1 % (Kimelman, 1994; Briner et al., 2003). The patient who has a sense of smell often takes it for granted, but should it be lost, there are likely to be bitter recriminations. By assessing it, not only will you be able to document whether it is already absent or reduced, but you will also be reminded to mention to the patient the risks of surgery to their sense of smell (Fig. 8.6). You might also discuss the possible benefits of surgery to their sense of smell if it is poor. It will also help you to get an idea about how important the sense of smell is to the patient. If there is a partial loss of smell, then surgery has the potential to improve it in approximately 70 % of patients. However, in severe polyposis, especially associated with late-onset asthma or sensitivity to nonsteroidal anti-inflammatory drugs, it is worth warning the patient that any improvement in their sense of smell may not be sustained—thus you may avoid disappointment.

Olfactory tests are many and varied. The use of smell bottles has not been validated, and the "leading" questions that often accompany them can give undesirable false-positive results. The 20-page UPSIT scratch-and-sniff test is good but is time-consuming and expensive, and many of the options for each card are not recognizable outside North America, for example, "root beer." The Zurich smell identification test (Briner and Simmen, 1999) has multi-use numbered pull-out capsules with cross-cultural visual options. This test is quick and the kit can be reused for more than a year. It has been validated, and a score of the eight smells offered can be recorded in the notes. A commercial test for olfactory threshold is available but is primarily used in research as it is time-consuming (Wolfensberger et al., 2000). Serial dilutions in "sniff" bottles can be made up relatively easily (Robson and Woolons, 1996), but these have not yet gained acceptance in clinical practice. A threshold olfactometer is used in research (Fig. 8.7).

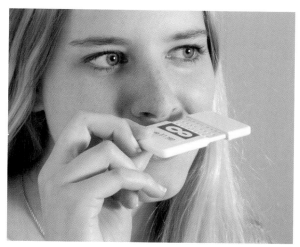

Fig. 8.**6** We strongly recommend that you test your patient's sense of smell before surgery.

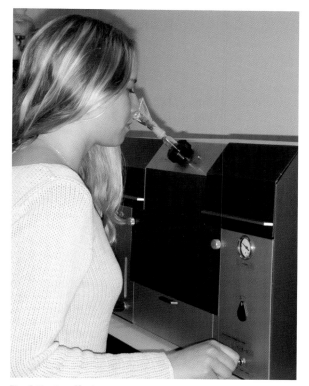

Fig. 8.**7** An olfactometer.

## Vision

It is worth, at the very least, asking the patient preoperatively whether they have any visual problems and whether any problem is with visual acuity or double vision. If there are any doubts, or if there is any question of proptosis, it is worth obtaining an orthoptic and/or an ophthalmological assessment. This de-

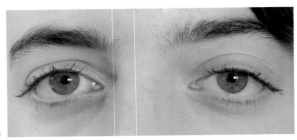
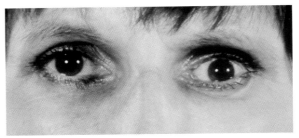

a                                                                                                          b

Fig. 8.**8**   **a** Left proptosis noticed incidentally; this needs an ophthalmological assessment. **b** Left enophthalmos due to   silent sinus syndrome—involution of the maxillary sinus with collapse of its roof (Beasley et al., 1995).

fines any problem preoperatively and will help to obviate any postoperative recrimination that surgery has led to a problem that in fact was already present (Fig. 8.8 a, **b**).

If there is any paranasal sinus pathology that impinges on the orbit, check for proptosis by going behind the patient and placing the end of your index fingers on the anterior surface of both closed eyelids; then compare them with the supraorbital margin and the zygomatic prominences. It is also important to look for any alteration in the axis of the pupils from the front because this is more frequently the cause of diplopia than is proptosis. Be sure to ask whether the patient has a dominant seeing eye owing to an astigmatism; this is important and common. The poorer-seeing eye may have much worse vision. This should be documented.

An inability to focus even when wearing glasses or when looking through a pinhole (this avoids any problem with acuity and so provides a way of testing a patient's eyesight when they have mislaid their glasses) means that there is a significant problem and an ophthalmological opinion is required. The loss of color discrimination, particularly of red, is a worrying symptom of pressure on the optic nerve, and this requires urgent treatment. For any orbital surgery, e.g., orbital decompression, an ophthalmological assessment is required. It is alarming if a unilaterally enlarged pupil like an Adie's pupil is only noticed during or after surgery. (An Adie's pupil reacts poorly to light but better for accommodation to near objects, and redilates slowly after constriction. It is sensitive to diluted pilocarpine 0.1 %, which constricts it though not to the size of a normal pupil. The condition is benign and not associated with significant neurological problems elsewhere, although there can be diminished ankle jerks.)

### ■ Review the Relevant Medical History

Document allergies to drugs such as penicillin and nonsteroidal anti-inflammatory drugs. If the patient is taking aspirin, it is advisable to ask them to stop taking it at least 14 days before the day of their surgery in order to reduce bleeding.

### ■ Preoperative CT Checklist

Like an airline pilot before preparing for take-off, you must go through a systematic check of the CT scan before surgery so as to avoid the surgical equivalent of a crash. Particular problems occur in the absence of the middle turbinate or where there is a hypoplastic maxillary sinus, a sphenoethmoidal air cell, or an asymmetrical skull base. It is vital to systematically check the CT scan. You must do this or you will be more likely to miss a danger area or a relevant variation in the anatomy (Fig. 8.9 a–d).

A systematic, five-step approach to examining CT scans will ensure that no problem is overlooked (Mason et al., 1998 b).

**Step 1.** When placing the scans on the viewing box, orientate the scan sequence from anterior to posterior and ensure that the sides are marked and placed as though as you are looking at the patient. Follow the cuts anterior to posterior; follow the septum, note any deviation, and look for the size and extent of the ethmoidal bulla, which is a relatively consistent landmark.

**Step 2.** Examine the lamina papyracea, uncinate process, and middle turbinate. See whether the lamina papyracea is dehiscent. It is important to define the site and insertion of the uncinate process and its proximity to the lamina papyracea so that a middle meatal antrostomy can be undertaken safely (Fig. 8.**10** a, **b**). Delineate the insertion of the uncinate process as it extends upward from the superior aspect of the inferior turbinate and establish whether

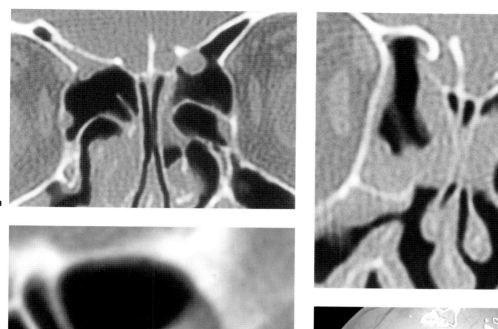

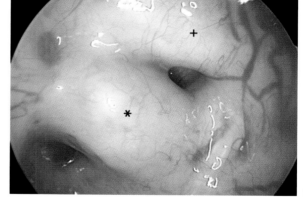

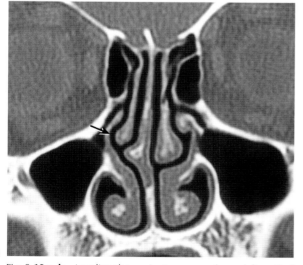

Fig. 8.**9**  **a** A polyp arising from the lamella lateralis. **b** Asymmetrical skull base. **c, d** CT (**c**) and endoscopic (**d**) views of de-hiscent optic nerve (+) and carotid artery (∗) in the sphenoid sinus, left side.

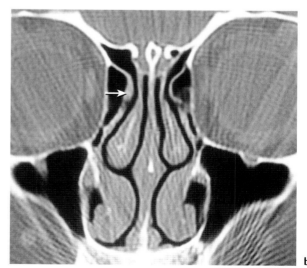

Fig. 8.**10 a, b**    Localize the uncinate process (arrow) from its free margin posteriorly and follow it anteriorly and upward.

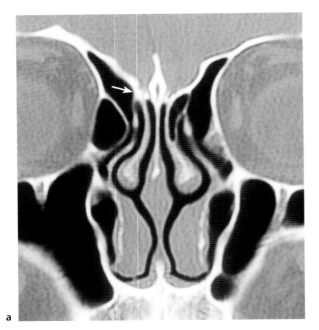

a

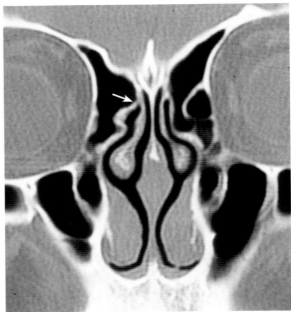

b

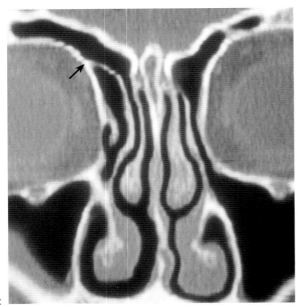

c

Fig. 8.**11**   **a** The uncinate process inserting into the skull base (arrow) on the right. **b** The uncinate process inserting into the middle turbinate (arrow) on the right. **c** The uncinate process inserting into the lateral nasal wall (arrow) on the right and the middle turbinate on the left.

it inserts onto the lamina papyracea, skull base, or middle turbinate (Fig. 8.11 a–c). In particular, determine the proximity of the uncinate process to the orbit and define the degree of aeration of any agger nasi air cells (Fig. 8.**12**). Ensure that the maxillary antrum is not hypoplastic because hypoplasia increases the risk of entering the orbit. Look for an infraorbital cell that may be entered during a middle meatal antrostomy and may be mistaken for the antrum itself (Fig. 8.**13** a, b). Examine whether there is a middle turbinate, as its absence is one of the main factors associated with complications involving the orbit and the skull base (Fig. 8.**14**). Define whether there is a concha bullosa or whether the middle turbinate is paradoxical.

**Step 3.** Examine the area of the frontal recess. The frontal recess lies anterior and superior to the ethmoid bulla. The infundibulum expands superiorly to form the frontal recess, but the way it does so varies. Ante-

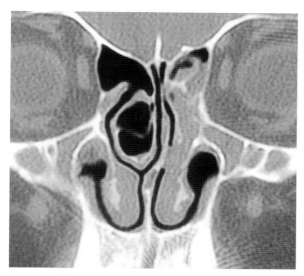

Fig. 8.**12**   The right uncinate process originating from the lamina papyracea.

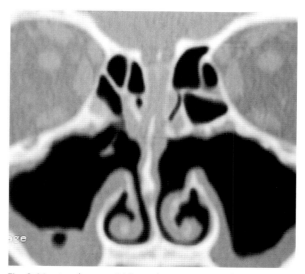

Fig. 8.**14**   An absent middle turbinate is a significant risk factor.

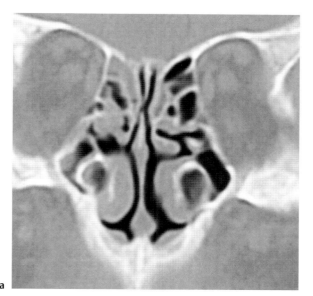

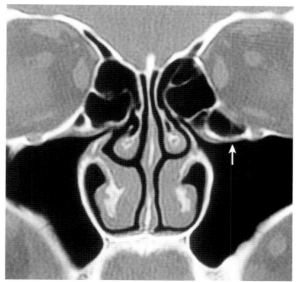

a

b

Fig. 8.**13**   **a** Hypoplasia of the maxillary sinuses. **b** A left infraorbital cell (arrow), whose roof looks thin.

rior ethmoid air cells can interrupt its path, and the degree of aeration of the agger nasi air cells will define how narrow the frontal recess is. If an agger nasi cell is well pneumatized and it extends into the frontal sinus, it is called a bulla frontalis. Sizable agger nasi cells may reduce access to the frontal sinus to leave a slit between the middle turbinate and the medial surface of the agger nasi cells. A key aspect of frontal recess surgery is to define the insertion of the uncinate process as this may also "guard" anterior access to the

frontal recess by forming a web if it attaches to the skull base or middle turbinate (Fig. 8.**15 a–d**).

**Step 4.** Determine the height of the skull base. Identify the relationship between the height of the cribriform plate and the fovea ethmoidalis (the roof of the ethmoid sinuses). Sometimes their relationship is flat, but sometimes the cribriform plate can be at a much lower level (Fig. 8.**16 a–d**). A well pneumatized supraorbital cell will cause the anterior ethmoid

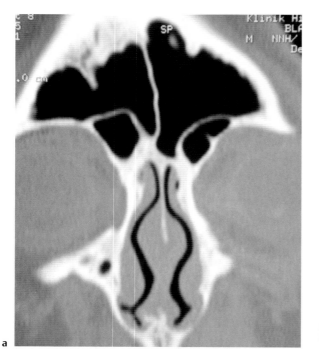

a

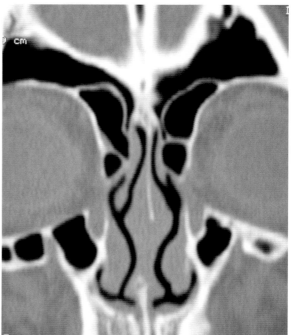

b

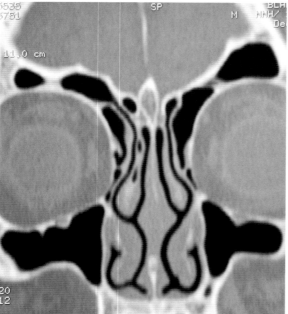

c

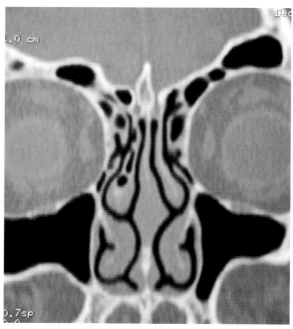

d

Fig. 8.**15**    Serial CT scans in the same patient. **a** Bilateral bulla frontalis. **b** Bulla frontalis and the start of agger nasi cells below. **c** The attachment of the uncinate process. **d** Bilateral suprabullar recesses and supraorbital cells.

artery to traverse the ethmoid in a separate channel below the ethmoid roof (Fig. 8.**17 a–c**). Damage to the anterior ethmoid artery may cause retraction into the orbit with subsequent immediate formation of an orbital hematoma and exophthalmos.

The medial aspect of the ethmoid roof joins the cribriform plate via a thin vertical strut, called the lateral lamella. This is particularly thin bone that can easily be traversed. The fovea ethmoidalis is asymmetrical in approximately 7 % of individuals, and it is important to

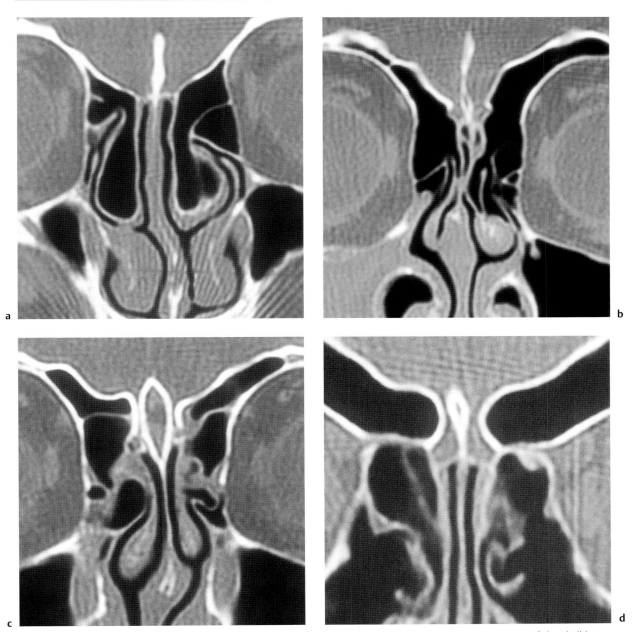

Fig. 8.**16 a–d**  Variations of the position of the cribriform plate that depend on the degree of pneumatization of the skull base.

look for this (Fig. 8.**18 a**, **b**). The height of the posterior ethmoid cells varies, and it can be estimated by examining the distance between the roof of the maxillary sinus in the posterior coronal cuts and the height of the posterior skull base. There are rarely more than two or three cells on either side in the posterior ethmoid sinuses. Approximately 18 % of patients have an Onodi (sphenoethmoid) air cell, which increases the risk to the optic nerve. An Onodi cell is a posterior ethmoid cell that is lateral to the sphenoid sinus (Fig. 8.**19 a–c**).

**Step 5.** Examine the sphenoid sinus. The perpendicular plate of the vomer always attaches to the midline and is a useful landmark. The sphenoid septum is frequently asymmetrical and may attach laterally to the prominence created by the internal carotid artery or the optic canal (Fig. 8.**20**). It is important to note whether the carotid artery is medially placed or dehiscent. The optic nerve indents the lateral wall of the sphenoid in up to 20 % of individuals (Fig. 8.**21 a–d**). Axial views are not done routinely in many departments because of the extra irradiation and time that it

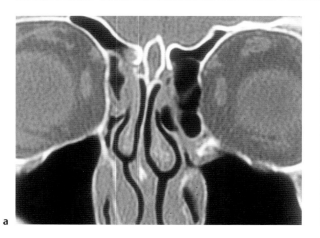

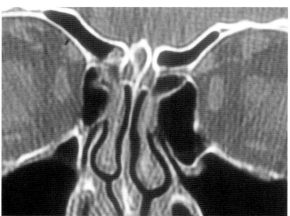

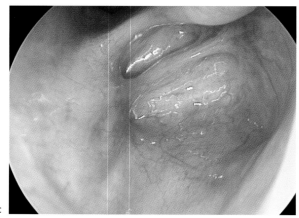

Fig. 8.**17 a**, **b**   Sequential CT scans showing the anterior ethmoid artery leaving the orbit across the ethmoid sinuses to the septum. **c** Endoscopic view of the anterior ethmoid artery, which travels anteriorly as it goes medially after leaving the orbit.

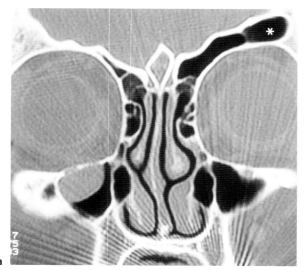

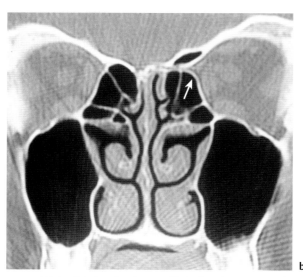

Fig. 8.**18 a**, **b**   These two CT scans show how the degree of pneumatization between the left and right side affects the exposure of the anterior ethmoid artery. The presence of a supraorbital cell (∗) makes it more likely that the anterior ethmoid artery is dehiscent (arrow).

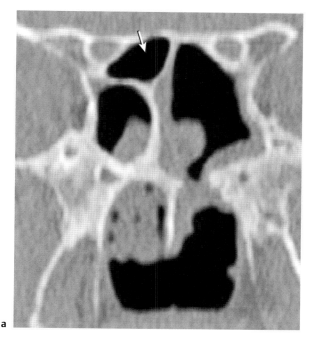

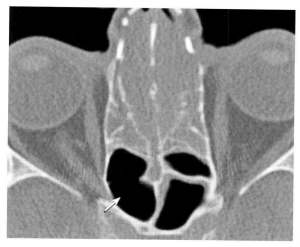

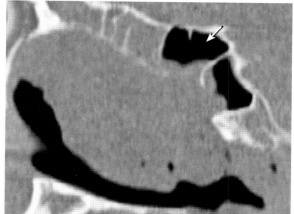

Fig. 8.**19** **a** Axial, **b** coronal, and **c** sagittal CT scans of sphenoethmoid air cells (arrows).

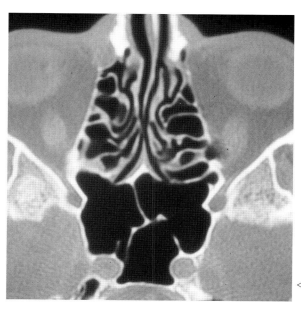

takes if a nonspiral CT scanner is used. Axial views are easily obtained from spiral CT data, and they are particularly desirable in cases involving malignancy or sphenoid pathology where disease involves the orbit. Check for any bony dehiscence (Fig. 8.**22 a–d**).

## ■ Planning and Staging the Procedure

Stage the extent of the disease and decide on the procedure. After examining the scans, stage the extent of the radiological changes. Surgical time and a strategy can then be planned and tailored to match the extent of the disease. The most popular staging system has been described by Lund and Mackay (1993) (Table 8.**1**).

◁ Fig. 8.**20** Sphenoid intersinus septum going to the carotid artery on both sides.

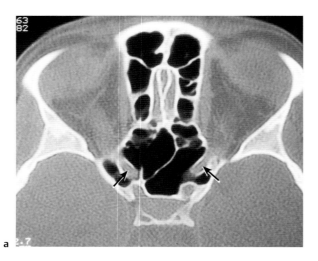
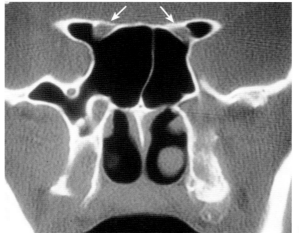
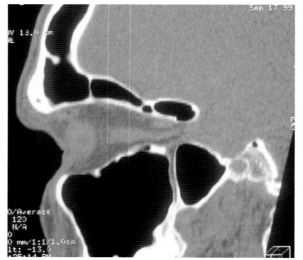
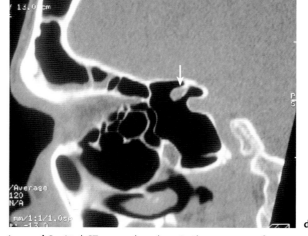

Fig. 8.**21** **a** An axial CT scan showing dehiscent optic nerves (arrow) in the sphenoid sinus. **b** Coronal CT scan showing dehiscent optic nerves (arrow) and thin bone over both carotid arter- ies. **c**, **d** Sagittal CT scans show how in the presence of a very large supraorbital cell the optic nerve (arrow) is likely to be exposed.

Table 8.**1** The radiological grading as part of the Lund and Mackay (1993) staging system, which also includes symptom, endoscopic appearance, anatomical variation, and surgical scores

| | Radiological grading (score 0–2)[a] | |
| | Right | Left |
| --- | --- | --- |
| Maxillary | | |
| Anterior ethmoids | | |
| Posterior ethmoids | | |
| Sphenoid | | |
| Frontal | | |
| Ostiomeatal complex[b] | | |
| Total | | |

[a] Each sinus group is graded between 0 and 2 (0 = no abnormality; 1 = partial opacification; 2 = total opacification).
[b] Ostiomeatal obstruction is either 0 for not obstructed or 2 for obstructed.

## ■ Informed Consent

It is important that the surgeon has an open two-way discussion with the patient when surgery is considered, both when the patient is visiting as an outpatient and whenever possible on admission before their surgery. The following issues need to be addressed.

● What are the options available to the patient?
● Specifically what would happen if no surgery were undertaken?
● What is the patient's prognosis with the various treatment strategies?
● What does the surgery involve?
● What are the complications of surgery? This should include complications occurring more frequently

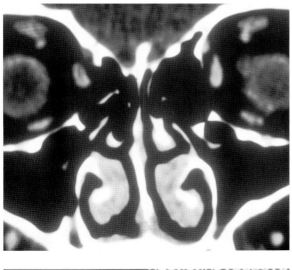

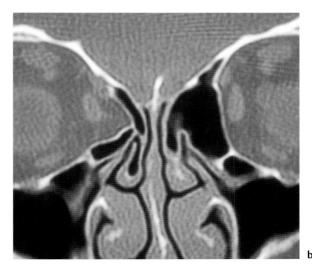

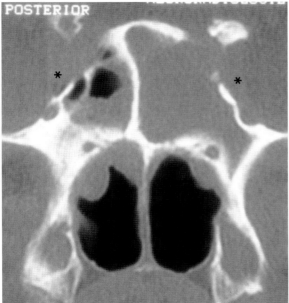

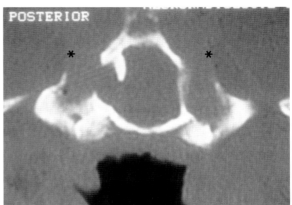

Fig. 8.**22**  **a** Soft-tissue window settings fail to show the medially placed orbital contents revealed in the high-resolution image of **b**. **c**, **d** Bony dehiscences on coronal (**c**) and axial (**d**) CT scans of the sphenoid sinus in polyposis, placing the cavernous sinus (∗) at risk.

than 1 in 100, and severe complications even if they are rare. (Having heard some of the rare but serious complications, some patients are understandably concerned, and we find it reassuring to say to the patient that we will do everything within our power to look after them and prevent these complications from happening.)

# 9 Patient Consent and Information

How much do we need to explain to our patients to properly gain their consent? The answer is as much as they can understand given their ability to make sense of the main points that are outlined below. The surgeon may feel that mentioning complications to the patient will frighten them unnecessarily, but it is possible to mention even serious complications in the right context without causing alarm, and it is our duty to do so. For example, one might say "Serious complications involving the eye have been described but these are rare and we will do everything that we can to look after you and avoid them."

Patients need to:

- Understand their diagnosis.
- Understand the context of their symptoms in the light of their diagnosis. For example, a patient who has persistent postnasal drip and who has late-onset asthma and polyps needs to understand that while surgery can aerate their sinuses, remove the bulk of the polyps to help breathing, and reduce the surface area that produces polyps, it will not stop all the mucus production from the lining of the sinuses. The mucus production is due to generalized inflammation of the mucosa of the nose that is like asthma, and surgery will not stop it.
- Understand the principles of the surgical procedure, the "thinking" behind the reason for operating, and the main technical aspects of the procedure.
- Be informed about complications that occur with any frequency as well as about severe ones—even if they are rare.
- Be informed about what they can expect in the postoperative period: the healing process, the symptoms they can expect, the medical therapy they should take, and the need for time off work.

Patient information leaflets support what has been said during the consultation. The patient information leaflets that we use are included as an Appendix at the end of this book. You may copy these for your patients.

## ■ How To Communicate the Benefits and Risks of Surgery to the Patient

It is very helpful to have the patient's CT scans with you to illustrate what is happening in their sinuses and what procedure is planned, and to show the proximity of the orbit and brain when discussing possible complications (Fig. 9.1). An alternative is to have a diagram of the sinuses available. We normally describe sinus surgery to patients who have little medical knowledge as "plumbing" of the sinuses. Another analogy that patients understand is describing the sinuses as 14 little rooms connected by corridors on either side, and sinus surgery as like these being converted into a big hall on each side (Fig. 9.2 a, b). We say that surgery helps drainage, reduces the surface area from which polyps can form, and allows access to topical nasal medication. However, it is important to emphasize that surgery is not always a "cure" for all of the patient's symptoms, particularly in the presence of allergic rhinitis or when the patient also has late-onset asthma.

Tempering patients' expectations is vital. If patients feel better postoperatively than they expected, they are often pleased and happy. However, if their progress does not meet their idea of what they thought would happen, they will often be unhappy. For example, in patients with late-onset asthma, severe nasal polyposis, and aspirin sensitivity, we emphasize that polyps often recur and that their condition is akin to "asthma of the nose." Surgery can help these patients, but it cannot eradicate their problems.

In other conditions, such as immune deficiencies, ciliary dyskinesia, or cystic fibrosis, it is important to temper the patient's expectations further and emphasize to the patient which, if any, of their symptoms are likely to be improved by surgery.

We normally specifically mention that symptoms of catarrh may not be eradicated. Although purulent catarrh and postnasal drip will hopefully become clearer with surgery, many patients who complain of these symptoms have a hyperawareness of mucus or a minor degree of globus pharyngeus, and it is wise to temper their expectations preoperatively.

While surgery can reduce the surface area that is capable of producing mucus, it often cannot reverse the mucosal pathology that produces the secretion of mucus. Notable exceptions are in fungal rhinosinusitis and bacterial rhinosinusitis, where there are no underlying cilial or immunological problems. In these patients, the likelihood of eradicating these symptoms is much greater.

As has been stressed before, it is important not to falsely raise patients' expectations that their sense of smell will be improved after surgery for marked polyposis (although by using the technique of preserving and gently "lateralizing" the middle turbinate, we have achieved mainly good results). In patients who have absolutely no sense of smell following previous polyp surgery, be cautious about promising any improvement because they have often had their olfactory mucosa removed or have synechiae obstructing their olfactory clefts. With anosmia secondary to other causes, such as trauma or a neuropathic virus, the sense of smell will not improve, and this should be stated before surgery.

### Time Off Work and Advice about Flying

It is wise to advise patients about the amount of time they will need off work to allow them to recover. After minor surgery, such as a limited anterior ethmoidectomy, patients could return to work after one week if they felt well enough. If they work in dusty or smoky environment, this should be extended by a further week so that the mucociliary function has time to recovere more. Patients who have had more extensive sinus surgery are advised to take 2 weeks off work; this suits most patients, although the occasional stoical individual will return to work sooner than this.

Advice differs as to how soon after sinus surgery it is safe for patients to fly. Some authorities have advised that it is wise to wait up to 6 weeks after surgery,

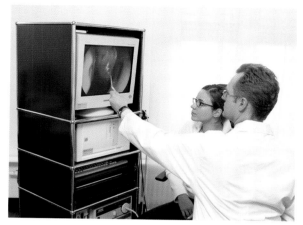

Fig 9.**1** Discussing complications with the patient.

but our view is that if patients are able to do a Valsalva maneuver and can readily inflate their ears, they may fly. We do advise them to liberally apply a topical nasal decongestant 20 minutes before landing in order to help eustachian tube function.

### Complications

Our aim is to inform the patient without alarming them unnecessarily. Having the patient's CT scan on view will help show the patient how the sinuses are separated by thin bone from the eye socket, the tear duct, and the brain. We mention that the only complications that occur with any frequency are adhesions that may need cleaning a week after surgery, bleeding that may require further packing, and periorbital bruising that can look alarming but will settle quickly. Bleeding requiring transfusion is extremely unusual.

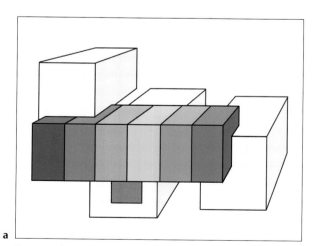

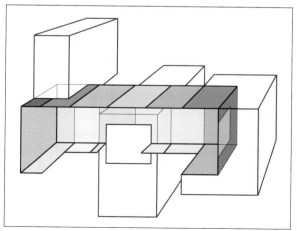

Fig. 9.**2 a**, **b**  Line diagrams to illustrate the different "rooms" of the sinuses that are converted onto one big "hall" after surgery.

Table 9.**1**   The incidence of complications in conventional and endoscopic surgery

| Complications | Conventional technique | Endoscopic technique |
|---|---|---|
| Adhesions | 2–8% | 4–6% |
| Bleeding | 0.9–2.65% | 0.48–0.6% |
| Periorbital bruising | 0.4–7% | 0.4–1.3% |
| Nasolacrimal injury | 0.1% | 0–0.5% |
| CSF leak | 0.1–0.6% | 0.07–0.9% |
| Anosmia | 0.1% | 0.4% |
| Frontal mucocele | Unknown | 0.08% |
| Retro-orbital hemorrhage | 0.3–3.4% | 0–0.4% |
| Extraocular muscle damage | 0–0.4% | Unknown |
| Optic nerve injury | Unknown | 0.007% |
| Pneumocephalus | Unknown | Unknown |
| Meningitis | 0.1% | 0.007% |
| Carotid artery injury | Unknown | Unknown |

We say that other more severe complications such as damage to the eye or to the "sac of fluid around the brain" have been reported but that they are uncommon and that we will do everything within our power to avoid them. We say that the reported risk of any moderate or serious complication is approximately 0.5% to 1%. On reviewing the world literature on the prevalence of complications associated with endoscopic sinus surgery, it is worth mentioning that these are no more common than with conventional surgery (Table 9.**1**).

Adhesions occur with approximately the same frequency in conventional and endoscopic sinus surgery. They can be minimized by avoiding mucosal damage to adjoining surfaces, and by making space between any tissue surfaces in order to reduce the chances of two damaged surfaces contacting one another and a fibrinous bridge forming. Gently "lateralizing" the middle turbinate after an ethmoidectomy can reduce synechiae in the olfactory cleft as well as improve ventilation to this area. Advising the patient to douche the nose postoperatively and reviewing the patient after one week, when gentle debridement of any bridges of fibrinous exudate may be required, will minimize the incidence of adhesions. Mucosal preservation, particularly in the frontal recess, is central to avoiding adhesions, fibrosis, and stenosis.

Damage to the nasolacrimal duct can be caused by overzealous removal of the uncinate process or enlarging the middle meatus too far anteriorly. Damage to the nasolacrimal duct has been reported to occur in up to 12% of patients peroperatively, but thankfully this is usually temporary. Epiphora occurs in only 0.02% in the longer term (Stankiewicz, 1987, 1989).

Contrary to most surgeons' perception, the next most frequent complication is a CSF leak. It is our practice to mention this complication but at the same time to say that should it occur, it can be repaired.

Most surgeons fear orbital complications. Periocular ecchymosis can occur when the lamina papyracea is traversed, but this normally disperses within 3–4 days without any problem. A more serious complication is bleeding within the posterior compartment of the orbit. This is usually produced by retraction and bleeding of the anterior ethmoidal artery. Unrecognized and untreated, this can cause blindness. Direct damage to the optic nerve has been reported to occur in approximately 0.007% of procedures.

If the surgeon has audited their complication rate, they may quote this to the patient. It is always wise to mention the potential complications described to show that the surgeon takes them seriously. This means that the unfortunate few who will experience problems will have been prepared and those who do not will be even more grateful afterwards that they do not have a problem.

## Specific Complications

### External Incision

When undertaking frontal recess surgery, and in particular revision surgery, or when a median drainage procedure is planned, it is worth mentioning the possibility of the need for an external incision. For vascular tumors of the lateral nasal wall, such as an angiofibroma, it is important to mention that an external approach such as a lateral rhinotomy or midfacial degloving may be required. In the management of mucoceles, it is important to mention the real chance of recurrence in both the short and long term. Although wide marsupialization is associated with good results, 100% success can by no means be guaranteed (Kennedy, 1989; Beasley and Jones, 1995b; Conboy and Jones, 2003).

### Inverted Papilloma

The removal of inverted papilloma justifies particular counseling. First, after removal of the lesion as completely as the surgeon is able to achieve macroscopically, histology may show the presence of atypia or malignancy. If this is the case, a further, more radical procedure may be required. Second, as the surgeon should aim to remove all the diseased mucosa (unlike in most other endoscopic sinus surgery procedures that preserve mucosa), there is an increased risk of stenosis, particularly in the frontal recess.

However, the incidence of malignant transformation in these tumors has been overstated. A review of the available literature shows that this is very rare indeed if there is no atypia or malignancy on thorough examination of tissue after the initial removal of the disease.

The incidence of recurrent disease is as high as 30%, and this should be explained to the patient prior to surgery (Lawson et al., 1989).

## Local Osteitis

A rare complication is local osteitis caused by exposure of bone. This is akin to a "dry socket" after a dental extraction. It produces a dull, severe nagging ache that lasts for 10 days before abating. Major analgesics are required, and local treatment appears to provide little help. Patients are particularly at risk of this in surgery for inverted papilloma where mucosa is not preserved.

## Infection

Infection following surgery is rare and can be minimized by giving perioperative antibiotics when purulent disease is present.

Surgical emphysema, caused by air being forced through a defect in the lamina papyracea, is avoided if the surgeon advises the patient not to blow their nose or to stifle sneezes for 4 days after surgery.

## Visual Complications

If a patient has significant proptosis or displacement of the axis of their pupils due to paranasal sinus disease (e.g., a mucocele), they may have adapted slowly to these changes over several weeks and not have any diplopia.

Occasionally, patients may have some temporary diplopia after surgery when this displacement is suddenly corrected, and it is worth mentioning this before surgery. Patients who undergo orbital decompression are at an increased risk of diplopia, although maintaining the medial–inferior strut of bone between the medial wall and floor of the orbit minimizes this risk. However, it should be mentioned as a possible complication, and it is wise to mention loss of vision in any surgery of this nature, given the reports of sporadic cases that have been attributed to reflex spasm or thrombosis of the retinal artery.

## Recurrent Polyposis

Lastly, when counseling a patient with nasal polyposis associated with late-onset asthma or aspirin sensitivity, it is wise to mention that, in spite of good surgery and postoperative medical treatment, the majority of patients will have a recurrence of their polyps. This will avoid the return of a disgruntled, rather than an informed patient.

# 10 Perioperative Aids

While it is vital for the surgeon to have a thorough knowledge of the anatomy and pathophysiology of the paranasal sinuses and to have practiced endoscopic surgery under supervision, advances in technology are providing instruments to complement these skills:

- Local anesthesia
- General anesthesia
- Operating room setup
- Ancillary staff
- Camera-guided surgery
- Instruments
- Computer-aided surgery

## ■ Anesthesia

### Local Anesthesia

The advantages of performing endoscopic sinus surgery under local anesthetic are:

- It can be done as a day-stay procedure.
- The surgeon has to be gentle with tissue, thereby encouraging preservation of mucosa.
- Whether owing to the instillation of local anesthetic agents with a vasoconstrictor or to endogenous epinephrine, there is less peroperative bleeding.
- In a patient who is deemed to be unfit for a general anesthetic, a moderate amount of endoscopic surgery can be done under local anesthesia.
- It is possible to monitor vision, and the risk of orbital complications is reduced as the patient will notice if the surgeon enters the orbit.

The disadvantages of local anesthesia include:

- More extensive procedures such as surgery in the posterior ethmoids, frontal recess, or sphenoid are uncomfortable with local anesthesia, even with nerve blocks and sedation.
- Under local anesthesia a moderate degree of sedation may be needed. Under these circumstances, even if there is only a little bleeding, it may result in coughing and spluttering if the cough reflex has partially been suppressed.
- In some cultures, patients have come to expect a general anesthetic as a right; they have faith in general anesthesia and wish to minimize any discomfort or awareness of their surgery.

- For most patients having extensive surgery done under local anesthesia, an anesthetist, is required to provide controlled sedation.

### Local Anesthetic Technique

Either cophenylcaine (a mixture of lignocaine and norepinephrine) or a 6–10 % solution of cocaine can be placed on a patte or thin ribbon gauze in the nasal airway for several minutes before replacing it in the middle meatus and nasal airway more posteriorly (Fig. 10.**1a**, **b**). Although an initial spray of the solution can be used, much of it ends up in the oropharynx. This produces an unpleasant sensation for the patient, making them feel there is something there and that they have to continually try to swallow it away. After 5 minutes the patte can be removed and local anesthetic injected using 1–2 % lignocaine with norepinephrine 1 : 200 000 using a dental needle. Bending the end can help to deliver it at the correct angle. We inject less than 1 ml into the lateral nasal wall just behind the anterior lacrimal crest. We do not inject the inferior turbinate.

Nerve blocks in both the sphenopalatine area (just below and lateral to the base of the middle turbinate) and, where posterior surgery is indicated, in the greater palatine foramen, can help supplement local infiltration. It often helps to leave the cophenylcaine-soaked patte in position while you move on to work in another area or the other side in order to maximize both anesthesia and vasoconstriction.

### General Anesthesia

The advantages of using general anesthesia are:

- The surgeon is freed from worrying about whether the patient feels discomfort from the surgery.
- It is possible to access areas that are not readily anaesthetized with local anesthetic, for example, the frontal recess and the sphenoid.
- It is worth giving local anesthesia at the same time in order to help reduce the amount of general anesthetic required and limit immediate postoperative pain. It also helps reduce bleeding as it usually also contains a vasoconstrictor.
- If bleeding is moderate or marked, it can be sucked out as the patient is not distressed by having to repeatedly spit out blood.

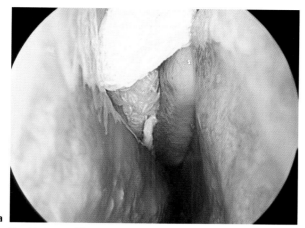
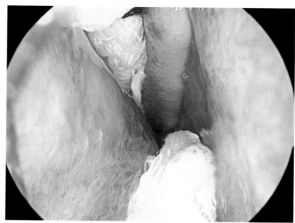

a    b

Fig. 10.**1**    **a** Ribbon gauze deep in the middle meatus and **b** nasal airway.

- In infected cases, local anesthetic works poorly and general anesthesia has a distinct advantage; for example, it is difficult to anesthetize a patient with acute sinusitis using local anesthetic even for a minor procedure such as a maxillary antral washout.
- The patient is unaware of unpleasant sensations, even when these do not cause pain, for example, vibrations from a drill.

The disadvantages include:
- Attention to detail and respect for the mucosa is no longer encouraged by the complaints of a conscious patient.
- The patient no longer provides an early warning to indicate that the orbit has been breached or entered.
- There are general risks associated with a general anesthetic, immediate postoperative recovery, and the likelihood of requiring an overnight stay.
- There tends to be more mucosal bleeding than under local anesthesia. This may in part be due to less local vasoconstrictor having been used, or to a reduction in the amount of endogenous epinephrine.

### General Anesthetic Technique

A topical vasoconstrictor such as xylometazoline can be given on the ward 20 minutes prior to surgery. A vasoconstrictor on a swab/pledget or as liquid can be placed in the nose in the same way as under local anesthesia.

If a liquid is applied, the patient is positioned with their head extended and their shoulders being supported by a pillow. In this position with the head very extended, the solution inserted will bathe the spheno-

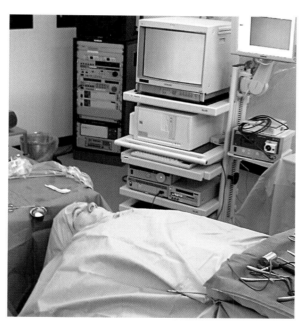

Fig. 10.**2**    Positioning of the patient in the operating room. Some more head-up tilt of the patient on the table helps reduce bleeding by lowering their venous pressure, and this should be done after the vasoconstrictor has been in position for several minutes.

palatine artery; this appears to reduce the amount of peroperative bleeding. Whether cophenylcaine, or 2 ml of 6% cocaine with 8 ml of saline, or Moffatt's solution (2 ml of 6% cocaine, 1 ml of 1:1000 epinephrine, 1 ml of sodium bicarbonate 8%, made up with 6 ml of saline to 10 ml overall) is used depends on the surgeon's preference. It is best left in position for at least 5 minutes to have its maximum effect (Fig. 10.**2**).

We find that placing tampons on either side of the laryngeal mask is preferable to inserting wet gauze, which is far more abrasive on the soft palate, and the use of tampons is associated with less postoperative discomfort. Tampons are provided with their own inserters and a little sterile jelly placed on the end will ease their insertion.

If there are extensive polyps, it may not be possible to introduce the solution. In this case, the solution can be used to soak ribbon gauze or pattes and these can be inserted instead. They can be reinserted after a few minutes when the polyps have shrunk in order to get a better result. The longer the vasoconstrictor is left in position, the better the effect. If bleeding remains a problem, either through the amount lost or because of restricted visibility, it is best to place a pack with 1 : 10 000 epinephrine and wait, or move to operate on the other side. More concentrated epinephrine often has a sympathomimetic effect on the heart; occasionally it can affect the pupil through the sympathetic reflexes on the carotid in the sphenoid sinus. During the procedure, if there is a moderate amount of bleeding, you should use a larger sucker to remove the reservoir of blood in the nasopharynx before reinserting the other instruments as this minimizes the amount of time spent removing blood.

A key point regarding general anesthesia is for the anesthetist to reduce cardiac output primarily by ensuring that there is bradycardia. Oral metoprolol given the day before and on the morning of surgery can be used when there are no contraindications, for example, asthma. Smooth induction helps and a laryngeal mask produces less stimulation and is now our main method of protecting the airway. It also produces less stimulation on extubation, with less coughing, and this reduces the bleeding on waking in recovery. Having the patient 20° body-up reduces the venous pressure. Vasodilators should not be used to reduce the blood pressure as these cause more bleeding.

We are not anesthetists, but we have observed several aspects of anesthetic technique that provide a better operative field:

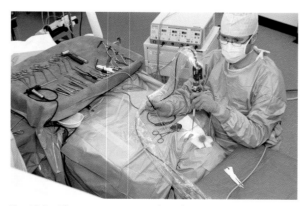

Fig. 10.**3**   The surgeon is seated, with arm support to reduce fatigue and stabilize the arm holding the camera.

- A smooth induction, peroperative anesthesia, and reversal leads to less bleeding. Coughing on a cuffed tube will result in a great deal of bleeding. If this happens, it is best to wait until the patient has settled.
- Position the patient 20° body-up during surgery.
- The use of topical vasoconstrictors (and allowing sufficient time for them to work).
- Do not rely on vasodilatation to induce hypotension as this will result in more bleeding.
- If hypotensive techniques are used, it is best to keep the mean blood pressure between 65 and 75 mmHg.
- The use of a laryngeal mask reduces stimulation to the airway, particularly on extubation.
- Beta blockers need to be used with extreme care, and not in asthmatics.

## ■ Operating Room Setup

### Operating Table

The main features to look for are that the table can be tilted to have the patient angled with the head of the table raised so that the body is at an angle of about 20°, and that the head can be flexed at the neck. It should also be possible to place one's legs under the table, to allow the surgeon to sit down during surgery.

### Surgeon's Seat

An adjustable seat allows the surgeon to find a comfortable position that will reduce fatigue and neck problems (Fig. 10.**3**).

### Position of the Anesthetist

The anesthetist sits at the foot of the table so that they are not fighting for space with the surgical assistant.

### Setup for One Surgeon

We prefer to operate from the screen on the video stand that is positioned directly opposite the surgeon at a level just above the plane of the surgeon's visual axis. This is good for posture, in particular for the neck. One of the authors prefers to sit down during the procedure with his left elbow resting on a secure table alongside the patient. This allows the left arm to hold the endoscope and camera steadily in a vertical axis for an extended period (Fig. 10.**4a–c**).

One of the authors used a beamsplitter for many years but has found that this is not only more tiring during the procedure but can cause long-term prob-

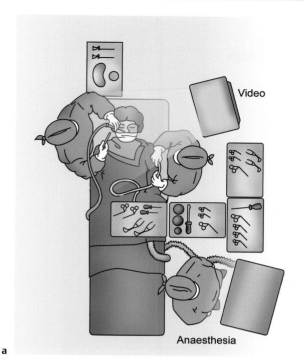

a

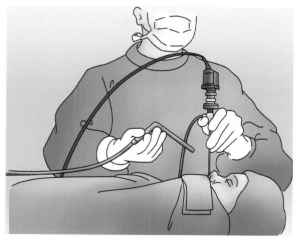

b

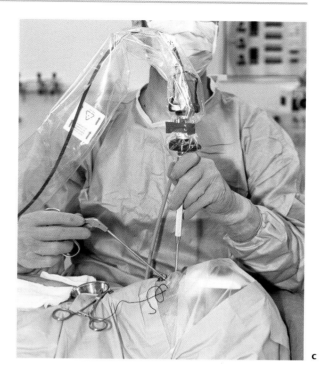

c

Fig. 10.**4 a–c** Setup for one surgeon.

lems with posture. Even the best beamsplitter reduces the reflected light that is picked up by the camera and produces a poor image.

## Setup for Two Surgeons

The advantage of having two surgeons is that one can hold the camera while the other has two hands free (Fig. 10.**5 a–c**). This means that for very vascular tumors it is possible to suck and operate at the same time and, where navigational surgery is critical, that a guiding instrument can be used at the same time as operating. It also allows the operator to place traction on tissue and cut at the same time, thus allowing more delicate surgery. The surgeon holding the camera sits at the head of the table with the endoscope and camera steadied by both hands. Both surgeons can see the video screen, which is positioned a little further back.

## Video Stack/Cameras

The screen should be positioned at a level that makes the surgeon raise their head just a little, as this will encourage good posture. A larger screen with high resolution is worth investing in. Ideally the stack will hold

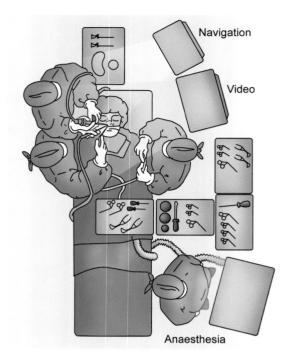

a

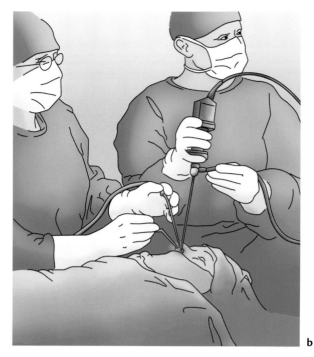

b

the majority of the accessory instruments in order to reduce the time needed to set up the equipment and reduce wear and tear on the equipment. A good light source is one of the most critical factors in obtaining a good image. The quality of the camera system determines the detail that the surgeon is able to see and is extremely important. A three-chip camera gives a much better image. The stack may also hold the drive for powered instrumentation and an image recording system (Fig. 10.**6**a, **b**).

## Cables

Cables can get in the way and their weight can tire the surgeon. The light cable and camera lead should be clipped to the drapes so that their weight going to the stack does not pull on the surgeon's supporting hand. Take a minute to organize where the leads go before starting so that there is a free area for the operating hand to introduce instruments without tripping over other cables (Fig. 10.**7**a, **b**). Other cables from powered instrumentation such as suction and navigation should be lined up parallel on the surface top. It is important that the scrub nurse gives and takes each set of instruments so that they are kept separate and do not become entangled.

c

Fig. 10.**5**a–c   Setup for two surgeons.

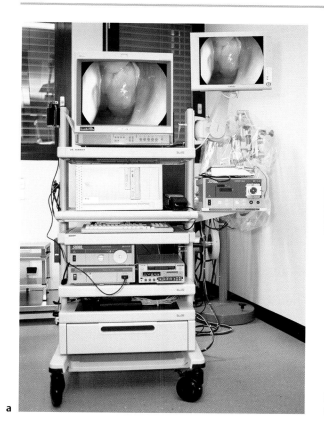

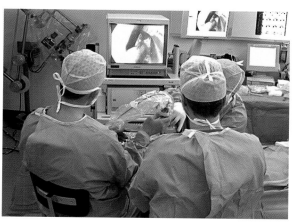

Fig. 10.**6a**, **b**   The stack system is positioned in front of the surgeon.

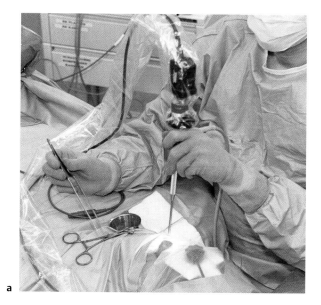

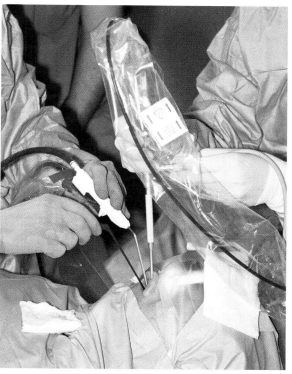

Fig. 10.**7a**, **b**   The cables can be arched over the surgeon's operating hand or held toward the patient's head so that they are not in the way.

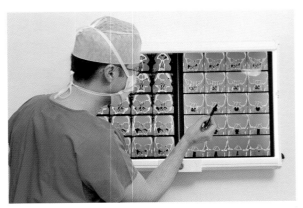

Fig. 10.**8** The CT scans must be in the operating room and should be inspected before operating.

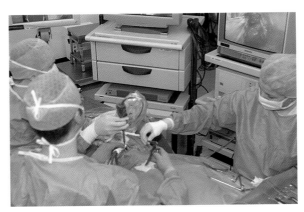

Fig. 10.**9** The scrub nurse should be strategically positioned to pass instruments.

## Lighting

For optimal viewing, the screen should have a relatively dim background. Do not have a bright window behind it or a bright ceiling light above reflecting onto the surgeon.

## Radiograph Screen

The CT scans must be placed in order on a screen for the surgeon to inspect before and during the procedure (Fig. 10.**8**).

## Ancillary Staff

The value of a good surgical assistant cannot be overestimated (Fig. 10.**9**). To be passed the correct instrument to fit the hand at the right moment saves time, particularly when there is a moderate amount of bleeding with limited time between maneuvers until further suction is required. Having the correct instrument placed in the hand saves the surgeon turning their head to look away from the screen. Often when the surgeon turns away from the screen the endoscope will move and become smeared with blood and then has to be removed and cleaned. A conscientious assistant who looks out for any movement of the eye when the surgeon is operating on the lateral nasal wall can save damage to the patient's eye. Care of the instruments is important. The ends of instruments will fail to come together if there is any debris left in or around the hinge of the jaws. It is easy for the surgeon to become frustrated and annoyed and vent their feelings on the nearest person (the scrub nurse); this is unfair and will not help. We try to build up a team who together will win the day for the patient.

## ■ Instruments

### Endoscopes

The majority of surgery is best done using a 0° 4 mm endoscope, which allows good illumination. Even in a child or a narrow nose it is easier to operate with this than with a 2.7 mm scope. A 4 mm scope is also more robust. The use of a 0° scope means that the operator is working in line with their normal visual axis and is less likely to veer off course. The light cable also comes off at any angle, and this allows it to be positioned out of the way of the operating field. Most of the paranasal sinuses can be visualized with a 0° scope, with the exception of the lateral, medial, and inferior walls of the maxillary sinus. It is best to do as much surgery as possible using the 0° scope. (Fig. 10.**10 a**, **b**).

Even the frontal recess can be approached using a 0° scope, but you need to remove the front of any agger nasi air cells. A 45° scope provides superior access and visibility that helps conserve mucosa around the frontal recess. A 30° scope can provide a better view than a 0° scope, but a 45° scope is far better at providing visibility of the varied anatomy around the frontal recess. The 45° scope has excellent optical properties and a wide angle of view, making it an essential piece of equipment. The attachment for the light cable can come off at 90° or at 180° from the axis of the scope. The 90° version is best as this keeps the cable out of the way of the operating hand. A 70° scope is more difficult to use but allows visibility of much of the maxillary sinus and high into the frontal recess. A handle holder is available to improve comfort and helps the operator to stabilize the endoscope.

### Camera Systems

The three-chip camera gives a superlative image that allows detailed surgery of the paranasal sinuses. A good camera and light source are required because redness of bleeding from the rich blood supply to the nose absorbs much of the light and it is difficult to get definition and a sense of depth with a poor image. Operating with the naked eye down an endoscope does provide a good image. There is, however, a dear price to be paid for this, and that is that the operator may develop neck problems over time. If others wish to view the image, a split beam can be used, but this reduces the quality of the image. Overall we recommend operating from the screen. **DVD** 1, 2

## Suckers

A straight-ended sucker with a bend two-thirds down its shaft with a fenestration is good for most purposes. The bore needs to be wide enough to cope with moderate bleeding; otherwise, the operator will spend most of their time trying to aspirate blood rather than operating. The fenestration is useful because, without it, if the sucker is introduced into the nose with a collection of blood, it can suck it with such force that the blood can splatter over the end of the endoscope. If the fenestration is uncovered and the sucker is introduced into the pooled blood posteriorly and then the fenestration is covered, this will not happen. A 2 mm diameter sucker is ideal for locating the sphenoid sinus adjacent to the septum about 1 cm above the posterior choana. A sucker with a larger diameter will often fail to find the area of thin bone in this area that enables the sphenoid sinus to be located safely (Fig. 10.**11 a**, **b**).

## Curved Olive-ended Suckers

There are several olive-ended suckers with different angles, and these are useful. Their rounded ends minimize mucosal trauma and they can have a dual purpose to explore and gently find out whether there are spaces behind partitions and to quantify them so that through-cutting forceps can safely be used to remove the partitions. They are often too wide to access the frontal sinus except when marked polyposis has expanded it. The right-angled version is useful for initiating the "lazy way" middle meatal antrostomy that bypasses the dissection of the uncinate process. The more obtuse sucker has a role in some patients in expanding the frontal recess where it has been defined. The thin walls of high agger nasi air cells can be lateralized by gently pushing the mucosa and the thin bone to one side (an alternative technique is to remove the bone submucosally with a ball probe, but bleeding does not always make this an easy task) (Fig. 10.**12**). The curved suckers also allow suction of the maxillary contents and they can be used to palpate to discover whether there are any polyps in the sinus out of view, or loculations of pus. A version with nonfatigable metal that allows it to be bent is available.

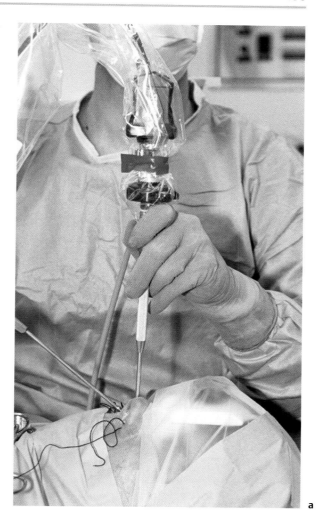

a

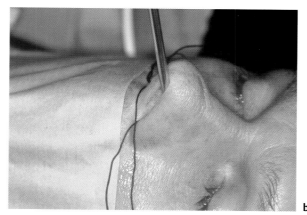

b

Fig. 10.**10 a**, **b**   It is often better to have the endoscope positioned high in the nostril to allow other instruments to be introduced from below.

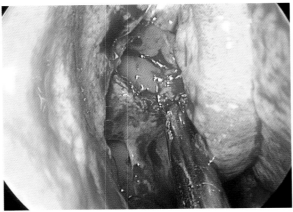
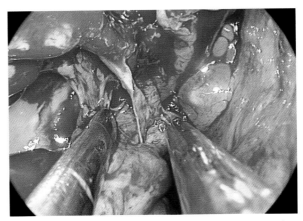

a

b

Fig. 10.**11**　**a** A single fenestrated sucker in the right middle meatus. **b** Having an assistant holding the camera allows bimanual instrumentation.

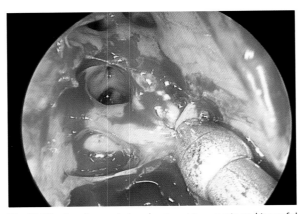

Fig. 10.**12**　An olive ended sucker is not traumatic and is useful when the frontal recess has been identified.

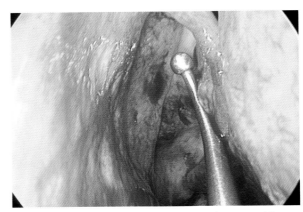

Fig. 10.**13**　A ball probe is valuable as a probe—a sensitive extension of the fingertips.

## Ball Probes

These are among the cheaper of all the instruments but some of the most valuable. They can be used as a probe (not as a prodder) to find the frontal recess (Fig. 10.**13**). Their shape and thinness makes them ideal for this purpose. In addition, they can be used to dissect the mucosa that forms the frontal recess off the bone of a high agger nasi air cell so that the mucosa is preserved. There is a ball probe with a reversed end to allow bony fragments that occasionally become inadvertently pushed up into the frontal recess to be retrieved by getting above them with the probe and then pulling them backward—like retrieving a foreign body from the nose.

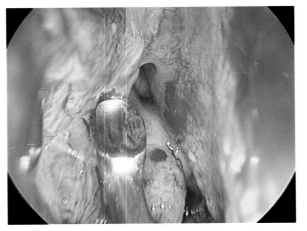

Fig. 10.**14**　A curved Kuhn–Bolger curette for removing more resilient ethmoid cells in the frontal recess. Every effort is made to preserve mucosa around the frontal recess.

## Curettes

A curved Kuhn–Bolger curette allows firm fragments of bone in the frontal recess to be removed, submucosally if possible, when a ball probe is not strong enough for this (Fig. 10.**14**). Its shape means that it has

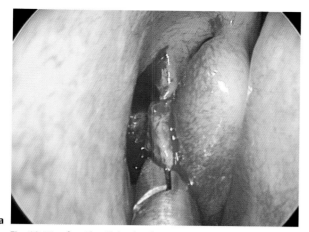

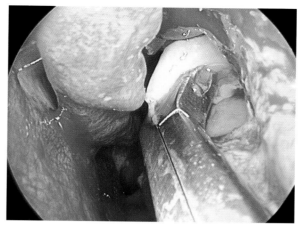

Fig. 10.**15 a**, **b**   The Blakesley forceps are useful for removing mobilized tissue or polyps. Try not to tear tissue with them.

to be fed into the nose in a "scooping" fashion. It is important not to prod with it, but only to place it where it will go without any pressure, and ideally under direct vision. A straight curette is used for removing the knuckle of the crista ethmoidalis that guards the posterior branches of the sphenopalatine artery. Its shape allows the controlled and accurate removal of bone or mucosa when this is indicated.

## Blakesley Forceps

Blakesley forceps have the advantage of providing the surgeon with a delicate sense of how much pressure is being exerted between the ends of the forceps (Fig. 10.**15 a**, **b**). This is very important around the skull base to obtain a sense of the structures you are dealing with. These forceps are useful for getting hold of loose fragments of bone. However, they normally result in some degree of tearing of the mucosa.

Blakesley forceps are useful for punching a hole into the ethmoid bulla, then opening the forceps within it, and then pulling back with the jaws open. This will help open the hole further and expose the bulla's lining (Fig. 10.**16**). They should be used with care as their sharp end can easily puncture the lamina papyracea or skull base. They are strong enough to tear part of the middle turbinate off the skull base inadvertently. If they are used to remove bone or mucosa, it is best to use their sides. Even then, they run the risk of tearing mucosa and leaving denuded bone. The 90° forceps should be used with particular care; their use almost implies that their ends are to be placed out of view, so they should only be used where the operator can be certain that they are not going to cause any harm.

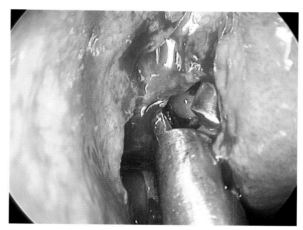

Fig. 10.**16**   The straight and angled Blakesley forceps are useful in penetrating the ethmoid bulla.

## Through-cutting Instruments (Rhinoforce Blakesley/Mackay–Grunewald Forceps)

These are invaluable because they allow the controlled removal of tissue without tearing mucosa (Fig. 10.**17 a**, **b**). Mucosal tears not only result in more bleeding but they often leave bone exposed. There are straight and 45° through-cutting forceps and they are best used with the "jaw" that opens being placed behind the piece of bone that needs to be removed. This allows the surgeon to gauge the depth of the space that lies behind that bone, and then the jaws are opened and slipped either side of the bony partition. The larger 45° through-cutting forceps are useful high in the frontal recess if there is a supraorbital cell, as the division between it and the frontal sinus is best "clipped" without tearing the mucosa. With through-cutting forceps, removal of tissue is more controlled and there is less bleeding and less trauma to the mucosa.

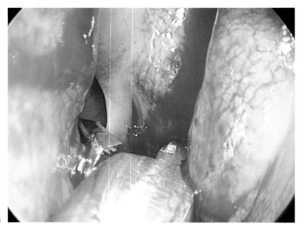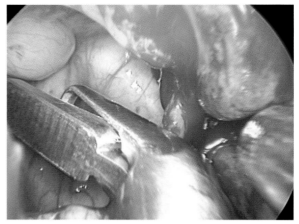

a                                                                                                          b

Fig. 10.**17 a**, **b**    Through-cutting instruments allow the precise removal of tissue.

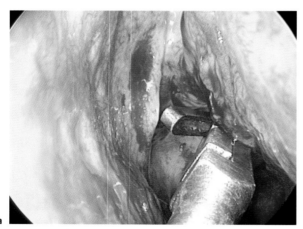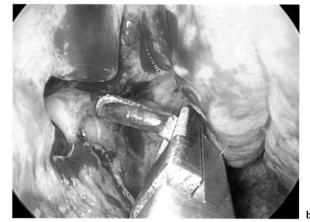

a                                                                                                          b

Fig. 10.**18 a**, **b**    The Rhinoforce Stammberger antrum punch being used to remove the inferior part of the uncinate process.

### Rhinoforce Stammberger Antrum Punch ("Back-biters")

There are left, right, and intermediate "back-biters". It is best to have the left and right ones, otherwise the handle of the instrument can hit the light attachment of the endoscope as the operator tries to get it in the correct position. The back-biting blade is best introduced closed for undertaking an uncinectomy and then the end of the instrument rotated into the middle meatus under the middle turbinate. The instrument is then rotated and its blade is opened almost vertically, just posterior to the edge of the uncinate process. The blade can then be slipped behind the uncinate process and rotated down into the infundibulum. It is possible to take two to three bites with these back-biters before they need to be removed and cleaned (Fig. 10.**18 a**, **b**).

### Hajek–Kofler (Rotating) Punch

The Hajek is a safe instrument because it cannot go through a bony structure but can only remove bone that its leading beak can get around. The micro-Hajek is even more precise than other punches and is particularly helpful along the skull base (Fig. 10.**19 a**, **b**).

The rotating locking mechanism allows its end to be angled in any direction and then locked with a rotating cuff. This helps to avoid its handle hitting the endoscope and means that one instrument will do for most circumstances. This is also a good instrument for removing the majority of the anterior lacrimal crest in order to minimize the amount of bone that needs to be drilled in an endoscopic dacryocystorhinostomy.

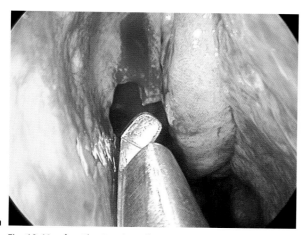
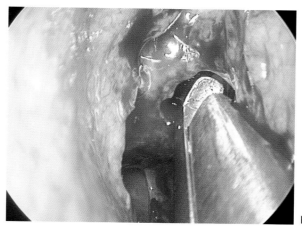

Fig. 10.**19 a, b**    The Hajek–Kofler punch is very good and safe at removing segments of bone and mucosa when there is space behind it.

## Stammberger Cutting Mushroom Punch

The Stammberger mushroom punch allows the sphenoid ostium to be opened safely and incrementally, although several bites are needed instead of only two or three with the Hajek punch (Fig. 10.**20**). There is an angled mushroom punch for the frontal recess, to nibble the remains of bony fragments in this area.

## Kerrison Antrum Punch

The size and angle of the end of this punch are ideal for getting around the anterior lacrimal crest and removing it in a controlled way in an endonasal dacryocystorhinostomy.

## Freer Elevator

This is useful for gently medializing the middle turbinate to get a view of the middle meatus and the uncinate process. Alternatively, it can be used to gently lateralize the middle turbinate in order to find the sphenoid ostium by walking up the anterior wall of the sphenoid from the posterior choana (Fig. 10.**21 a**, **b**). When doing this, it is the blunt midsection that should contact the middle turbinate and not its sharp end.

## Sickle Knife

This is used for incising the uncinate process but, as mentioned, care needs to be taken in order to avoid entering the orbit (Fig. 10.**22**). It can also be used to incise a concha bullosa if the surgeon wants to remove its lateral half (the medial half should be left intact as it contains valuable olfactory fibers). The concha bullosa having been opened, the lateral segment can be incrementally removed with straight-through cutting instruments.

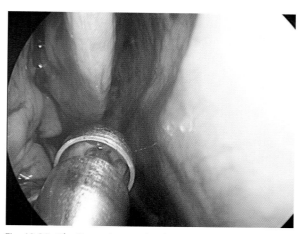

Fig. 10.**20**    The Stammberger circular cutting mushroom punch.

## Belluci and Zurich Scissors

These are for delicate cutting such as creating anterior and posterior flaps in the opened sac in a dacryocystorhinostomy. They can be used to cut tags of mucosa that remain attached to the uncinate process in an infundibulectomy in order to avoid pulling and tearing mucosa (Fig. 10.**23**).

## Stammberger Side-biting Punch Forceps

These essentially help to open a middle meatal antrostomy inferiorly (Fig. 10.**24**). These are useful if an extensive ethmoidectomy has been done and it is desirable to lateralize the middle turbinate and open up the olfactory cleft. This particularly applies if there are polyps medial to the middle turbinate, either coming off it or off the septum. This creates an antrostomy with an exit that will be below the inferior level of the

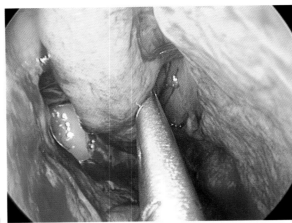
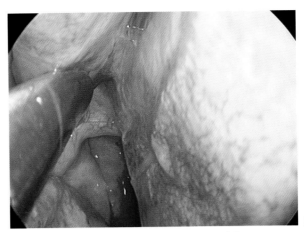

a  b

Fig. 10.**21 a**, **b**   The Freer elevator is being used to gently lateralize the middle turbinate to open the olfactory cleft.

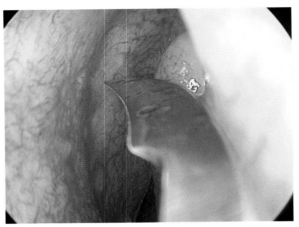

Fig. 10.**22**   A sharp-ended sickle knife.

lateralized middle turbinate. If too much is taken off, it can bite through the base of the inferior turbinate. That is not a problem in itself, although it can catch a branch of the sphenopalatine artery coming through it.

## Heuwieser Antrum Grasping Forceps

These are useful for debulking polyps in the maxillary sinus (Fig. 10.**25**). They have relatively sharp ends, so it is not possible to avulse polyps in the maxillary sinus. This is desirable, as it is best to leave a relatively intact lining in the sinus; otherwise, cilial regeneration will take many months.

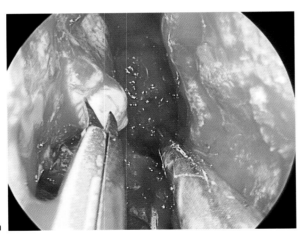
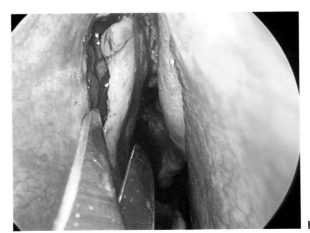

a  b

Fig. 10.**23**   **a** Small Belluci scissors and **b** slightly larger Zurich scissors.

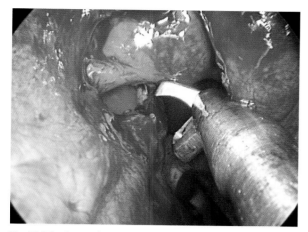

Fig. 10.**24**   Stammberger side-biting punch forceps enlarging a maxillary ostium inferiorly.

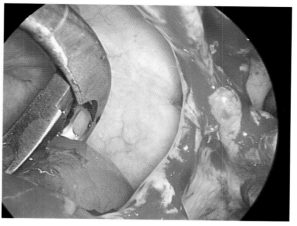

Fig. 10.**25**   A Heuwieser antrum grasping forceps debulking a polyp in the maxillary sinus.

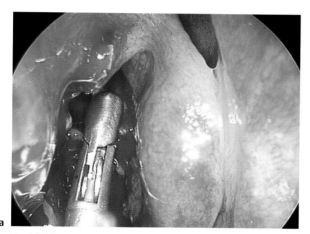

a

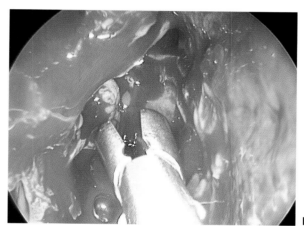

b

Fig. 10.**26**   **a** Anterior-posterior and **b** side-grasping giraffe forceps in the frontal recess.

## Giraffe Forceps (Kuhn–Bolger)

These are shaped to retrieve fragments of bone high in the frontal recess that cannot be reached by any other instrument (Fig. 10.26 a, b). They should be introduced in a "scooping" motion in order to avoid hitting the mucosa. There are forward and side-grasping cups; each has its own use depending on the position of the bone that needs to be removed.

## Powered Shavers

There are two main uses for these instruments: the first is for the removal of polyps and redundant mucosa; the second is to remove bone as well. It is important not to forget to send any collected material for histological examination. These instruments have the advantage of cleanly cutting through soft tissue, which reduces the amount of bone that is left exposed at the end of the procedure (Fig. 10.27). The versions that can remove bone need to be used with the utmost care in order to avoid very serious complications. It is safest to remove bone around the orbit or the skull base with instruments that provide more feeling and information about the quality of the tissue in that area.   *DVD* 6

## Drill

The long-shanked drill with extra-long burrs allows drilling to be done within the nose without scuffing or abrading the surrounding mucosa. It delivers irrigating fluid near the end to stop the burr from heating up. Extra-coarse diamond burrs have been produced to help removal of bone where it is thick, for example, the beak of the frontal recess or the anterior lacrimal crest. Using these burrs, it is possible to expose the orbital periosteum or dura without tearing them (this is helpful in endonasal tumor surgery) (Fig. 10.28). A finer di-

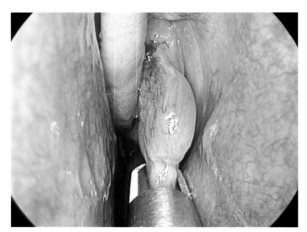

Fig. 10.**27** The shaver sucking and about to shear off a polyp.

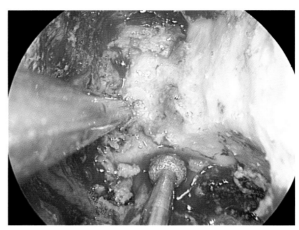

Fig. 10.**28** An irrigated coarse diamond burr removing fibrous dysplastic bone at the orbital apex.

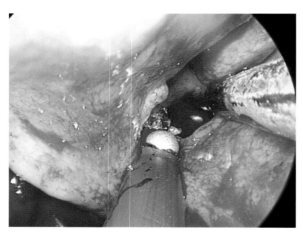

Fig. 10.**29** Unipolar suction diathermy cauterizing the septal branch of the sphenopalatine artery.

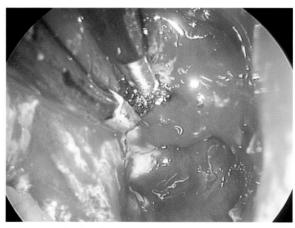

Fig. 10.**30** The bipolar suction diathermy forceps are easiest to use in the anterior half of the nose.

amond burr is indicated for work over the optic nerve, but otherwise a coarse diamond burr is the one of choice.

### Unipolar Suction Diathermy

Unipolar suction diathermy allows blood vessels to be cauterized safely. A suction channel helps to remove any smoke and also blood at the same time (Fig. 10.**29**). It is helpful when coagulating any branches of the sphenopalatine artery or when there is marked bleeding in tumor surgery. The coagulating ball-shaped end lies above the suction channel in order to allow good visibility. **DVD** 12

### Bipolar Suction Diathermy

The advantage of bipolar suction diathermy forceps is that they can be used with outpatients as the current is limited to the tissue between the ends of the insulated forceps (Fig. 10.**30**). The disadvantage is that the suction channel is easily blocked by coagulated blood.

### ■ Computer-aided Surgery

The principle of computer-aided systems is to provide the surgeon with a direct interactive link with the preoperative CT (or MRI) images (Fried and Morrison, 1998). This is achieved by reformatting patient specific CT (or MRI) images acquired preoperatively and displaying them on the screen in the coronal, sagittal, and

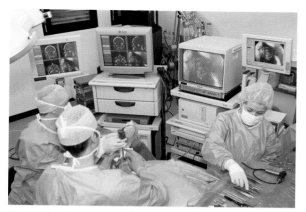

Fig. 10.**31**   Theater setup for computer-aided surgery.

axial planes. During the operation, the system tracks the position of specialized surgical instruments and identifies these positions on the preoperative images (Fig. 10.**31**).

At present an intraoperative accuracy of 1–3 mm can be achieved (Fig. 10.**32**). Anatomically, computer-aided surgery is most useful in the sites that are associated with an increased risk of causing orbital or intracranial complications. Relevant procedures include opening the frontal sinus when normal landmarks have been altered, clearing sphenoethmoid cells, median drainage procedures, the excision of lesions of the skull base, and pituitary surgery. Other applications include optic nerve and orbital decompression (Anon et al., 1997). **DVD** 8

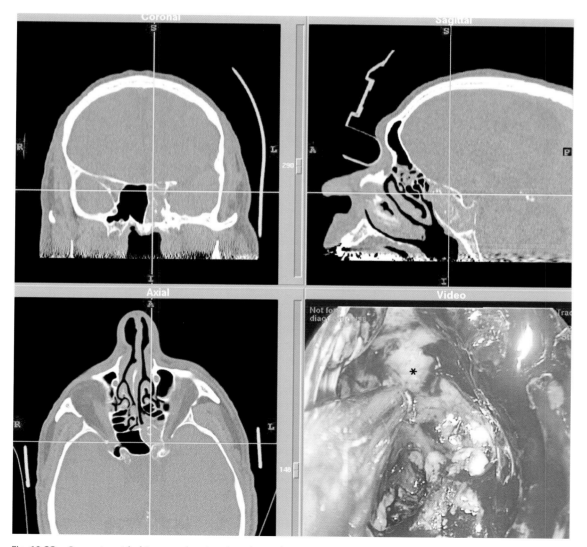

Fig. 10.**32**   Computer-aided images showing that the probe is in a sphenoethmoid air cell at the skull base (∗).

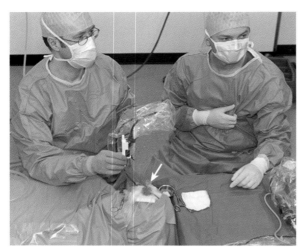

Fig. 10.**33** Checking the reference points for accuracy on the patient's headset (arrow) during registration.

View the information provided critically in the light of your clinical judgment, as it is dangerous to rely on this information alone. Always remember that you are the "pilot" and that the image-guided system cannot "fly" on its own; it is just an instrument. Year by year the technology supporting these techniques is improving. The accuracy, the speed of setting up, and the cost are all getting better (Uddin et al., 2003).

**Advantages:**
- Navigational surgery helps the surgeon build up a 3D image.
- It is a valuable teaching tool for the trainee surgeon.

**Disadvantages:**
- Computer-aided surgery is more expensive.
- Extra time is required in the set-up.
- The operator must not rely on navigational systems alone.
- The displayed image only shows the preoperative CT scan and does not take into account the tissue that has been removed.
- Added radiation results when finer CT cuts are required.

Computer-aided surgery adds a "third dimension" by allowing the surgeon to point to a specific structure in the surgical field and view its location on the pre-loaded CT images on the computer monitor (Olson and Citardi, 2000). However, these systems are no substitute for a thorough knowledge of paranasal sinus anatomy as, at present, the reformatted images only help the surgeon to confirm the position and they are not reliable enough to be used on their own (Simmen, 2000). It must be remembered that they do not account for tissue that is removed during surgery as they are based on the preoperative anatomy.

## Preoperative Work-up

If a decision is made to use computer-aided surgery, a CT (or MRI) scan is done preoperatively using axial slices of 1 mm thickness at 1 mm intervals. The format often depends on the manufacturers' specification. Some systems require a headframe to be worn during the preoperative CT scan. The CT data can be transferred to the computer in the operating room on a magnetic/optical disk or digital tape. Calibration of the instruments is mandatory and each instrument is checked prior to the operation to verify its accuracy (Caversaccio et al., 1999).

## Modeling

The data from the preoperative axial image is reformatted to reconstruct images in the coronal, sagittal, and axial planes at the same time. CT is the imaging modality that presents least problems for current computer technology; MRI has problems due to distortion of magnetic field lines (Klimek et al., 1998).

## Positioning of the Patient, Surgeon, and Equipment

The patient is placed supine on the operating table and the headset is applied. During surgery, the surgeon faces the computer workstation monitor and observes the CT projections and endoscopically navigated pictures. While these can be displayed together, the surgical endoscopic view is of better quality on a larger, separate screen and the operator primarily uses this and only refers to the CT projections to confirm the position of the instruments. **DVD** 2

## Registration

It is important to check that the instrument in the surgical field and the CT images correlate well. The correlation of the $x$, $y$, and $z$ coordinates in the three orthogonal image planes to the actual position of the probe defines the accuracy of the system (Fig. 10.**33**).

A number of techniques for registration have been described. One method is to register artificial reference points that are stuck onto the skin or are included in the headgear during both the preoperative CT scan and the operative procedure. A malleable registration mask with nickel fiducial markers has recently been described (Albritton et al., 2001) and it is likely that processes such as these will be simplified as well as being made more accurate.

Natural landmarks can be used to perform "surface registration" that allows preoperative scanning without any headset or patient-mounted fiducials. This involves the surgeon touching a finite number of

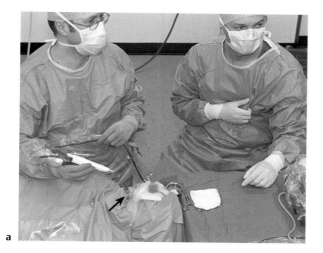

discrete points on the patient with a probe and registering the corresponding points on the three-dimensional model depicted on the computer display (Anon et al., 1994; Fried and Morrison, 1998). Four reference points are usually chosen and may include the following: the tragi, lateral orbital rims and lateral canthi, medial canthi, the deepest part of the glabella, the columellar–labial angle, and the nasal alar rims. Once registration has been completed, the surgeon should perform an anatomical check with known structures to evaluate positional accuracy and estimate target error. With the electromagnetic system, once the headframe has been applied, registration is quickly checked using the spine, origin of the middle turbinate, and anterior lacrimal crest, and posteriorly the base of the middle turbinate and root of the vomer. This gives excellent accuracy (Fig. 10.**34** a, b).

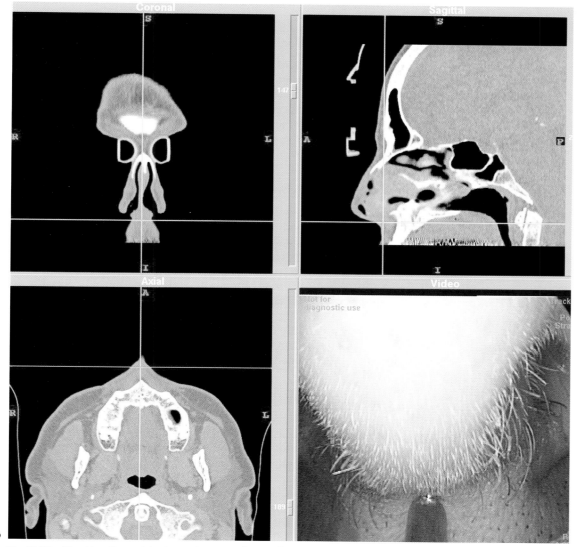

Fig. 10.**34**   Checking the registration points on **a** the nasal spine (arrow) and **b** the navigation screen.

## Methods of Localization

The localization system is used to translate the position of an instrument in the surgical field into coordinates superimposed on the preloaded preoperative CT images displayed on the computer monitor. The critical component of this localization system is the digitizing sensor or tracker. Four different types of tracking technology have been used: electromagnetic, optical, electromechanical, and sonic. At present the optical and electromagnetic systems are the only two in widespread use.

### Electromagnetic Systems

Low-frequency magnetic fields recognize the position of an instrument via ferromagnetic probes that detect gradients in the magnetic field. The influences of these probes on the magnetic field can be calculated to work out their position. The equipment comprises a headframe with an electromagnetic transmitter and a suction device with an electromagnetic receiver in its handle. Be aware that any ferromagnetic or paramagnetic object in the surgical field, such as aluminum, can distort the magnetic field. This is rarely a problem, however. The identical headframe needs to be worn for the preoperative CT scan and the operative procedure. This system is easy to use and is widely accepted.

### Optical Systems

There are two types of optical tracking systems: one active, the other passive. In the active system, the headframe and the instrument have infrared-emitting diodes that are detected by the cameras. These utilize a number of infrared imaging diodes attached to the operating probe or instrument in a distinctive geometric pattern. This system needs the hand-held instrument to be connected by a wire. A passive system does not need a wire as it depends on markers attached to the instrument that are detected by the infrared cameras. A three-camera array system positioned 2 meters from the headset detects the position of these diodes and detects the position of the probe (Klimek et al., 1998; Anon et al., 1997). The headset, which does not need to be worn during the preoperative scan, contains a sterile keyboard that is used intraoperatively. The headset also contains diodes and is therefore crucial for registration of each instrument.

The disadvantage with this system is that a clear line of sight must be maintained between the instrument sensor, the headset, and the camera array. It is vital that the headframe does not slip during the procedure. Instruments available at present do not have infrared imaging diodes placed in a variety of positions

that enable them to be used and detected by a camera in one position. This particularly applies to working in the frontal recess. This means that the camera and stand have to be moved so that the signal can be picked up.

### Electromechanical Systems

Electromechanical systems rely on detectors located within the joints of a table-mounted, position-sensitive, articulated multijoint robotic arm. The position of the probe tip that is connected to the arm is calculated from the arm geometry and information from the joint detectors (Klimek et al., 1998). Problems with this system are that movement of the patient's head affects registration and therefore the head has to be immobilized. The device is also bulky and takes up considerable space in the operating room (Fried and Morrison, 1998).

### Sonic Systems

Sonic systems are based on measuring the time for the sound emitted from several locations to be detected by several microphones. However, temperature differences and humidity affect the speed of sound, and echoes, airflow, and convection currents may diminish the reliability of the system (Anon et al., 1997; Klimek et al., 1998).

## Display of Images

The working computer display screen for computer-aided endoscopic sinus surgery is divided into four quadrants. Three quadrants simultaneously show grayscale two-dimensional coronal, sagittal, and axial sectional images reconstructed from the preoperative CT scan (Anon et al., 1997; Klimek et al., 1998). The tip of the probe is depicted by crosshairs on these images (Fig. 10.**35**). The fourth quadrant can be used to display the endoscopic image or alternatively, in newer systems, it can show a three-dimensional reconstructed model.

## Accuracy

Inaccuracies can originate from the CT scan and its reconstruction, the sensor device, movement of the headset, bending of the probe, its placement at registration, and patient motion. This reinforces the fact that the success of the operation still depends primarily on the skill and experience of the surgeon, which cannot be replaced by technology. However, generally accepted figures suggest an accuracy range of 0.5–3 mm with a mean of approximately 1 mm (Cartellieri et al., 2001).

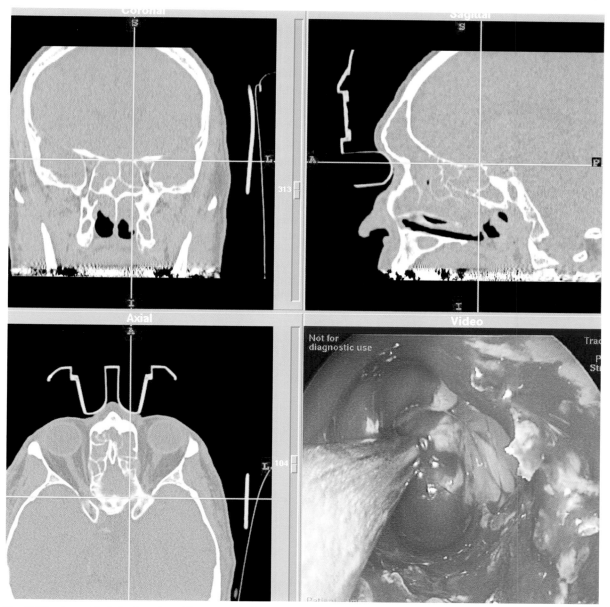

Fig. 10.**35**  Aspergillosis in the sphenoid sinus. Note that the CT images do *not* show that the sphenoid has been opened and its contents have been removed.

## Operative Time

Registration is the main factor that adds to the operating time using the optical system, although some would argue that, because it allows rapid identification of difficult anatomical areas, surgeons can operate faster (Metson et al., 2000).

## Economic Factors

In addition to the computer system, the costs of the optical disks, prolonged anesthetic time, and possibly the need for a larger operating room must be considered. A cost analysis by Gibbons and colleagues showed that computer-aided endoscopic sinus surgery provided significant benefits to the patient despite being more expensive and hence was "cost-effective" (Gibbons et al., 2001). Taking the above into consideration and given the higher precision of surgical dissection and improved surgeon confidence, most authors believe that the high initial costs of 3D navigation systems are justified in the long term (Cartellieri et al., 2001).

## Teaching

Computer-aided systems help trainees to appreciate paranasal sinus anatomy and are an excellent teaching tool. They have an invaluable role in helping the surgeon to build up a "real-time" 3D image in their mind. This technology should not give the trainee a false sense of security and they should not use it to justify operating outside the boundary of their experience.

## Real-time Computer-aided Surgery

Computer-aided surgery relies on preoperative imaging data rather than intraoperative imaging and hence does not reflect or compensate for tissue changes, volume shifts, or dissection during surgery (Olson and Citardi, 2000). The future of computer-aided endoscopic sinus surgery is for simultaneous or periodic real-time imaging using intraoperatively acquired MRI images to reflect these changes in anatomy (Anand and Kacker, 2000).

## Peroperative Monitoring of Optic Function

Analogously to facial nerve monitoring in parotid and mastoid surgery, attempts have been made to monitor visual evoked potentials during endoscopic and anterior skull base surgery. Monitoring of this nature would be of particular benefit when operating at the orbital apex, such as during optic nerve decompression or removal of disease in this area. While visual evoked potentials have the capacity to provide an early indication of reversible changes to the visual system, they are too variable to be reliable at present (Jones, 1997).

# 11 Hints

This advice comes as a result of our experience—which means what we have learnt from our mistakes.

## ■ In the Operating Room

Before starting the operation:
- Never be tempted to operate without the CT scans.
- Do not operate without the patient's records.
- Take your time. The saying "more haste, less speed" was never more true than in performing endoscopic sinus surgery. Being in a hurry may mean that you forget something on your checklist, that you do not give enough time for the topical decongestant to work, or that you introduce your instruments abruptly and scuff the mucosa in the anterior aspect of the nose. In the long run, any of these will slow you down.
- It is worth taking time to show that you appreciate the anesthetist and the nursing and supporting staff.
- Optimize your operating conditions by maximizing preoperative medical treatment. If there are no contraindications (e.g., asthma) an oral beta-blocker can be given the day before surgery as well as on the morning of surgery. Allowing enough time for topical vasoconstrictors to work requires patience, but it will be rewarded.

## ■ Anesthetist's Goals

Hints to reduce bleeding:
- A smooth induction and anesthetic (if the patient is coughing on the anesthetic tube, wait until everything has settled down or there is likely to be substantial bleeding).
- Bradycardia lowers cardiac output and bleeding.
- Avoid other methods of lowering the blood pressure, such as volatile agents, as this will result in peripheral vasodilatation and more bleeding.

## ■ Preparation

- Operate with the body 20° head-up to reduce venous engorgement in the nasal mucosa.
- Have the head flexed on the neck to make the plane of the anterior skull base more vertical. This will reduce the likelihood of traversing it.
- Do not tape the eyes, so that they can regularly be examined when you are operating on the lateral nasal wall. Also regularly ballotte the eyes with the lids closed to check whether there is any dehiscence of the lamina papyracea.

## ■ Surgical Hints

- This is not "smash and grab" surgery. Rather, it requires good preparation, analysis of CT scans, and a thorough knowledge of the anatomy and attention to detail in surgical technique.
- Stay back with the endoscope. By doing this you will maintain perspective and reduce the splattering of blood on the end of the endoscope.
- Introduce instruments ahead of the endoscope to avoid scuffing the anterior one-third of the septum. Care taken during the first 15 minutes of a procedure is a good investment as it will avoid the frustration of the scope becoming coated with blood every time it is introduced past an abraded anterior one-third of the nose.
- Endoscopy does not provide stereoscopic vision, so it is important to use landmarks (middle turbinate attachment, middle meatal antrostomy, frontal recess, roof of the sphenoid) and stay back with the scope to allow as many of these to be seen as possible.
- Stop if visibility is poor. Either work on the other side or place 6 mm ribbon gauze soaked with a vasoconstrictor (1 : 10 000 epinephrine) in position. If the bleeding is excessive, curtail the procedure.
- Do not remove or grab anything that you cannot see clearly (this also applies to the microdebrider).
- It is easier to use a 0° endoscope for most operating, as then you do not inadvertently operate where you do not want to. At the limits of the visual field via an angled endoscope, there is foreshortening and it is possible to be working much higher up than you

imagine. This is in part due to the excellent wide range of the new scopes that span approximately 30° outside the axis of the scope; for example, using a 45° scope you may be working at 75° (45° + 30°) from the axis of the endoscope.

- It is safer to initially stay medial to the medial wall of the maxillary sinus, below the take-off of the middle turbinate from the cribriform plate and below the level of the roof of the sphenoid sinus. This "block" of cells contains most of the sinuses, and it is safe to remove tissue in this area.
- If you have not removed any polyps for some time during the surgery, consider whether you are making progress or just increasing your chance of producing a complication.
- Do not instrument around the territory of the anterior ethmoid artery if there are polyps in that area and you cannot readily identify landmarks.
- Respect the mucosa of the frontal recess. Use through-cutting instruments rather than tearing or pulling mucosa. Preserve mucosa so that the result-ing cavity at the end of surgery is lined. This not only reduces cicatrization of the frontal recess, it also speeds up healing and the return of mucociliary function.
- Never push with a probe or a sound.
- Preserve all the olfactory mucosa if at all possible.
- Gently lateralize the middle turbinate after a thorough ethmoidectomy if there are polyps medial to the middle turbinate.

## ■ Objectives of the Operation

It is worth following the discipline of working out which specific sinuses you are going to operate on before picking up an instrument. It is then best to follow a predetermined plan and do no more, unless there are very good reasons. This prevents unnecessary "wandering" into areas that you do not need to be in, for example, the frontal recess.   *DVD* 6, 7, 8

# 12 Preventing and Dealing with Complications

Complications will always occur. We have a duty to try and minimize them and to take the most appropriate action to help our patient when they do occur. It is important not to ignore them or to hope that they will rectify themselves unaided (Table 12.**1**).

## ■ Peroperative Complications

### Bleeding

Bleeding can be minimized by maximizing preoperative medical treatment and removing tissue with through-cutting forceps or a shaver to avoid tearing the mucosa. The other main causes of bleeding, besides those caused by a coagulopathy, are related to the sphenopalatine artery and the anterior ethmoidal artery.

#### The Sphenopalatine Artery

The anterior branches of the sphenopalatine artery come through the lateral nasal wall horizontally, just above the attachment of the inferior turbinate. If the middle meatal antrostomy is opened widely posteriorly to come to a level in the coronal plane that is less than 0.5 cm away from the posterior wall of the maxillary antrum, a branch of the sphenopalatine artery will often be cut and require cautery. Alternatively, you can damage a branch that comes through the inferior turbinate, but this branch is rarely traumatized in endoscopic sinus surgery.

Another branch of the sphenopalatine artery comes through the middle turbinate, and if more than half of the anterior part of the middle turbinate is removed, this artery often bleeds.

The septal branch from the posterior tributary of the sphenopalatine artery runs across the anterior wall of the sphenoid. If the sphenoid ostium is opened lower than halfway up its height, this branch will be found and it can bleed substantially.

#### The Anterior Ethmoid Artery

Damage to the anterior ethmoid artery can have serious consequences. If the artery retracts into the orbit, this can cause a marked increase in pressure in the

Table 12.**1** Peroperative and postoperative complications (after Johnson and Jones, 2002)

| Peroperative | Postoperative |
|---|---|
| • Bleeding | • Bleeding |
| • Fat herniation | • Adhesions |
| • CSF leak | • Epiphora |
| • Retro-orbital hemorrhage | • Periorbital emphysema |
| • Medial rectus damage | • Anosmia |
| • Optic nerve lesion | • Frontal recess stenosis |
| | • Crusting |
| | • Infection |
| | • Osteitis |
| | • Neuropathic pain |

posterior compartment of the eye. This will compromise the vascularity of the optic nerve and retina and result in blindness if not recognized and dealt with. The main reasons for complications are poor visibility and blood on the lens. It is important not to operate, probe, remove, or grasp anything that you cannot see. Curved probes, giraffe forceps, and 90° forceps are all too easily placed where they should not be. If it is not possible to see—stop. If there is excessive bleeding, check that the patient is 20° body-up and that the arterial mean pressure is kept between 65 and 75 mmHg. Use a 6 mm ribbon gauze soaked in cophenylcaine or 1 : 10 000 epinephrine on the side with the bleeding and move on to work on the other side while the bleeding abates. It is possible to work from side to side, transferring the pack periodically.

If in spite of these measures there is still bleeding that cannot be controlled by diathermy, cleared with a larger sucker, or reduced by placing a catheter through the other nostril into the nasopharynx while it is on suction to remove the reservoir of blood, then stop operating. Normally with this amount of bleeding it is best to stop and have a further trial of medical treatment. It is surprising how often the patient is delighted and symptomatically improved although the surgeon feels that the ethmoidectomy that they have undertaken is incomplete. This does not matter as much as the patient's safety, which should be put first. It is good to recognize when little progress has been made during a procedure. In a polypectomy, for example, when little tissue has been removed in the previous 5 minutes, it may be worth stopping. Re-

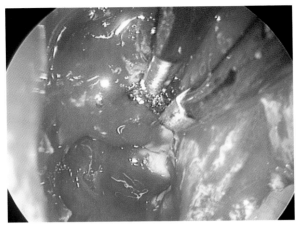

Fig. 12.**1**    Bipolar suction diathermy works well as the ends are not immersed in blood that dissipates the current.

member that most of the complications are likely to occur toward the end of the procedure when the surgeon is fiddling about clearing small areas of polyps on the skull base, which may in itself produce little benefit.

To stop bleeding from these discernible vessels, you can use either bipolar forceps (Fig. 12.**1**) or unipolar suction diathermy (Fig. 12.**2 a**, **b**). Some of the bipolar suction forceps now available help to remove the blood and smoke at the same time. The bulbous head of the unipolar suction device allows cautery of a sizable vessel anywhere in the nose, and its large suction channel is less likely to become blocked by congealed blood (Fig. 12.**3 a**, **b**). The anterior ethmoid artery is rarely responsible for postoperative bleeding but, if it is, this can be diathermied (Fig. 12.**4 a**, **b**).  **DVD**  12, 13

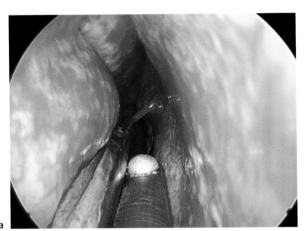
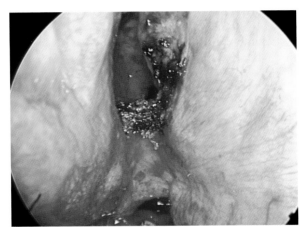

a                                                                                                b

Fig. 12.**2 a**, **b**    Unipolar suction diathermy being used to coagulate the septal branch of the sphenopalatine artery during a large sphenoidotomy.

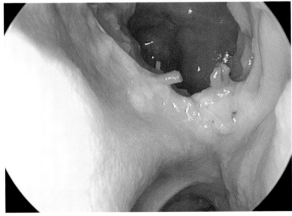
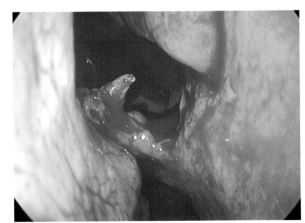

a                                                                                                b

Fig. 12.**3**    **a** A cadaver injected with latex to show the position of the septal branch of the sphenopalatine artery cut while enlarging the sphenoidotomy inferiorly and **b** a clinical case.

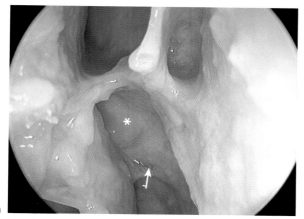
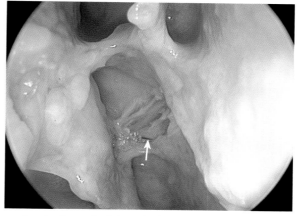

a

b

Fig. 12.**4a**, **b**   A cadaver injected with latex to show the position of the right anterior ethmoid artery (arrow). Note the sulcus terminalis on the left and a large supraorbital cell (∗) in front of the anterior ethmoid artery.

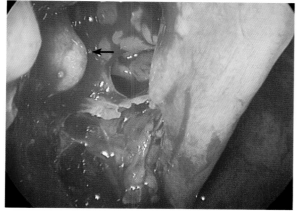
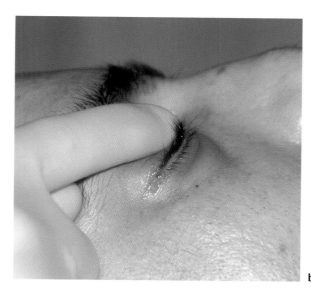

a

b

Fig. 12.**5**   **a** A peroperative view of fat herniating through a defect in the lamina papyracea (arrow). **b** Ballotte the eye so the surgeon can see whether there is a dehiscence of the lateral nasal wall.

If by some misfortune there is torrential bleeding because of trauma to the internal carotid artery in the sphenoid, then prompt packing of the sphenoid sinus is required with a firm gauze pack. The patient is then resuscitated and the help of an interventional radiologist is sought. Blood is sent for cross-matching and when there is sufficient blood available the pack may gently be removed to see whether the bleeding continues. If not, then the sinus is best repacked with fascia and fat followed by oxidized cellulose, and an antibiotic-impregnated pack is left in position for a week.

If bleeding continues when the pack is gently removed, the radiologist should be asked to do an occlusion study under EEG control. If that is not possible and the situation is not stable, then the patient must be transferred to a unit where this can be done. If there are no EEG changes after the occlusion, it is best to seal the artery using angioplastic techniques, otherwise the help of a neurosurgeon may be needed to undertake a transcranial approach. Tying off the internal carotid artery in the neck is not a good option because of the back pressure from the cerebral circulation.

## Fat Herniation and Violation of the Orbit

The orthodox anterior approach to an uncinectomy is potentially one of the most dangerous procedures in endoscopic sinus surgery and we now recommend a retrograde removal of the uncinate process for those who are just starting ESS. Not infrequently there are no ethmoid air cells to act as a cushion between the uncinate process and the lamina papyracea and an incision

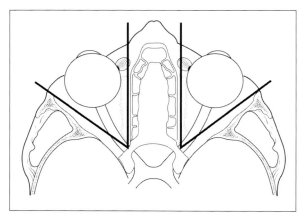

Fig. 12.**6**   A line diagram to show the plane of the medial walls of the orbits.

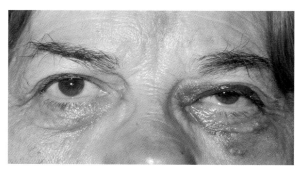

Fig. 12.**7**   Ecchymosis caused by traversing the orbital periosteum.

as little as 2 mm through the unciate process can also go through the lamina papyracea and into the orbit. Even if the uncinate process is ballotted to define its extent and the sickle knife is kept as near as possible to the sagittal plane to avoid traversing the lamina papyracea, it is easy to inadvertently enter the orbit. We have seen this happen with experienced surgeons and therefore advise a retrograde approach for beginners. When operating on the lateral nasal wall, it is best to have the eyes exposed and kept moist with simple eye ointment and to ask an assistant to look for any eye movement. We offer a bottle of the best champagne we can buy to an assistant who reports any orbital movement and is correct. This has certainly saved several patients a complication, as well as and our reputation! If the assistant says that they think there has been some movement when there has not, we do not ignore them or chastise as we want their threshold for alerting us to remain low.

Both at the start of a procedure and during it, it is worth asking the assistant to palpate the closed eye to see whether there is any dehiscence of the lamina

papyracea, as in this case the lateral wall will be seen to balloon medially (Fig. 12.**5 a**, **b**). Occasionally, you will be surprised and find that the orbital contents prolapse into the nasal cavity when the eye is ballotted. This can occur even in a patient who has not had any previous surgery, particularly if they have marked nasal polyposis.

Another danger area is the "armpit" where the lateral nasal wall joins the middle turbinate. Frequently, agger nasi air cells cushion the operator from the lamina papyracea, but sometimes the lamina papyracea and the uncinate process have already merged and it is possible to go straight into the orbit here. Remember that the orbits are not "carrot shaped" cylindrical structures whose long axis is sagittal (Fig. 12.**6**). The orbit's medial walls are sagittal and as long as you stay medial to the medial wall of the maxillary sinus you are likely to be safe. It is true that there are often cells lateral to the sagittal plane of the medial wall of the maxillary sinus that need opening, but these are best identified on CT and they are readily found and opened after the more medial cells have been exposed. Gentle palpation with a blunt-ended probe behind the remaining lamella will safely disclose most of these cells.

If the lamina papyracea is cracked or a segment is removed during the procedure, this may cause a minor ecchymosis (Fig. 12.**7**); this will settle spontaneously in 3–4 days. If the orbital periosteum is traversed, then orbital fat prolapses into the nasal airway. Although fat has a yellow hue, it can look remarkably like nasal polyps. Palpation of the closed eye by the assistant, or you, will tell whether it is orbital fat as it will move abruptly with this maneuver. If it is fat, do not panic; there is a temptation to push it back into the orbit (this will fail), to pull it out (this will make the damage to the orbit worse), or to cauterize it. None of these is necessary and they may cause more harm.

If powered instrumentation is being used, this should be stopped because the suction can easily remove the fat, which is then sheared off, and this makes matters worse. If the surgeon has the experience to carry on, placing a moist neurosurgical patte over the fat can protect this area while the rest of the procedure is completed. As long as the only damage done is opening the periosteum, the only problem will be some periorbital ecchymosis. The surgeon who has performed an extensive orbital decompression and widely decompressed and incised the periosteum, allowing the fat to prolapse medially without creating a problem, will realize that this is not a major complication/difficulty as long as it is recognized and the orbit is not entered further.

The patient should be advised to avoid blowing their nose and or stifling any sneezes for 4 days in order to avoid surgical emphysema and it is best to give prophylactic antibiotics to avoid the theoretical risk of orbital cellulitis (Fig. 12.**8**). The tension within the orbit should be monitored by gently comparing it with the other eye to ensure there is no bleeding or pressure building up in the posterior compartment. If the globe is tense and proptosed then decompression may be required. The axis of the pupils should be checked. If it is altered, this may indicate that a considerable amount of the orbital contents have been removed or proptosed into the airway, or that the medial rectus has been damaged. Under these circumstances, an urgent ophthalmological opinion should be sought.

The pupils' light reflexes should be checked with the "swinging flashlight test" (Mason et al., 1998 a) (Fig. 12.**9** a–c). This will show whether there is an afferent pupil defect. As an example, if there is concern

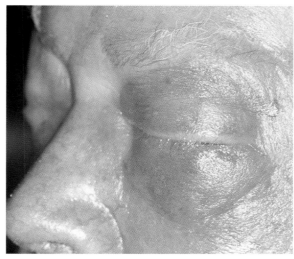

Fig. 12.**8**   Postoperative periorbital cellulitis.

---

Left pupil dilated during endoscopic sinus surgery but has a **NORMAL** swinging flashlight test.
Therefore no optic nerve damage - pharmacological dilatation + full recovery likely.

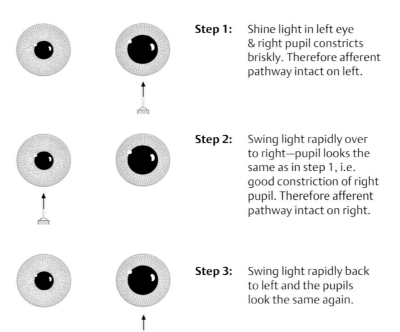

**Step 1:**   Shine light in left eye & right pupil constricts briskly. Therefore afferent pathway intact on left.

**Step 2:**   Swing light rapidly over to right—pupil looks the same as in step 1, i.e. good constriction of right pupil. Therefore afferent pathway intact on right.

**Step 3:**   Swing light rapidly back to left and the pupils look the same again.

In other words, no matter which eye the light shines in, the pupil of the right eye remains responsive to light. (The left pupil is sluggish or non-responsive because of pharmacological dilatation or damage to the oculomotor nerve on this side [rare].)

a

Fig. 12.**9 a**   The swinging flashlight test to check for an afferent optic nerve defect.
Fig. 12.**9 b, c**   ▷

Assistant notices tugging movement of left eye
during endoscopic sinus surgery. Swinging flash light
test shows left afferent pupil defect. Therefore optic nerve damage.

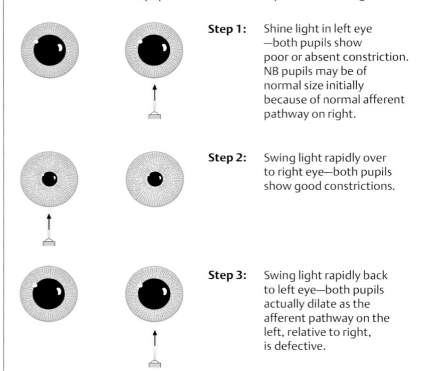

**Step 1:**  Shine light in left eye
—both pupils show
poor or absent constriction.
NB pupils may be of
normal size initially
because of normal afferent
pathway on right.

**Step 2:**  Swing light rapidly over
to right eye—both pupils
show good constrictions.

**Step 3:**  Swing light rapidly back
to left eye—both pupils
actually dilate as the
afferent pathway on the
left, relative to right,
is defective.

b

Fig. 12.**9 b**, **c**   Eye signs in
various clinical situations.

## Unilateral Dilatation

1. Pupillary dilatation due to trauma to the oculomotor nerve.
2. Pharmacological dilatation of the iris, e.g. cocaine spilled into eye.
3. Reduced conduction of the third nerve caused by cocaine on the inferior
   division of the oculomotor nerve as it passes through the superior orbital
   fissure, in close proximity to the sphenoid/ethmoidal sinus (local anesthetic
   affect).

## Unilateral Constriction

Pupillary constriction is caused by damage to the sympathetic supply
to the iris (Horner syndrome).

c

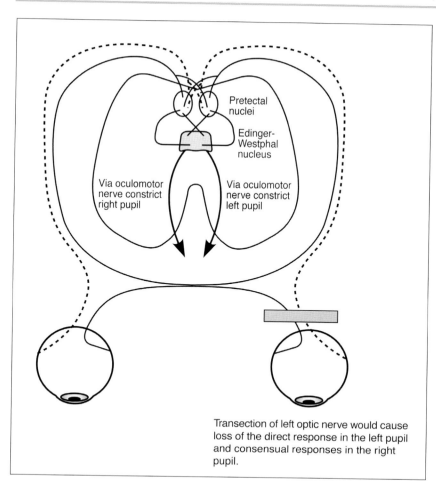

Fig. 12.**10**   A line diagram of the optic and oculomotor pathways.

**Pretectal nuclei**

**Edinger-Westphal nucleus**

**Via oculomotor nerve constrict right pupil**

**Via oculomotor nerve constrict left pupil**

Transection of left optic nerve would cause loss of the direct response in the left pupil and consensual responses in the right pupil.

about left optic nerve damage then the light is shone in the left eye. If there has been damage to that optic nerve, then if light is shone in that eye both pupils will show poor or absent constriction (the pupils may be normal size initially because of a normal afferent pathway on the right). The light is then swung rapidly over to the right eye, and both pupils should show good constriction. The light is then swung rapidly back to the left eye, and if both pupils dilate then this indicates that the afferent pathway on the left is defective. This is the best way of checking to see whether there is an afferent pupil defect if the patient is anaesthetized. The appearance of the pulsation of the retinal vessels is not a reliable sign. The ultimate test is to wake the patient up and check their vision (Fig. 12.**10**).

The surgeon should not ignore any complication or potential complications (Fig. 12.**11 a**, **b**). The authors have sometimes been asked to comment as expert witnesses on events where the surgeons have realized that they have damaged the orbital contents and then failed to take the appropriate action.

If there is an orbital complication, the light reflexes, the pressure of the orbit, and, most importantly, the visual acuity should be checked. No harm comes from checking these, in particular the vision. If there is any concern about the integrity of the afferent pathway or the orbit, we recommend that the vision be checked every 15 minutes for the first hour, then every 30 minutes for 2 hours, and then hourly for a further 2 hours. If the pressure is raised within the orbit, requiring decompression, this should be done within one hour. To ignore this puts the patient's sight at risk.

Be sure to close the other eye when checking the vision of the eye in question. It is best to gently remove any excess eye ointment by wiping the eye while it is closed, otherwise acuity will be affected and this can alarm both the patient and the surgeon (Fig. 12.**12 a–e**).

## CSF Leak

The key points that need to be observed in order to prevent complications involving leakage of cerebrospinal fluid (CSF) are:

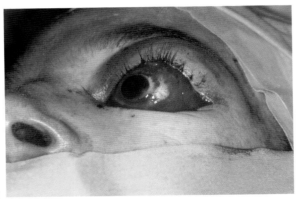

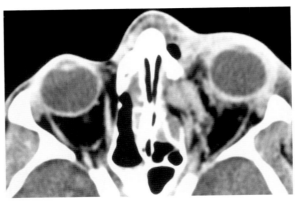

a

b

Fig. 12.**11** **a** A proptosed eye due to retro-orbital bleeding. **b** A CT scan of a patient who had bleeding into the left posterior compartment of the eye that was not decompressed and resulted in blindness.

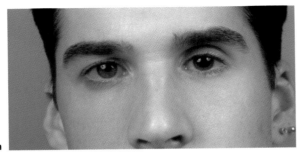

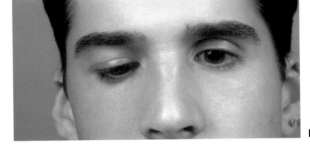

a

b

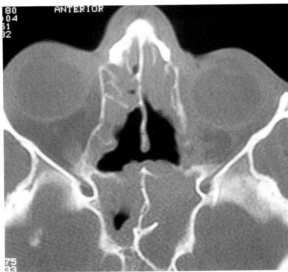

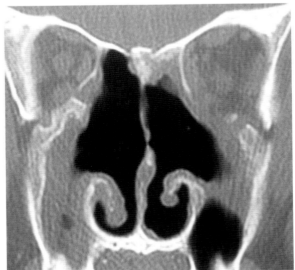

c

d

Fig. 12.**12 a**, **b** A patient who had left enophthalmos, ptosis, and a dilated pupil without blindness due to excessive removal of bone that included the floor of the orbit and damage to the oculomotor nerve. **c**, **d** Radiology showing the result of surgery.

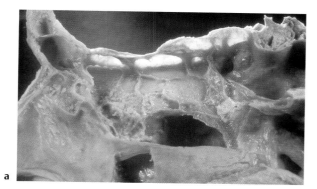

a

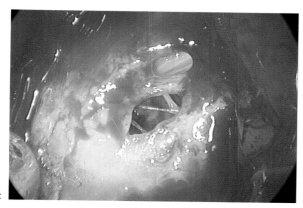

c

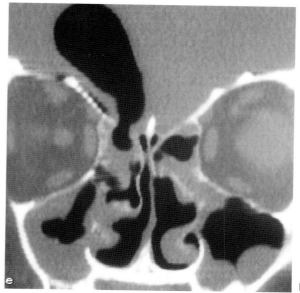

e                                                                    b

Fig. 12.**13**   **a** A transilluminated skull showing the thin bone of the anterior skull base. **b** A coronal CT scan showing pneumocephalus because the skull base has been traversed. **c** An endoscopic view of the defect.

- Follow the preoperative checklist.
- Do not fiddle around the attachment of the middle turbinate to the roof of the anterior skull base unless you are familiar with this area.
- It is safest to open the posterior ethmoid air cells once you have found the height of the roof of the sphenoid sinus: if you stay below this level you will not go through the skull base.
- Do not angle your instruments medially toward the lateral lamella as the skull base is extremely thin in this area and you are more prone to cause a leak.

The thinnest area of the skull base is adjacent to where the anterior ethmoid artery enters the anterior skull base at the lateral lamella of the cribriform plate (Fig. 12.**13 a–c**). The next most common area where CSF leakage occurs is where the middle third of the middle turbinate starts to attach more laterally from the skull base to the lateral nasal wall. It is here that it can inadvertently be grasped, twisted, or pulled and a defect created. The skull base tends to angle inferiorly as the surgeon works posteriorly, and the height of the posterior ethmoid sinuses varies. You need to have a good reason to be in the posterior ethmoid sinuses. This reason is often that there is severe polyposis with or without purulent disease.

The CT scan can help the surgeon decide the extent of surgery that is likely to be needed to remove dis-

eased mucosa and aerate the affected sinus. (NB Be careful if the CT scan was done during or shortly after a course of oral steroids as this can appreciably reduce the amount of mucosal swelling and the retention of secretions.) See whether there is a "black halo" of some air in the peripheral cells around the skull base (Fig. 12.**14 a, b**). This is an encouraging sign as it means that there is a cushion of normal cells that will be entered before reaching the skull base. A "white-out" on CT needs to be approached with more caution. First, it is worth judging the height of the posterior ethmoid sinuses on CT by examining the height from the posterior skull base to the roof of the maxillary sinuses on the posterior coronal cuts. Next, the surgeon should check for the presence of a sphenoethmoid air cell. Before starting any surgery it is worth flexing the head on the neck as this will place the skull base in a more vertical plane. This is particularly worthwhile as, following intubation, the patient is often positioned on the operating table with the head extended, making it more likely that the surgeon will enter the skull base if they go straight backward.

If there is a "white-out," one safe strategy is to enter the sphenoid sinus before the posterior ethmoid sinuses have been opened to find the height of its roof. As the roof of the ethmoid sinuses is never lower than the roof of the sphenoid sinus, this is a useful indicator of the level below which it is safe to operate. While the

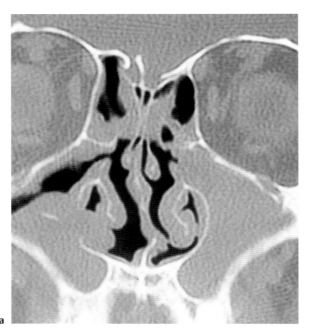

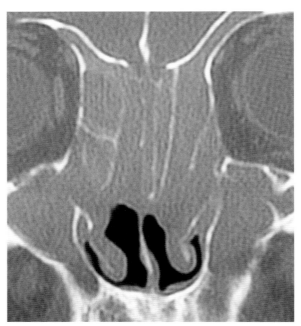

a

b

Fig. 12.**14** **a** A "black halo" of air on a CT scan showing that the surgeon will come across aerated cells before the skull base. **b** A "white-out" with no aeration of the sinuses.

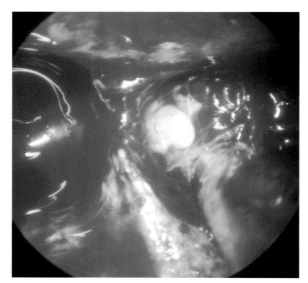

Fig. 12.**15** CSF coming out of a defect in the posterior wall of the sphenoid sinus.

posterior ethmoid sinuses can be higher than the roof of the sphenoid sinus, these cells are few and usually large, and just by opening them below the level of the roof of the sphenoid sinus it will become apparent where they are. A curved-ended sound, for example, the olive-shaped end of a curved sucker, can be used to feel whether there is a space behind any of the bony partitions so that these can be removed with through-cutting forceps or a Hajek punch.

### Dealing with an Intraoperative CSF Leak

Clear fluid may be seen emanating from a skull base defect (Fig. 12.**15**). It looks like a clear stream in a pool of blood and it often pulsates. Unless you are aware of this possibility you may miss it. Occasionally an ethmoid air cell full of mucus that is opened will produce a similar appearance, but then the stream stops almost immediately. The edges of the bony defect should be defined. Many graft materials have been used, ranging from a "bath plug" fat graft for small leaks (Wormald and McDonagh, 1997) to a free turbinate or conchal cartilage graft for larger defects (Marshall et al., 2001 a). It is best to place the graft above the defect so that it underlays the defect, but wedging it within the hole also works. This is then overlaid by a free mucosal graft from the inferior turbinate. We have found that a lumbar drain is unnecessary. The graft is supported by a dressing of oxidized cellulose to avoid it sticking to a pack such as a bismuth and iodoform impregnated gauze for 10 days. Both peroperative and postoperative prophylactic antibiotics are given for 10 days. The patient is nursed 30° or more head-up and asked not to strain (e.g., not to lift heavy objects and to avoid becoming constipated). Patients are discharged home after 36 hours. **DVD** 15

## Retro-orbital Hemorrhage

Usually the anterior ethmoid artery can be located one cell behind the frontal recess. The size of this cell varies: it can be small, it can be large. This cell is called a supraorbital cell (it is often an extension of the suprabullar recess) (Bolger and Mawn, 2001). The anterior ethmoid artery can often be seen on CT, particularly as it enters the orbit where it produces a fluted defect in the lamina papyracea. The more pneumatized the supraorbital recess is, the more vulnerable it is to damage (Fig. 12.**16**). Occasionally the ethmoid bulla attaches directly onto the skull base. In these patients, the anterior ethmoid artery lies within its roof and is one "undulation" behind the attachment of the anterior wall of the ethmoid bulla to the skull base. The anterior ethmoid artery lies above the level of the attachment of the anterior end of the middle turbinate to the skull base and it can be avoided by staying below this level. This is yet another reason for not instrumenting the frontal recess unless there are good reasons for doing so. However, if the frontal recess does require opening, it is best approached anteriorly, away from the anterior ethmoid artery if the landmarks are poor owing to previous surgery or bleeding. As the anterior ethmoid artery is sometimes dehiscent, it is wise not to grasp polyps in this area if you are unable to identify the anatomy clearly. If visibility is good and the ethmoid bulla has not previously been opened, then, after inspecting the CT scan to check for the presence and position of agger nasi/bulla frontalis cells, the frontal recess can be found by following the anterior wall of the ethmoid bulla superiorly.

The anterior ethmoid artery is dehiscent at some point in the majority of patients (Lang, 1989). It is important to avoid damaging it; while tearing it can cause marked bleeding, the main concern is that if it is transected and it retracts back into the orbit, this can cause a marked increase in the pressure in the posterior compartment of the eye and place the retinal artery and its supply to the retina at risk. If it is torn, gentle bipolar diathermy will arrest the bleeding, but do this with great care in order to avoid transecting it by burning the remaining segment of the artery.

If there is significant bleeding into the posterior compartment of the eye, the eye will proptose, the orbit will become very firm, and after a few minutes the swinging flashlight test will reveal an afferent defect. A patient who is awake will mention discomfort and a loss of vision. If this is recognized immediately, an orbital tourniquet should be tried. This involves placing cotton wool over the closed eyelid and applying an orbital tourniquet (the ophthalmological equivalent of a sphygmomanometer) over the cotton wool and around the head, and then inflating it to systolic pressure. This should be done for one minute and then

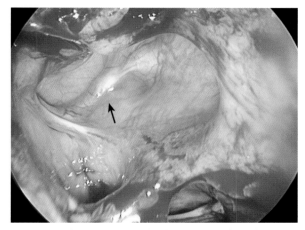

Fig. 12.**16**    The ridge created by the anterior ethmoid artery is clearly seen (arrow) because of the degree of pneumatization of the skull base.

it should be removed and the pupil reflexes and/or the vision checked. If the vision or pupil reflex has improved, the optical tourniquet should be reapplied and the process repeated every minute for up to 5 minutes. If this is done soon after the injury, it may be sufficient to stop bleeding into the orbit and it can arrest the process.

It is wise to monitor the vision for 6 hours afterwards to ensure that no further bleeding into the posterior compartment occurs. If this maneuver is not possible or does not work, the orbit must be decompressed. It is the authors' preference to do a lateral canthotomy and inferior cantholysis as this is both quick and efficient and is associated with minimum morbidity (Fig. 12.**17**). While some evidence suggests that the optic nerve can withstand ischemia for up to one hour, it is best to decompress the orbit as early as possible (Jones, 1997). You should not wait for an ophthalmological colleague to arrive unless they will do so well within one hour. Assessing the vascular supply of the retinal vessels with an ophthalmoscope is inadequate and should not be relied upon.

## Lateral Canthotomy and Inferior Cantholysis

It is important to have practiced this procedure on a cadaver in order to have the confidence to do it in vivo. Local anesthetic should be placed around the lateral canthus of the eye. Small straight scissors should be used to divide the lateral canthus down to the bone of the orbital rim and to the depth of the lateral sulcus of the conjunctiva. It is important to protect the globe in order to avoid a corneal abrasion or conjunctival damage (Fig. 12.**18 a–d**). The lower lid is then retracted downward to expose the substance of the lower lid; the scissors are angled at 45° to the horizontal axis and

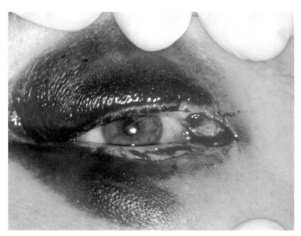

Fig. 12.**17** A patient who has just had a lateral canthotomy and inferior cantholysis for a retro-orbital hemorrhage.

the lateral ligament and septum are divided. The globe and contents of the orbit will then prolapse forward. A little blood-stained exudate will come out, but do not expect much bleeding and do not probe into the posterior compartment of the eye. The pupil reflexes, the

pressure of the orbit, and vision should all be checked. Over the next 2–3 days, the orbit will retract to its normal position and the incision will normally be almost imperceptible as it fades into the crowsfoot of the eye. It does not require suturing at any stage.

This procedure is normally sufficient to decompress the posterior compartment of the eye. If it is inadequate, a medial decompression should be undertaken as well. This can be done either endoscopically by removing the lamina papyracea widely and incising the orbital periosteum or externally via a Lynch–Howarth incision; the choice depends on the surgeon's experience. Do not be frightened about making an external incision if you are most comfortable with that approach. Preserving vision takes priority and comes before any embarrassment you may have about producing an external scar. In any event, an external incision normally heals well as long as the line is broken with a seagull shaped incision, as this will minimize the chance of webbing. If the orbit is decompressed by an external approach, the anterior ethmoid artery will not be found as it will have retracted into the substance of the orbit. It should not be sought, as this would cause more disruption and damage to the orbit.

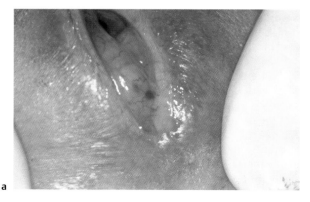

a

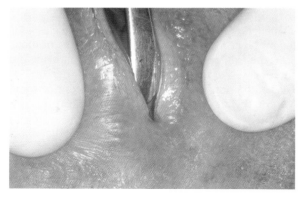

b

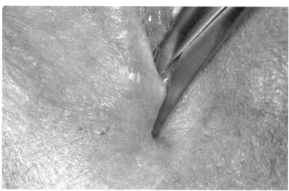

c

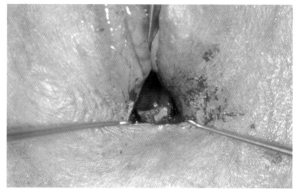

d

Fig. 12.**18 a–d** A lateral canthotomy and inferior cantholysis. Expose the lateral canthus, protect the conjunctiva, incise through all layers down to the orbital margin, and then cut the lateral ligament off the orbital rim.

## Medial Rectus Damage

Medial rectus damage occurs through inattention: if the orbital periosteum is traversed, the assistant should notice movement of the globe. The operator should be very cautious while operating on the lateral nasal wall in this area and ask the assistant to repeatedly ballotte the eye. Damage to the medial rectus normally occurs through deeper penetration into the orbit (Fig. 12.**19**). Unfortunately, even if it is recognized at the time, it is very difficult to prevent the scarring and diplopia that are likely to occur (Flynn et al., 1979). Even expert strabismus surgeons have difficulty in trying to improve the problems that are caused by damage to the medial rectus.

## Optic Nerve Lesion

The optic nerve can be damaged by penetration of the orbit through the lamina papyracea (Fig. 12.**20**). If the assistant looks out for eye movement when the surgeon is operating on the lateral nasal wall, it is unlikely that the nerve could be damaged before it was noted that the orbit had been entered.

The other means by which the optic nerve can be traumatized is if it is exposed in a sphenoethmoid air cell (Fig. 12.**21 a, b**). A sphenoethmoid air cell should be sought on the CT preoperatively and care should be taken in removing polyps or cells lateral to the sagittal plane of the medial wall of the maxillary sinus. In these circumstances, it is particularly advisable to find the sphenoid sinus medially first of all and then work forward. The optic nerve can be prominent in 20% of patients in the upper half of the lateral wall of the sphenoid sinus, but it is rarely dehiscent. The carotid lies in the lateral and inferior aspect of the sphenoid sinus and it is therefore advisable to avoid the lateral wall of the sphenoid, unless there is good reason (e.g., optic nerve decompression). If a powered shaver is placed in the sphenoid sinus, its suction port should be directed medially to minimize the risk of damaging the structures in the lateral nasal wall.

## ■ Postoperative Complications

### Bleeding

For minor general oozing, sitting the patient 30° head-up at the end of the procedure will often suffice. There is temporarily more bleeding during coughing when the patient wakes up as this will increase the venous pressure. For more than minor oozing, a pack can be soaked in 1 : 10 000 epinephrine if there is no contraindication. This can be removed in recovery or left in position for 12 hours if the oozing continues. If packs

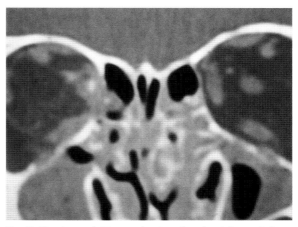

Fig. 12.**19**   Coronal CT scan showing that the right medial rectus has been damaged.

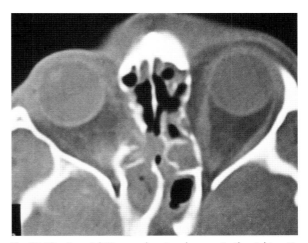

Fig. 12.**20**   An axial CT scan showing damage to the right optic nerve.

need to be left in position for more than 24 hours, a prophylactic antibiotic should be given because the dressings become fetid unless they contain an antibiotic ointment. Rarely, torrential reactionary bleeding can occur from these vessels in the first 12 hours. It is thought that this is due to these vessels initially going into spasm at the time of surgery when a platelet plug and clotting factors block them, but with time either relaxation of the artery or fibrinolysis reverses this process and bleeding starts. Apart from resuscitating the patient, if necessary, it is best to define endoscopically the site of bleeding. Normally a local pack with a vasoconstrictor and local anesthetic will control this situation and allow bipolar cautery of the offending vessel if necessary. If it is not possible to visualize the vessel and/or gain control of the bleeding by this method, a nasal pack and/or balloon may be necessary

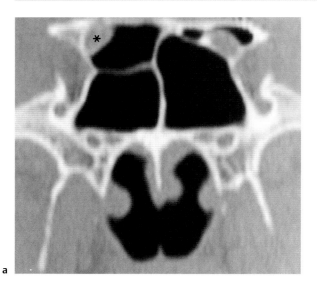

a

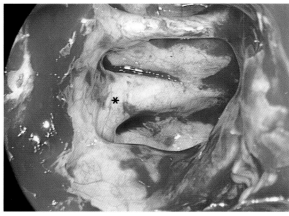

b

Fig. 12.**21**  **a** A coronal CT scan and **b** operative view of a large sphenoethmoid air cell with the optic nerve (✳) exposed within it.

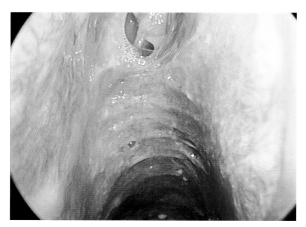

Fig. 12.**22**  Severe adhesions obstructing the olfactory cleft due to mucosal damage on adjacent surfaces.

to tamponade the bleeding until the sphenopalatine artery can be ligated under general anesthesia. If there has been a large sphenoidotomy, then the bleeding probably originates from damage done to the septal branch as it crosses the anterior wall of the sphenoid.

## Adhesions

Adhesions are the consequence of mucosal damage to adjacent surfaces (Fig. 12.**22**). They can be minimized by creating space, treating mucosa with care, opening the olfactory cleft where there has been mucosal damage on both surfaces, asking the patient to douche vigorously three or more times a day, and reviewing the patient at one week and anesthetizing the mucosa with cophenylcaine and removing any strands of

fibrous exudate that are starting to form. We have not found that splints or steroid creams improve matters, as they often appear to cause more local mucosal damage and stimulate fibrosis. Similarly, earlier debridement appears to delay healing and stimulate more fibrosis. If adhesions are present preoperatively, they need more than sectioning in order to avoid them reforming. A segment of the adhesion needs to be removed with a through-cutting punch and more space created, followed by douching and debridement at one week.

## Epiphora

The uncinate process is attached anteriorly to the bone around the nasolacrimal duct and if a middle meatal antrostomy is extended too far anteriorly the lacrimal sac or nasolacrimal duct is damaged (Fig. 12.**23 a**, **b**). The best way to avoid this is to not enlarge the ostium anteriorly. If the middle meatus needs to be enlarged anteriorly to allow improved access or drainage, then the uncinate process is best removed retrogradely with back-biters. If the back-biters require anything other than minimal force to remove the uncinate process, then it is likely that the bone around the nasolacrimal duct is also within the jaws of the biters and you should not continue to grip the instrument. If a patient complains that their eyes are watering in the days after surgery, it is best not to intervene as it will often resolve of its own accord. If epiphora persists, an endonasal dacryocystorhinostomy will resolve the problem.

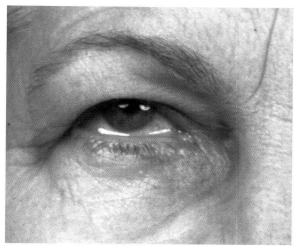

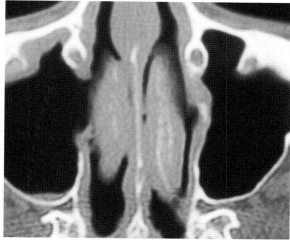

a

b

Fig. 12.**23**   Epiphora due to damage to the right nasolacrimal duct (**a**) shown on CT scan (**b**).

## Periorbital Emphysema

If a breach in the lamina papyracea occurred at surgery and the patient has blown their nose in the first 4 days or stifled a sneeze (this dramatically increases the intranasal pressure), this can force air into the soft tissues around the eye (Fig. 12.**24**). If the surgeon recognizes that there is a defect in the lamina papyracea, the anesthetist should be advised to take care after extubating the patient and not to use too much force if the patient needs to be ventilated with a facemask (in other words, do not have a fixed valve on the circuit). If emphysema occurs, it will resorb, provided the patient does not blow any more air into the area. Prophylactic antibiotics are given in order to avoid periorbital cellulitis.

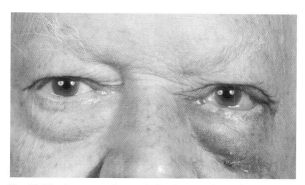

Fig. 12.**24**   Postoperative periorbital surgical emphysema.

## Anosmia

The importance of the sense of smell and taste to the psychological wellbeing of patients is often underestimated. Imagine if all you could taste was salty, sweet, bitter, and sour and that you could not smell your partner's perfume, aftershave, or pheromones! Smell is a precious sense, and every effort should be made to preserve or improve it (Fig. 12.**25**). This essentially means *total* respect of the olfactory mucosa that extends from the cribriform plate to cover almost all the medial side of the middle turbinate, and not only the same area on the septum but usually a little further inferiorly.

To avoid damaging this mucosa, it helps to give preoperative oral steroids (unless there are contraindications), especially if there are polyps medial to the middle turbinate visible at endoscopy when the patient is assessed as an outpatient. When polyps re-

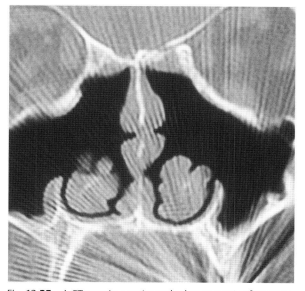

Fig. 12.**25**   A CT scan in a patient who has anosmia after resection of the olfactory mucosa.

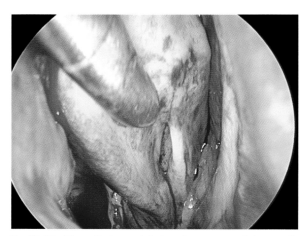

Fig. 12.**26** The olfactory cleft has been opened by gently lateralizing the middle turbinate after an ethmoidectomy.

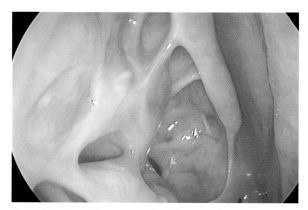

Fig. 12.**27** Frontal stenosis after this area has been instrumented in the past.

main medial to the middle turbinate at surgery, it is best to perform a thorough ethmoidectomy and then gently lateralize the middle turbinate to open up the olfactory cleft (Fig. 12.**26**). It is not a problem if the anterior end of the middle turbinate becomes adherent to the lateral wall provided the middle meatal antrostomy has been extended inferiorly below the inferior limit of the middle turbinate. Under these circumstances, visibility of the frontal recess in outpatients may be limited using a 2.7 mm 0° scope; it can be seen with a 30° scope, although this is rarely necessary. The recovery of mucosa in the olfactory cleft using this technique, even with large polyps in this area, needs to be tried to be believed. The technique also minimizes the risks of adhesions in this area and allows better access to topical nasal steroids. If a patient has hyposmia or anosmia after surgery and the middle turbinate is adherent to the septum, it is worth resecting these and lateralizing the middle turbinate as an elec-

tive procedure when any mucosal edema has settled down.

## Frontal Recess Stenosis

Most frontal sinus disease is the result of previous surgery, and it is important not to instrument this area unless there is a good reason. The frontal sinus is often opaque on CT in nasal polyposis, but this is not a reason to operate on the frontal recess as it is normally due to retained mucus. It is rare to find polyps within the frontal sinus. Simply opening the middle meatus and debulking polyps in the region below the frontal recess with a shaver or through-cutting forceps, followed by douching and topical nasal steroids, will often be enough to allow the patient's disease, and their symptoms, to be controlled.

The key point is not to denude the frontal recess of its mucosa since this runs the risk of causing stenosis (Fig. 12.**27**). If there is purulent disease within the frontal sinus causing symptoms, then it is best to open the recess, preserving as much mucosa as possible. This is best done by dissecting the mucosa off the agger nasi air cells with a ball probe and then pulling the probe down on the shell of the cell and removing the fragments of bone—being careful to preserve the mucosa. Any loose fragments of mucosa are best left alone, as to grab them and pull them will tear off the mucosa like tearing loose wallpaper from a wall, leaving bare bone that runs the risk of cicatrization. If there are large fragments of redundant mucosa that cannot be approximated to the walls around the frontal recess, these can be trimmed using a shaver or through-cutting forceps. If there is a bony partition between a supraorbital cell and the frontal recess or a high frontal cell, the partition between them should be removed submucosally, or a hanging partition can be punched with a through-cutting instrument. This will leave an almost intact covering of mucosa (Fig. 12.**28 a**, **b**).

When operating in the frontal recess, a 45° endoscope is invaluable. If you cannot locate the frontal sinus with a probe by the methods described, it is best not to probe with any force or remove tissue in the hope that you will find the recess, as this is how CSF leaks, orbital damage, or frontal stenosis are produced. Because of this complication, always ask yourself why you need to be in the frontal recess. Does the patient have genuine frontal sinusitis, or do they have tension-type headache? Frontal symptoms in nasal polyposis are uncommon and it is equally unusual for chronic frontal symptoms to be due to genuine rhinosinusitis.

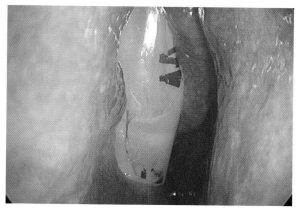
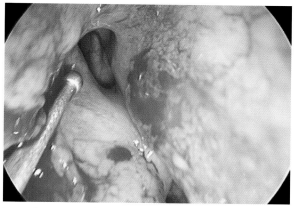

Fig. 12.**28**    **a** Granulation tissue surrounds a stent in the frontal recess and this may stenose when the tube is removed. **b** Open- ing and preserving the mucosa of the frontal recess is less likely to result in stenosis.

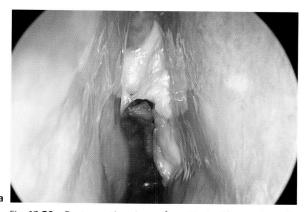
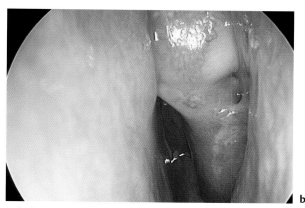

Fig. 12.**29**    Postoperative views of a patient with ongoing infection **a** before and **b** after douching along with antibiotic ointment.

## Crusting

Crusts result from mucosal damage. If there is full-thickness mucosal damage, the mucus produced stagnates because there are no functioning cilia to clear it and it may take up to a year for the cilia to start to function synchronously again. Mucosal damage should be minimized and a full-thickness defect should be avoided at all cost.

## Infection

Superficial infection of stagnant mucus is common and usually resolves with douching. Occasionally, staphylococci multiply in a sump of mucopus that collects in the maxillary sinus and this is slow to clear with douching alone (Fig. 12.**29 a**, **b**). Topical nasal mupirocin ointment sniffed up liberally after douching six times a day for 3 weeks can make a dramatic difference in these patients.

Infection spreading into the soft tissues is rare. If the patient has increasing pain 1–3 days after surgery associated with periorbital edema, parenteral antibiotics are required and the pain usually starts to settle within 2 days.

## Osteitis

A rare complication is severe pain caused by a local osteitis that is at least in part due to exposure of bone (Fig. 12.**30**). This is like a "dry socket" after a dental extraction. The patient complains of a severe, dull, nagging ache in the area where bare white bone is exposed. It produces a very dull, severe, crippling, nasty ache that brings tears to the patients' eyes. It is very distressing for the patient and worrying for the surgeon. The patient scores the pain as 9–10 out of 10. The pain lasts for 10 days before abating, whatever action is taken. Major analgesics are required and local treat-

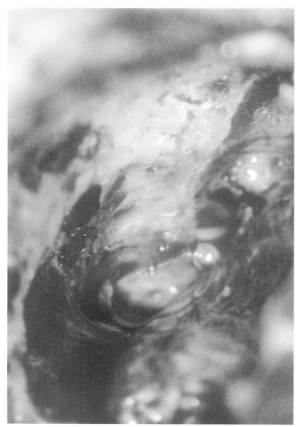

Fig. 12.**30**   Bone exposed at surgery is more liable to result in osteitis as well as crusting.

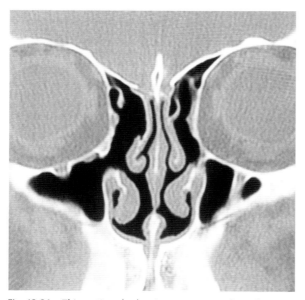

Fig. 12.**31**   This patient had pain postoperatively and no evidence of disease at endoscopy. We would not recommend a CT scan in this situation as there is always some mucosal thickening that is normal after surgery, but one had been done. The patient had midfacial segment pain.

ment appears to provide little help. Patients are particularly at risk of this in surgery for inverted papilloma where mucosal preservation is not practiced.

## Neuropathic Pain

Trauma or surgery causes pain that is mediated by myelinated A delta and unmyelinated C fibers. Prolonged stimulation of these can activate N-methyl-D-aspartate (NMDA) receptors and can cause central sensitization. In a small proportion of patients, an alteration in central processing can then lead to an alteration in pain thresholds, producing hyperalgesia, or even lead to spontaneous firing of neurons and may produce reverberating circuits. Trauma can be an initiating factor by either altering the fibers within the trigeminal nucleus or altering its somatosensory input, thereby altering nociceptive fibers to or within the caudal nucleus of the trigeminal nerve (Fig. 12.**31**). These patients are rarely helped by nonsteroidal anti-inflammatory drugs. They often respond to amitriptyline 10 mg at night, increasing it after 6 weeks by 10 mg every 2 weeks if necessary and up to 100 mg if necessary. Otherwise, carbamazepine, again built up slowly in order to minimize the side effects of nausea and dizziness, or gabapentin may help. All these need to be tried for at least 6 weeks at a dose within the therapeutic range before judging how effective they are, as they need that length of time before the neuronal junctions within the trigeminal nucleus are stabilized. The successful drug should then be given for 6 months before withdrawing it. It appears that this time of stability is needed; otherwise, the pain is more likely to return. The treatment of pain following surgery should primarily be with neuroactive pharmacological agents, which are effective in many patients (West and Jones, 2001; Jones, 2001 a; Khan et al., 2002).

# 13 Postoperative Management

We will have aimed by this point to have explained to the patient enough about their disease process that they will understand that their treatment is a combined effort from both the medical team and themselves to try to improve their symptoms. The patient should *not* feel that their treatment and surgery is something that the surgeon has done *to* them as a passive recipient. As part of an effort to improve their symptoms, they need to know that they also must take some action.

The key issues are:

- The need to irrigate stagnant mucus and altered blood and stop it from collecting on the lining of the paranasal sinuses until ciliary function has returned.
- Local medical treatment is usually needed to reduce inflammation present in the mucosa. (This may be the result of an unresolved preoperative infection, allergy, or nonspecific inflammation resulting from the persistent production of cytokines.)
- The patient should be aware that local debridement of their nose may be needed at about one week after surgery in order to avoid adhesions and to hasten recovery of the mucosa.
- Removal of a nasal dressing is often very unpleasant for the patient because of a dragging sensation or the moderate discomfort that pulling it out causes. The patient needs to be prepared for this. If the patient is aware that it is likely to be uncomfortable, if the staff are sympathetic, and if moderate analgesia is given beforehand, this problem can be reduced.
- Patients should be aware that after sinus surgery it is important to continue to look after the lining of their paranasal sinuses. The lining of the sinuses is like a lawn and often weeding, or even a weed-killer (organic!), is needed.
- Compliance with medical treatment is needed to maximize the benefit that surgery can offer through helping drainage, reducing the surface area, allowing access for topical treatment, and debulking diseased tissue.
- Pain control is vital for the patient's short-term and long-term wellbeing. All trauma, whether it is surgical or through injury, alters a patient's peripheral and central pain perception through neuroplasticity. Thankfully, in most cases the repair processes

mean that after a few days the patient's pain subsides. In a small proportion of patients, the pain persists. It is worth controlling patients' postoperative pain so as to minimize the possibility that their trigeminal nucleus may become "sensitized" and their postoperative pain perpetuated (Sessle, 2000; Romer, 2001; Khan et al., 2002).

## ■ The Postoperative Course

In the first few days, the nasal airway can collect a fibrinous exudate that sets like jelly in a mold. We encourage our patients to sniff and douche in order to avoid this (Fig. 13.1 a, b). The postoperative recovery period can be plagued by the repeated formation of crusts, which result from mucosal damage. Mucosal damage may be superficial, partial thickness, or full thickness (Shaw et al., 2001). Most nasal dressings cause superficial mucosal damage that results in mucus stagnation as there are few remaining functioning cilia that remain to clear any secretions (Shaw et al., 2000). If there is full-thickness mucosal damage it may take up to a year for the cilia start to function synchronously again (Shaw et al., 2001). With superficial mucosal damage it may take 2–3 weeks for the mucosa to recover. Similarly, if there has been a marked infection, (e.g., *Staphylococcus* within the mucosa—in these patients pus can be seen oozing out of the mucosa minutes after it has been cleaned and irrigated), it may take months of douching before the cilia start to work well. Continued douching is needed to clear the stagnant mucus otherwise it will become superinfected and the bacterial toxins produced will further damage the cilia and produce a self-perpetuating cycle of stagnation.

## ■ In the Hospital

### Nasal Packs

The most uncomfortable experience for the patient is that of having a nasal pack removed; accordingly, if packs can be avoided, it is best to do so. If there is a moderate amount of bleeding at the end of surgery, then a pack soaked in 1 : 10000 epinephrine can be

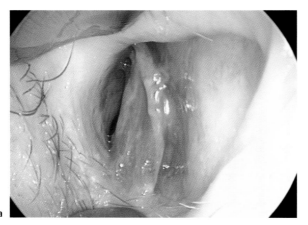
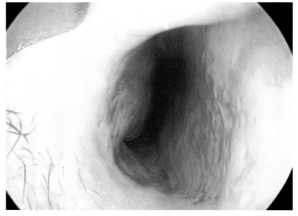

Fig. 13.**1**   **a** Fibrinous exudate that sometimes remains at 7 days and requires removal in order to avoid adhesions forming.

**b** The same patient one month later after suction toilet and douching.

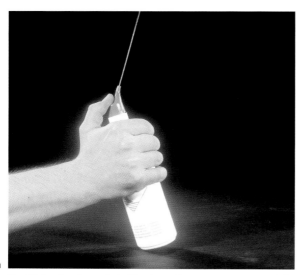
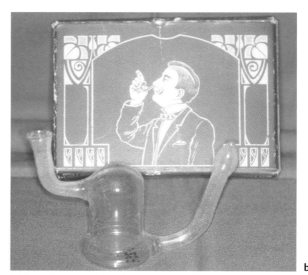

Fig. 13.**2 a**, **b**   Several sterilized nasal sprays are commercially available and many methods exist to help douche the nose.

placed and then removed in the recovery room just before the laryngeal mask is taken out. If there is a little oozing, it will usually stop when the patient is placed 30° head-up after extubation. The bleeding often increases temporarily when the patient wakes up and coughs, as this raises the venous pressure. Any more marked bleeding is best dealt with before the end of surgery; it is usually due to one of the branches of the sphenopalatine artery and is best stopped using suction diathermy.

## Douching

Ideally, patients are supervised in the douching technique before they are discharged. It is well worth spending some time with the patient to make sure

they know how to douche, both to see that they are doing it properly and to help them through the first time they do it (Fig. 13.**2 a**, **b**). This will greatly help compliance. Most patients are advised to douche at least twice daily for 2 weeks and particularly before taking any topical medication (see instruction sheet for the patient on page 285–286). Often patients are advised to douche four times a day in the first week if the mucosa is very unhealthy. In patients with severe polyposis, or those who have had a long history of infective rhinosinusitis, it may take weeks or months for the cilia to recover and protracted douching over this period may be required (Fig. 13.**3**). In patients who have ciliary dysmotility or cystic fibrosis, douching is needed in the long term. Some studies have shown that adding antibiotics such as tobramycin to the douching can help patients with cystic fibrosis.

It is interesting that studies have shown that douching, in its own right, helps relieve the symptoms of rhinosinusitis and the endoscopic appearance of mucosa (Taccariello et al., 1999; Heatley et al., 2001).

## Medical Management

Patients who have evidence of purulent secretions at surgery are advised to take a broad-spectrum antibiotic with anaerobic cover for 2 weeks, unless a culture suggests a different spectrum of sensitivity. Patients are advised that they may have loose stools toward the end of the course of treatment. Women are warned that they may get vaginal thrush toward the end of treatment and require an antifungal pessary. They are also warned that antibiotics can interfere with the absorption of the contraceptive pill.

Patients with allergic rhinitis are advised to continue their topical nasal steroid therapy after douching and to follow their preoperative treatment strategy (e.g., allergen avoidance, antihistamines).

Nasal drops enter the frontal sinus best if they are given with the patient lying flat and with their head cocked back over the edge of the bed. It is often difficult for a patient to gauge how many drops they have instilled in this position and it can be helpful to keep the drops in the fridge, so as to provide more sensation when they are put in. As with all patients with allergic rhinitis, the importance of compliance should be explained. In patients with nasal polyposis, topical nasal steroids are given for 3 months and then reduced if the mucosa looks healthy (Fig. 13.**4**). In patients with allergic aspergillosis or invasive aspergillosis, itraconazole is preferable to amphotericin as it is associated with fewer side effects. Nevertheless, liver function and morning cortisol levels should be monitored monthly.

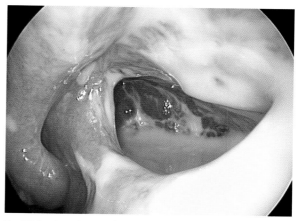

Fig. 13.**3** A patient with a persistent, purulent discharge who needs weeks, if not months, of douching and medical treatment.

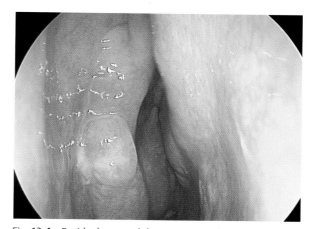

Fig. 13.**4** Residual mucosal disease at 2 weeks. We emphasize the importance of taking regular topical nasal steroids.

## ■ Outpatient Visit at One Week

### Debridement

In the early days of endoscopic sinus surgery, debridement was advocated in the first few days after surgery. This has not been shown to help, and patients dislike it (Fig. 13.**5 a–d**). We do as little suction and instrumentation to patients as possible as they find it very uncomfortable. It is our practice to see patients after one week and not to remove any eschar unless adhesions are starting to form between two adjacent surfaces. Under these circumstances, the nasal airway is anaesthetized with a topical local anesthetic and the adhesions are divided; the patient is encouraged to douche more frequently and enthusiastically. We find

that inserting cotton wool soaked in cophenylcaine for 3 minutes and then gradually advancing it is a good way to anaesthetize the nose and clear the eschar with a minimum amount of bleeding. Sometimes huge casts of altered blood can be removed to the satisfaction of the patient, as their airway is immediately improved. A further appointment in the following week may be indicated if there are concerns that adhesions may reform, so that any fibrinous strands can be cleared. Normally a further appointment at 6–10 weeks is given to check the state of the mucosa.

We reinforce the need for douching and advise that patients should continue this until their airway feels clear and they have not irrigated out any debris for several days. We are happy for patients to blow their nose after approximately 4 days. Patients with ciliary disorders will have been told preoperatively that they will need to douche in the long term.

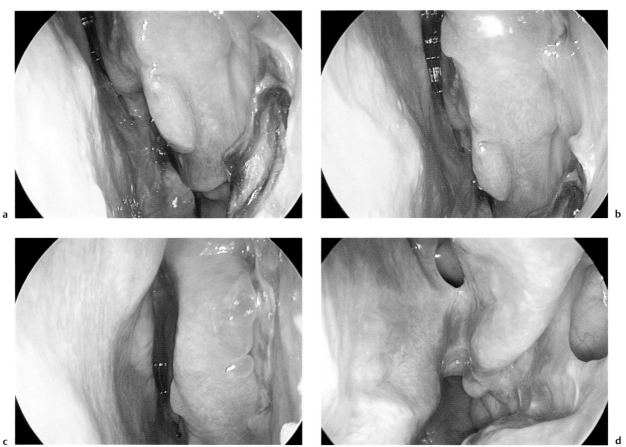

Fig. 13.**5 a–d**  Postoperative appearance of the left nasal airway and olfactory cleft in the same patient at 7 days, 14 days, 3 weeks, and 2 months.

## Medical Management

We are aware that some surgeons give steroids post-operatively to complement their surgery. We like to give them preoperatively rather than postoperatively in order reduce the extent of surgical manipulation and mucosal damage. For the first few days after surgery the patient will be more blocked than if they have postoperative steroids, but after that they will recover better because a smaller surface area of mucosa has been damaged.

## ■ Postoperative Problems

### Crusting

Where mucosa has been removed, it may take months for the cilia to return and any mucus that is produced will dry and collect. In this case, the following measures may help: regular douching, staying well hydrated, facial saunas or steam inhalations (advise patients to leave boiled water to stand for 5 minutes before inhaling as otherwise the steam will be too hot and will cause damage), and humidifying the environment (placing a damp flannel on a radiator in the bedroom or having a hot bowl of water in one corner). In a small proportion of patients, particularly those who have had several procedures or who live in a dry and dusty climate, areas of mucosa can become dry and atrophic. These patients may need to follow all of the above advice for an extended period. Various ointments have been used to stop the lining drying out. It is our experience that a greasy ointment such as petroleum jelly works best. Glucose and glycerin drops disperse too quickly, as do water-miscible agents. Patients who have had radiotherapy or who have ciliary dyskinesia will need to douche indefinitely.

### Bleeding

It is normal for the nose to produce blood-stained mucus for several days after surgery.

## Pain

The postoperative discomfort that patients experience is normally from bony damage; a combination of a nonsteroidal anti-inflammatory drug with either acetaminophen or codeine phosphate helps. The regular combination of these may be needed for a few days. It is good to give the nonsteroidal anti-inflammatory drug as a suppository or parenterally on induction so that it is active before the patient wakes up.

## Nasal Obstruction

In the first few days after surgery, the accumulation of secretions and dried mucus tends to fill any airway that remains after the swollen turbinates have encroached on it. Douching can help considerably, but in a moderate proportion of patients the eschar builds up no matter how much douching the patient does. Local sympathomimetic sprays can provide some help for an hour or two, but it is important to tell patients not to take these for more than a few days in order to avoid habituation developing in the turbinate vasculature. Douching and humidification are the mainstay of treatment until mucosal edema settles. Oral steroids in the postoperative period may help reduce the edema that results from surgery, but the risk–benefit analysis of this strategy remains uncertain. A patient with the stress of surgery, and possibly with a reduced appetite for a day or two, may be more liable to gastric erosions if they take oral steroids. There is insufficient evidence available for the authors to have a clear idea whether the benefits of taking postoperative oral steroids outweigh the risks.

Patients with allergic rhinitis, whether they have hay fever within season or perennial allergic rhinitis, will be helped by taking antihistamines up to and after surgery, in order to reduce the amount of secretions they produce and the amount of mucosal swelling following surgery.

# 14 Selected Procedures

This chapter is divided into specific procedures and surgical approaches to anatomical and pathological conditions. The use of the endoscope in providing improved access and visibility to manage pathology of the paranasal sinuses and their surrounding structures is expanding, as is the instrumentation that is being developed. The most useful procedures are discussed:

- Dacryocystorhinostomy
- Management of the sphenopalatine artery
- Management of the anterior ethmoid artery
- Median frontal sinus drainage procedure
- Orbital decompression
- Optic nerve decompression
- Choanal atresia surgery
- Medial maxillectomy
- Pituitary surgery

## ■ Dacryocystorhinostomy (DCR)

### Terminology and Classification

A DCR is the creation of a fistula from the lacrimal sac into the nose. Its main use is when there is distal outflow obstruction to the nasolacrimal system. It is important that with the history and examination—including syringing and probing—the correct diagnosis is made.

### Indications

One of the most important aspects of this surgery is to first make sure that the primary pathology is due to distal obstruction of the nasolacrimal system (Fig. 14.1 a, b). If there is proximal obstruction, then surgery will fail. Often distal obstruction is mixed with a varying degree of proximal obstruction and this needs to be taken into consideration when counseling the patient about their expectations from surgery. Syringing and probing is the main way to define the site of obstruction.

A dacryocystogram is indicated if there is any mass within the sac. Scintigraphy helps to define a functional problem. A bloody discharge from the punctum is a symptom that needs investigating to exclude malignancy in the sac. The common symptoms are epiphora, recurrent dacryocystitis, or swelling from a mucocele (Fig. 14.2). Epiphora causes not only tearing but an al-

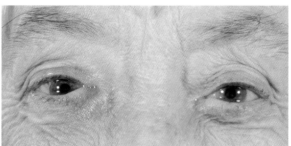
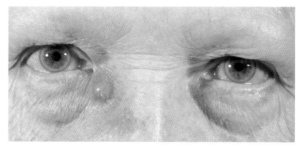

Fig. 14.**1**    **a** Right dacryocystitis. **b** A right lacrimal mucocele.

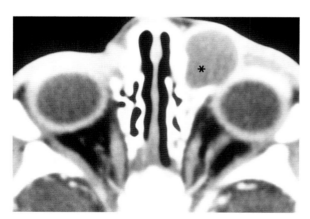

Fig. 14.**2**    An axial CT scan in a neonate with a congenital nasolacrimal mucocele (∗).

teration in refraction that requires the patient to repeatedly blink or wipe their eye. Its prevalence is much more common with aging. It is unusual for intranasal pathology to be responsible, but conditions such as Wegener granulomatosis and sarcoidosis can affect this (Fig. 14.3 a). Nasolacrimal duct obstruction can occur

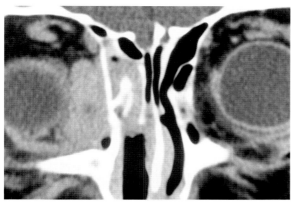

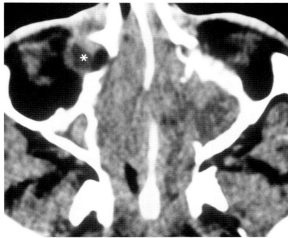

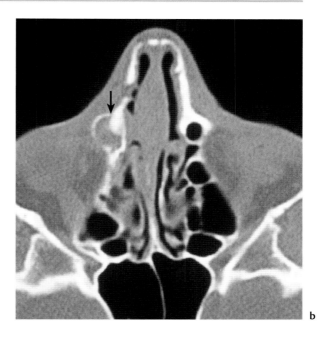

Fig. 14.**3**  **a** Wegener granulomatosis causing nasolacrimal duct obstruction as well as a mass in the orbit. **b** An axial CT scan showing a bony spicule going into the sac following a facial fracture (arrow). **c** An axial CT scan showing stenosis of the nasolacrimal sac (∗) caused by excessive bony resection for nasal polyposis.

following a middle-third facial fracture (Fig. 14.**3 b**). When this is the case, it can pose a surgical problem as the bone in the region of the lacrimal fossa may be thicker owing to callus formation or a concertina effect of the facial bones. Distal nasolacrimal obstruction can also occur secondary to endoscopic sinus surgery if back-biters used to remove the uncinate process are used too far forward (Fig. 14.**3 c**). A contraindication to DCR is the presence of a benign or malignant lesion in the lacrimal system or the surrounding tissues and active Wegener granulomatosis.

## Surgical Anatomy

The lacrimal system comprises the lacrimal gland and its drainage system, which starts with a punctum in each eyelid at right angles to the lid margin. After 1 mm, this continues as the upper and lower canaliculus, which run parallel to the lid margin and then join to form a common canaliculus that drains into the lacrimal sac. Inferiorly, the sac forms the nasolacrimal duct, which drains into the inferior meatus

about 1 cm posterior to the anterior end of the inferior turbinate. In the inferior meatus, a fold of mucosa called the valve of Hasner marks its drainage site, and this can be seen. The lacrimal sac sits in the lacrimal fossa, which is made of very thin bone (Fig. 14.**4 a**, **b**). However, its anterior margin, the anterior lacrimal crest, is made of very dense bone. In about 8 % of patients, an anterior ethmoid air cell, the lacrimal cell, lies medial to the lacrimal fossa. This has to be traversed before a rhinostomy can be created.

## Assessment

First, topical anesthetic drops such as amethocaine are placed in the eye. The upper and lower puncta are dilated. When instrumenting the canaliculi and the lacrimal system, it is important to do so gently in order to avoid inducing adhesions, stenosis, or a false passage. The puncta are best found by placing some tension on the lids laterally to stabilize them. The puncta are initially dilated with the instrument perpendicular to the lid margin, rotating it for the first 1 mm with the

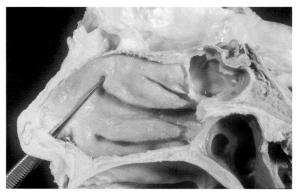

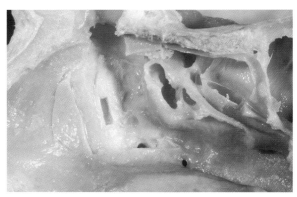

a

b

Fig. 14.**4**   **a** The right lateral nasal wall showing the position of the fundus of the lacrimal sac. **b** The relationship of the lacrimal sac to the most anterior ethmoid cells and the infundibulum of the frontal sinus.

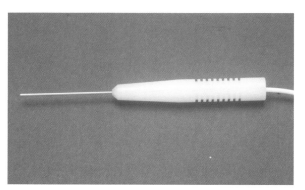

Fig. 14.**5**   A rigid light-pipe.

lid margin taut, before turning it medially parallel to the lid. Following dilation of the puncta, a "0" Bowman probe is placed through the dilated punctum and angled medially. As the probe enters the common canaliculus, slight resistance may be felt—the "soft stop"—and then as it touches the medial wall of the sac there is a hard stop. At this point the probe is angled vertically down to feel whether there is any sac pathology or distal obstruction. Rigid 0.7 mm dacryocystocopes, which are currently largely experimental, have allowed inspection of the fine obstructing membranes that can be found at the medial aspect of the upper and lower canaliculi (Jones, 1998 a). These proximal membranes are the main cause of proximal obstruction, and a DCR is not indicated if this is the site of the obstruction.

Pressing on the sac can squeeze tears out of Hasner's valve: this will help localize it although it is not routinely examined. Distal obstruction is diagnosed by probing and then syringing to see whether the fluid can initially be passed through the canaliculi into the nose. If it refluxes through the other punctum, this indicates that there is distal obstruction. If there is reflux through the same punctum, then there is

canalicular or common canalicular stenosis, and this can be confirmed by gentle probing. The most common site of distal obstruction is where the sac becomes the duct. As mentioned, a DCR is primarily done for distal obstruction, but in many patients there is also some degree of proximal obstruction. If that is the case, gentle probing and dilation along with a DCR and insertion of stents can be offered. The results, however, are not as good as if there is pure distal obstruction. Some surgeons will offer a DCR to patients with a functional blockage where there is free flow on syringing but on scintigraphy the pump system does not work. This is an area of contention, but the results rely on gravity to drain the tears, and this is often insufficient as they are not sucked into the sac and the pump system is the primary problem. Ninety percent of tears are drained via the inferior canaliculus and if there is pathology at this site a Lester–Jones tube that bypasses the whole system is often required.

## Surgical Technique

Endonasal DCR can be done under local or general anesthesia. It is possible to open the lacrimal sac endonasally with either conventional instruments or a laser. The laser procedure has the advantage that it can be done more readily as a day-stay procedure as there is a minimal amount of bleeding. The disadvantages of the laser are its expense, the precautions that need to be taken, and the fact that the results are not as good as with conventional instruments.

One technique that will help the operator to find the site of the lacrimal sac and the lacrimal bone is to insert a rigid light-pipe through the upper punctum and canaliculus and angle it down into the sac (Fig. 14.5). The site of the lacrimal fossa can then readily be identified endonasally by seeing the discrete pinpoint of light, and this will help the operator define where the bone is thinnest in the lacrimal fossa

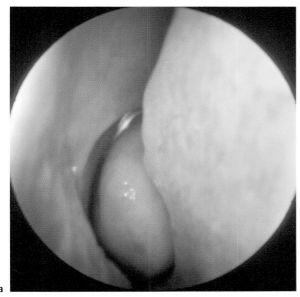
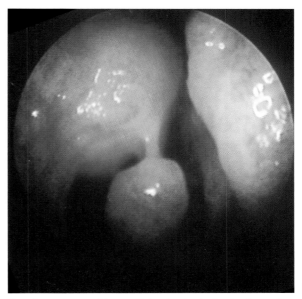

a

b

Fig. 14.**6**   **a** Light transmitted from a light-pipe in the lacrimal sac. **b** Light transmitted from a light-pipe in the lacrimal sac when there is a large agger nasi cell present.

(Fig. 14.6 a, b). In approximately 8% of patients there is an agger nasi cell in this area and the light will be more diffuse. Very occasionally, the light is difficult to see and then the light on the endoscope can be turned off to help define where the bone is thinnest. If the light is diffuse and there is an agger nasi air cell, it will be necessary to open this up and go through it before going through the lateral wall and the lacrimal bone into the sac. It is best not to open the sac very high up without also opening it inferiorly, as a sump can form that collects mucus and can predispose to recurrent infection. If the procedure is done under local anesthesia, amethocaine drops are placed in the eye, followed by a nasal pack (1 cm ribbon gauze or a patte soaked in cophenylcaine or 6% cocaine) and an injection of 1% lignocaine injected through the surface of the conjunctiva around the sac. The latter may look alarming to the novice, but the conjunctiva is well anaesthetized with topical anesthetic drops. Discomfort can be minimized by injecting slowly to avoid pressure and by warming the local anesthetic to near body temperature. Local anesthetic is injected around and not into the lacrimal sac. After 2 minutes, a subcaruncular injection will help anaesthetize the bone around the lacrimal fossa. This is followed up 5 minutes later with an injection of 1% lignocaine and 1:200000 epinephrine intranasally where the rhinostomy is to be made.

## Endoscopic Marsupialization of the Sac with Conventional Instruments

The best way to expose the lacrimal sac with conventional instruments endoscopically is to incise the mucosa on the lacrimal crest, producing a posteriorly based flap (Fig. 14.7 a, b). The anterior lacrimal crest is thick white bone, and the surgeon may recognize it as being the hard bone that they first approached with a sickle knife when they tried to perform a conventional uncinectomy and found that they could not incise this area (Fig. 14.8 a–c).

When a mucosal flap has been reflected, the white hard bone of the anterior lacrimal crest is readily seen and palpated. It is possible to remove this using a Kerrison or sphenoid punch, which can remove the greater part of it in three or four bites. In order to obtain a large ostium, the upper part of the lacrimal crest also needs to be removed. In a child this can be removed with a sphenoid punch, but in an adult a coarse diamond burr is needed to remove it as it is very thick (Fig. 14.9 a, b). This exposes the lacrimal sac more widely, to the extent that the common canaliculus can often be seen. Just posterior to the hard lacrimal crest lies the uncinate process, and just lateral to that the thin bone that forms the medial aspect of the lacrimal fossa. The very thin bone over the lacrimal sac can easily be removed as it is paper thin. The sac has a magenta hue, and it can be divided vertically with either a sickle knife or a 45° beaver scalpel (Fig. 14.10 a, b).

Placing a probe within the sac will help tense it medially and make incision into it easier (Fig. 14.11). Mi-

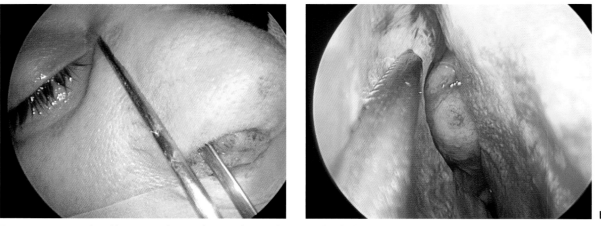

a

b

Fig. 14.**7** **a** External and **b** intranasal views showing forceps being used to help locate the lacrimal sac. This can help the novice to confirm the right area to expose.

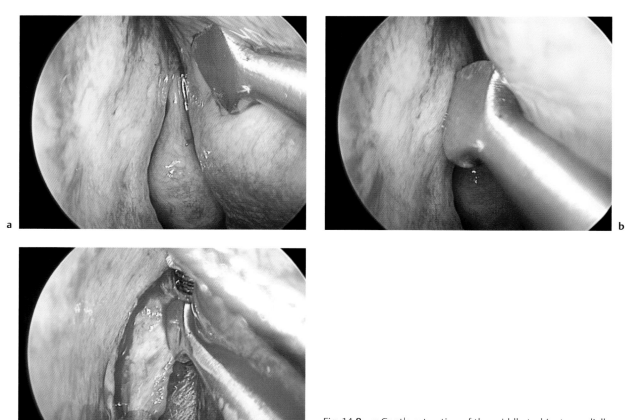

a

b

c

Fig. 14.**8** **a** Gentle retraction of the middle turbinate medially often helps access. **b** Incising the mucosa over the anterior lacrimal crest. **c** Elevating a flap to expose the white bone of the anterior lacrimal crest.

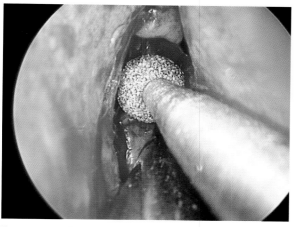

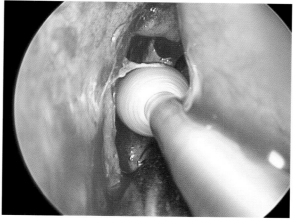

a

b

Fig. 14.**9**  **a** Palpating the anterior lacrimal crest with a coarse diamond burr. **b** Drilling the anterior lacrimal crest exposes the magenta-colored sac.

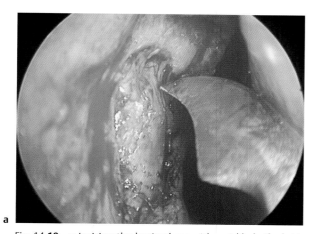

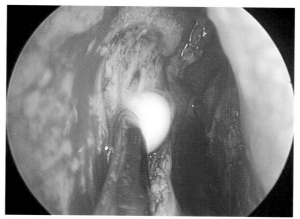

a

b

Fig. 14.**10**  **a** Incising the lacrimal sac with a sickle knife. **b** Mucopus being released from an infected lacrimal sac.

croscissors can be used inferiorly and superiorly to create anterior and posterior flaps from the lacrimal sac. Alternatively, a punch can be used to enlarge the rhinostomy (Fig. 14.**12 a**, **b**). These flaps of sac mucosa can then be placed in continuity with the mucosa of the nasal wall in order to avoid cicatrization and help maintain a patent rhinostomy (Yung and Harman-Lea, 1998). Stents are placed in position for 6–8 weeks (Fig. 14.**13**).  **DVD** 18

## Laser DCR

The laser is first used to ablate mucosa around the area where the light-pipe is most readily seen. The bone is then ablated over an area of 0.5–0.8 cm (Fig. 14.**14**). It is important to be guided by the light in the sac and not to follow the reflection of the aiming beam, which could potentially lead to the creation of a false passage.

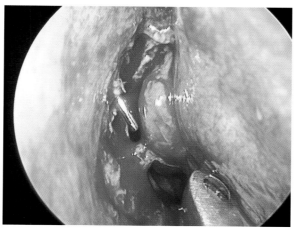

Fig. 14.**11**   A lacrimal probe is placed within the sac; this will help "tent" it medially to help incise the length of the exposed sac.

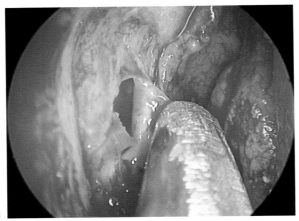

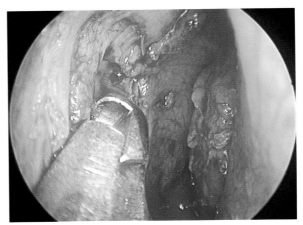

a

b

Fig. 14.**12**    **a** Suction reveals the opening in the sac. **b** A Hajek punch enlarges the rhinostomy and flaps are raised using mi-

croscissors. It helps to improve patency rates if part of the medial wall of the sac is removed.

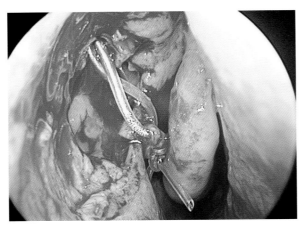

Fig. 14.**13**    Stents after a right dacryocystorhinostomy.

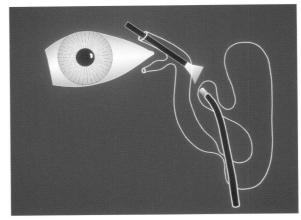

Fig. 14.**14**    A line diagram representing a right laser dacryocystorhinostomy.

Contact with the bone maximizes ablation as delivery of laser energy through a fiber does not deliver parallel light and its energy dissipates the further the fiber is from the tissue. Fumes can be sucked out with a sucker placed in the nose, or there are delivery devices that have a suction channel alongside the port that delivers the laser fiber. If bony ablation is suboptimal, it can leave a residue of charcoal. The laser will not be able to ablate charcoal, and charcoal will dissipate energy, causing damage to the surrounding tissue. If charcoal collects, it is best to curette it away; this is easily done with a chalazion curette or House curette.

Once the sac is exposed, the light-pipe should be withdrawn from the sac so that the laser does not puncture a hole in its metal sleeve, which may then become rough and can potentially tear the common canaliculus when it is withdrawn. A lacrimal probe is placed to help tent the sac medially and this will help

open it up with the laser. The sac is opened, being sure not to cause damage to its lateral wall. Once the sac has been opened to form a rhinostomy of 0.5–0.8 cm, silastic stents can be placed in the lower and upper canaliculi and retrieved in the nose before they are passed through a Watskie sleeve (Fig. 14.**15**). A knot is tied in the stents to stop the sleeve slipping off. The loop should not be so tight that the sleeve is pressing on the rhinostomy as this produces more granulations and the stent may "cheese-wire" through the canaliculi. Cheese-wiring destroys the pump system and should be avoided at all costs.

Silastic stents are supplied with metal introducers, and these can be bent and passed through the canaliculi. An alternative technique is to pass the stents through an introductory cannula; we believe that this causes less mucosal damage to the canaliculi and common canaliculus. The cut 3 cm end of the sleeve of an intravenous cannula can be passed through each canaliculus in turn over a 1/0 probe. The probe is then removed and the stent is passed through the abbocath and retrieved in the nose. When this is repeated through the other canaliculus, both the stent and the cannula are retrieved. The cannula is then removed before a silastic sleeve is fed over the stents and a knot is made to help secure the loop of tubing (Barki et al., 1998).

**Advantages of laser DCR:**
1. There is no external scar.
2. It can be done as an outpatient procedure.
3. It can be done in those who are not fit for general anaesthetic, e.g., with severe cardiovascular disease or on warfarin.
4. There is minimal bleeding and primary and secondary hemorrhage rates are low.
5. Short operating time.

**Disadvantages of laser DCR:**
1. Laser precautions are required.
2. The laser equipment is expensive.
3. There is a higher failure rate. (It is not easy to compare the results of external DCR or conventional endoscopic DCR with laser endonasal DCRs because the selection criteria used in the reported series differ, e.g., in the incidence of co-existing proximal block and the criteria for success. Many studies define "success" as the patient not returning: this is not satisfactory. Review of the evidence that is available suggests that laser DCR may induce more scarring and have a 10% lower success rate at approximately 12 months, so the relative advantages and disadvantages of this technique need to be presented to the patient to help them decide which operation to have.)

## Principles of Surgical Technique in DCR

Many different ways of creating a rhinostomy have been described, but the main objectives are:
1. To create a rhinostomy from the sac through the lateral nasal wall.
2. To create a rhinostomy that is about 5 mm wide (Figure 14.**16a**, **b**).
3. To minimize trauma to the lacrimal system and sac.
4. To minimize damage to the mucosa around the rhinostomy site.
5. To avoid a high rhinostomy, as this can produce a sump syndrome.
6. To avoid collateral mucosal damage in the nose, to minimize the formation of adhesions.

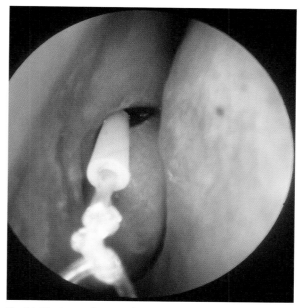

Fig. 14.**15**   Looped stents that pass through each cannaliculus and are fed over a Watskie sleeve before being tied.

## Alternative Surgical Techniques

1. The mucosa can be ablated with diathermy or laser, removed using power tools, or incised and reflected.
2. The bone can be ablated with a holmium laser, a Starpulse KTP laser, a chisel, forceps, or a drill. An external DCR can be done making a low Howarth incision. The sac is defined and retracted, with a rhinostomy being created into the nose. Flaps are then made from the sac, but these are difficult to suture to nasal mucosa because the sac itself gets in the way. The success rates reported using this technique are over 90% in series from specialist centers in patients with pure distal obstruction. It may not be possible to extrapolate from these to most individuals, as in practice many patients have some minor degree of common canalicular pathology.

## Stents

Some surgeons do not insert a stent, while others leave a stent in for several months. In our hands, the success rate of a laser DCR has been worse if we have removed the stents within 8 weeks. If we leave the stents in for longer than 3 months, the incidence of granulations around the tube is increased. In an endoscopic DCR using conventional instruments, the rhinostomy requires no stents if it is wide open.

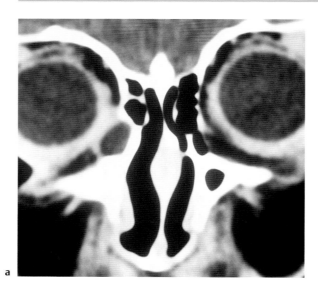

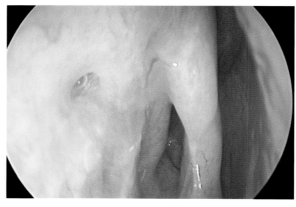

Fig. 14.**16**   **a** Preoperative coronal CT scan of a right lacrimal mucocele. **b** Postoperative right rhinostomy site.

### Useful Instruments

- Crocodile forceps to retrieve the end of the stents before tying them over a sleeve.
- Lacrimal probes of all sizes and a punctal dilator.
- A vitreoretinal light-pipe.
- A chalazion or House curette to remove charcoal if bony ablation has been suboptimal.
- A Kerrison antrum punch to remove the bone of the anterior lacrimal crest.
- A long-shanked drill with a rough diamond burr to remove the upper part of the lacrimal crest.
- A sickle or beaver knife to incise the sac.
- Bellucci microscissors to create flaps once the sac has been opened.

### Revision DCR

This is ideal for an endonasal laser approach as the bone should have been removed and only the thin membrane of mucosa that has formed at the rhinostomy site needs to be removed. This can easily be done under local anesthesia. However, we have frequently found that in revision DCRs not enough bone had been removed at the first operation or that an agger nasi air cell had been entered and not the nasal airway.

### Common Canalicular Pathology

It is now possible to view common canalicular pathology with a rigid fiberoptic 0.7 mm endoscope. Trials attempting to laser common canalicular pathology are under way but have yet to be of proven benefit. If the proximal pathology is severe, a Lester–Jones tube can be placed after a fistula is created from the medial inferior sulcus of the lid into the lateral wall of the nose. This can be done by placing a needle through the deepest medial part of the sulcus of the lower lid and passing it into the nose. It is then possible to laser around the needle and sleeve to create a fistula up to the sulcus in the lower lid. It is vital to protect the eye from the laser; the flange of the sleeve helps this, but a metal guard must be placed over the sclera. After an incision is made in the conjunctiva next to where the needle was placed, a ceramic Jones tube is then passed through the fistulous tract and sutured in place with a 7/0 Vicryl looped around it three times and sutured through the lower lid. The results of this technique await medium-term evaluation.

## ■ Management of the Sphenopalatine Artery

### Terminology and Classification

The sphenopalatine artery has several branches and in many texts the descriptions of its ligation only include its anterior branch. It is important to differentiate between ligation of the anterior branch of the sphenopalatine artery and ligation of all its branches. They all come out through the sphenopalatine foramen (Fig. 14.**17** a–c).

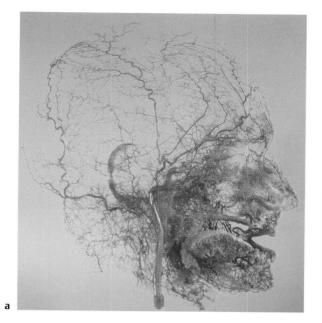

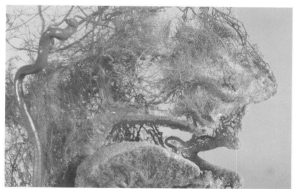

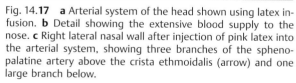

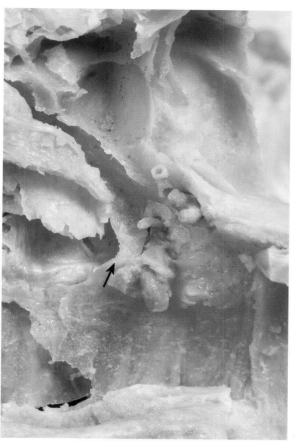

Fig. 14.**17**   **a** Arterial system of the head shown using latex in-fusion. **b** Detail showing the extensive blood supply to the nose. **c** Right lateral nasal wall after injection of pink latex into the arterial system, showing three branches of the spheno-palatine artery above the crista ethmoidalis (arrow) and one large branch below.

## Indications

If it is not possible to stop a nosebleed by outpatient inspection and cautery (ideally using endoscopy and suction bipolar diathermy forceps) or packing, then sphenopalatine artery ligation should be considered. Another indication is a posterior bleed from the lateral nasal wall. Conventionally, if there is a posterior bleed in the presence of a septal deviation, a submucous re-section and packing was done. However, it is better to ligate the sphenopalatine artery at the same time as doing septal surgery as this will not only minimize the need for nasal packing but also deal with the likely vessel near the site from which the bleeding is coming

(Rudert and Maune, 1997). The vast majority of nose-bleeds that do not come from the anterior part of the septum originate from one of the branches of the sphenopalatine artery. One of the few exceptions is when there is profuse bleeding after a nasoethmoid fracture, as this is likely to come from the anterior eth-moid artery.

## Anatomy

The sphenopalatine artery has three or four branches coming out of its foramen that lie at least 0.5 cm deep to the mucosa on the lateral nasal wall. The vessels split up as soon as they leave the foramen. The fora-

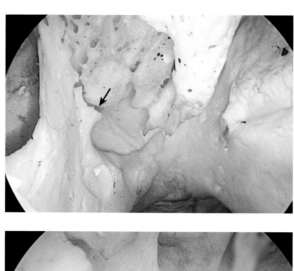

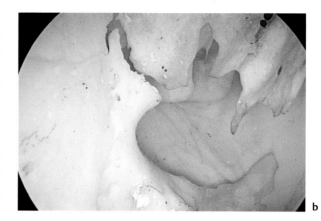

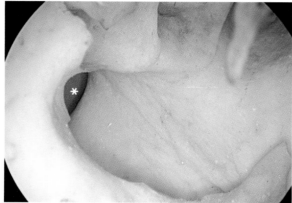

Fig. 14.**18**  **a** Right endoscopic view in a skull showing the crista ethmoidalis (arrow). **b**, **c** Closer views showing the sphenopalatine foramen ( * ) lying more laterally.

men becomes a slit whose anterior margin is a lateral "knuckle" of bone called the crista ethmoidalis (Wareing and Padgham, 1998). The crista ethmoidalis comes off the lateral nasal wall near the root or posterior–inferior base of the middle turbinate (Fig. 14.**18** a–c). The anterior branch of the sphenopalatine artery comes around the crista and can be found as it runs forward in the lateral nasal wall over the posterior fontanelle.

### Surgical Technique

A vertical incision is made through the mucosa over the posterior fontanelle, or a middle meatal antrostomy is enlarged posteriorly to come near the posterior wall of the maxillary sinus. Then the mucosa is elevated to the crista ethmoidalis (Fig. 14.**19** a–h). The crista needs to be curetted away or drilled with a coarse diamond burr to expose the other branches. These branches vary in number and course. They are often convoluted. It helps to make a good wide plane between the mucosoperiosteum and the lateral wall and not to "tunnel" too deeply as this will reduce visibility and access (Simmen and Heinz, 1998). Medial

traction on the mucosoperiosteum is needed to place the vessels under tension and help define them.

Some surgeons place clips, but we prefer diathermy to cauterize these vessels and then cut them. There are often one or two branches passing superiorly and another that goes backward around the posterior wall of the nasopharynx just above the posterior choana to supply the septum. This posterior branch may be cut if a large sphenoidotomy is done (Fig. 14.**20** a, b). If the Ligaclips come off, and this can happen as you are

Fig. 14.**19**  **a** Right endoscopic view in a cadaver, incising the ▷ mucosa over the posterior fontanelle. **b** Elevating the mucosa reveals a branch of the sphenopalatine artery. **c** Bipolar diathermy. **d** Unipolar suction diathermy to the anterior branch of the sphenopalatine artery. **e** Cutting the anterior branch of the sphenopalatine artery with microscissors. Note the crista ethmoidalis in front of the artery. **f** Drilling of the crista ethmoidalis to expose the foramen of the sphenopalatine artery. **g** The crista ethmoidalis has been removed to reveal several branches of the artery. **h** Note two cut branches of the sphenopalatine artery and an intact higher septal branch that will run on the anterior wall of the sphenoid.

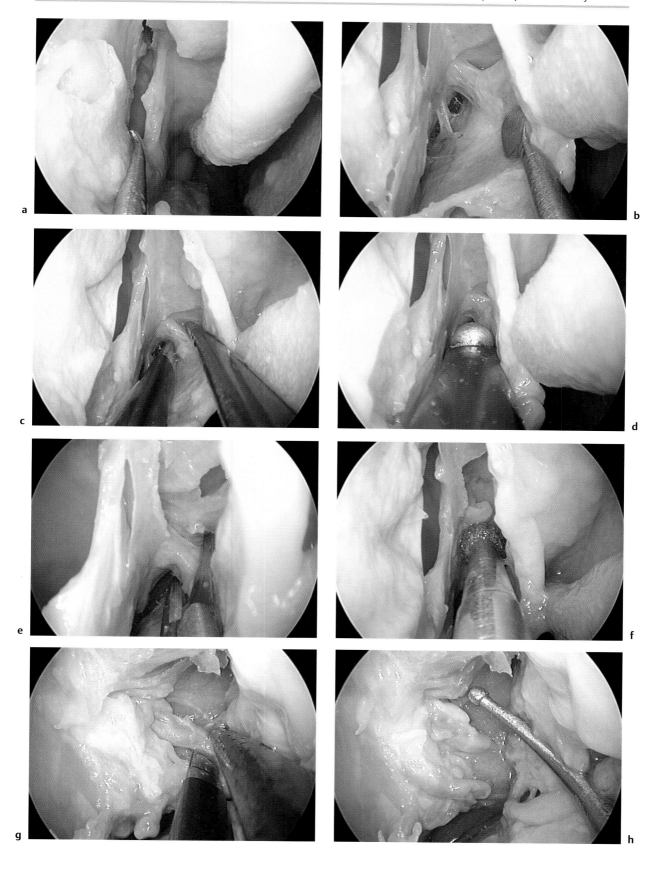

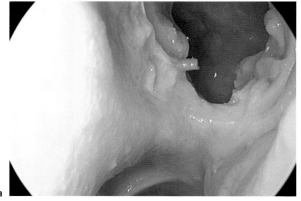

a

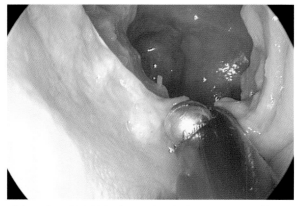

b

Fig. 14.**20    a** A large sphenoidotomy has cut the septal branch of the sphenopalatine artery as it runs across the anterior wall of the sphenoid. **b** Unipolar suction diathermy is most effective when there is a lot of bleeding.

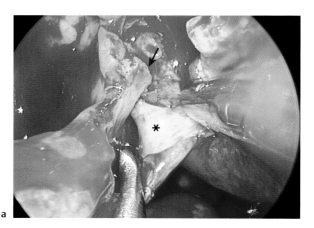

a

b

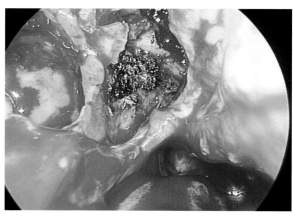

c

Fig. 14.**21    a** A peroperative view of the crista ethmoidalis (arrow) and the anterior branch of the sphenopalatine artery (∗). **b** The stump of three cut branches of the sphenopalatine artery (1, 2, 3). **c** Unipolar suction diathermy was used to cauterize the vessels.

looking for the other branches, then diathermy should be used (Fig. 14.**21 a–c**). In severe posterior epistaxis, always check the septal branch of the sphenopalatine artery that is posterior to its other branches (Fig. 14.**22 a, b**). **DVD** 12, 13

## Alternative Surgical Techniques

Before the introduction of the endoscope, packing with an anterior and/or posterior balloon or pack, sometimes in conjunction with a submucous resection, was often done. Failing that, maxillary artery ligation has also been advocated, via a Caldwell–Luc ap-

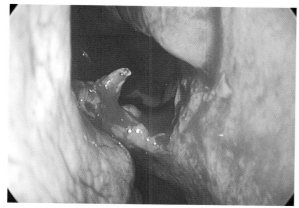

a

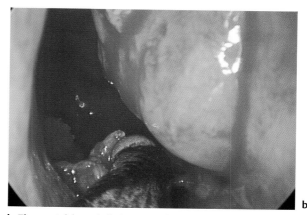

b

Fig. 14.**22** **a** Peroperative view of a bleeding septal branch of the sphenopalatine artery exposed during a sphenoidotomy.

**b** The septal branch being coagulated with unipolar suction diathermy.

proach. Other alternatives include embolization. Ligation of the external carotid artery is now avoided wherever possible because it limits access for interventional radiology should this be required at a later date and because of the rich cross-circulation from the other side. Ligating the artery that is at a distance from the responsible bleeding point is less effective than ligating the artery near where it is bleeding. The aim should be to minimize risk and morbidity and to deal with the bleeding as near to its site as possible. This normally means doing a sphenopalatine artery ligation.

## Useful Instruments

- A coarse diamond drill with a long-shank handpiece helps to remove the crista ethmoidalis without traumatizing the mucosa or vessels.
- An alternative is a straight curette.
- Suction diathermy forceps or unipolar suction device.
- A Ligaclip applicator.

## ■ Management of the Anterior Ethmoid Artery

### Terminology and Classification

The anterior ethmoid artery can be ligated, clipped, or diathermied for epistaxis. This might be necessary if, as a complication of surgery, it is partially torn.

If the artery has been divided and has retracted into the posterior compartment of the eye, this is a different situation as it can raise the intraorbital pressure and impair vision. Under these circumstances, no attempt should be made to find and tie the artery. This will cause more damage as the anterior ethmoid artery has retracted within the substance of the orbit and be-

tween septations of fibrous tissue that support the fat within the orbit. If the artery has retracted into the orbit, the posterior compartment usually needs to be decompressed (see section on Peroperative Complications, p. 171).

### Indications

The anterior ethmoid artery is often partially dehiscent as it runs in the roof of the ethmoid sinuses, and if a hole is made in it then cautery can be applied or a clip can be placed (Woolford and Jones, 2000). If profuse epistaxis follows a nasoethmoid fracture, bleeding often originates from the anterior ethmoid artery. The anterior ethmoid artery is rarely the cause of epistaxis under other circumstances and it is best to deal with the sphenopalatine artery first.

### Surgical Anatomy

The anterior ethmoid artery is a branch of the ophthalmic artery and therefore it originates within the orbit before traveling medially through the bone of the anterior skull base—the fovea ethmoidalis (the part of the frontal bone that forms the roof of the ethmoid sinuses). It is normally enclosed to a large extent within a bony canal, but often part of this is very thin or dehiscent. It can often be located just behind the supraorbital cell that is an extension of the suprabullar recess (Fig. 14.**23 a**, **b**). If the roof of the ethmoid bulla is attached to the skull base, the artery is found as the next undulation in its roof behind the attachment of the anterior wall of the bulla. Occasionally it can be accessed directly, medial to the medial wall of the bulla, between it and the middle turbinate high in the skull base. It may travel in a coronal plane, but often it is oblique, traveling more anteriorly as it goes medially. It gives off branches to the septum, the lateral nasal wall, and intracranially. How exposed it is depends in part on

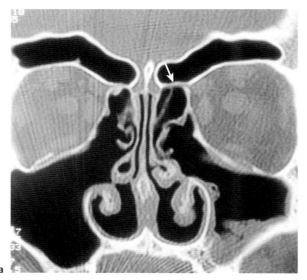

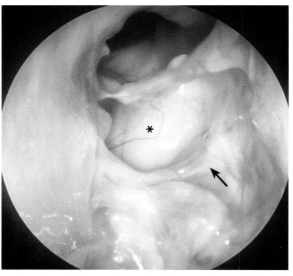

Fig. 14.**23**   **a** Coronal CT scan showing a free anterior ethmoid artery (arrow) in a well-pneumatized sinus system. **b** An endo- scopic view of the anterior ethmoid artery (arrow) behind a supraorbital cell (∗).

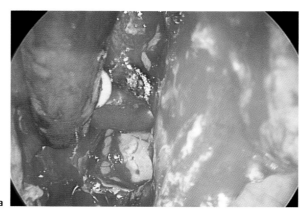

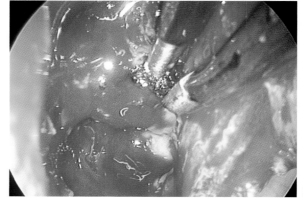

Fig. 14.**24**   **a** Unipolar suction diathermy being used to arrest hemorrhage. **b** Bipolar suction diathermy on a bleeding anterior ethmoid artery.

the degree of pneumatization of the sinuses and how "deep" the cribriform plate "dips" into the nasal airway. If there is little pneumatization of the paranasal sinuses and the cribriform plate is level with the fovea ethmoidalis, it is more likely to travel in a small bony undulation or be hidden within the bone. If there is considerable pneumatization with a large supraorbital cell, it is more likely to be exposed and vulnerable.

In an external frontoethmoidectomy, the anterior ethmoid artery lies approximately 2.4 cm posterior from the anterior lacrimal crest next to the frontoethmoid suture line.

## Surgical Technique

Careful scrutiny of the CT scans is required preoperatively to familiarize yourself with the anatomy of the skull base and the possible position of the artery (Fig. 14.**23 a**). The artery is usually seen as a funnel-like appearance passing medially through the upper-medial wall of the orbit (Fig. 14.**23 b**). The uncinate process is removed using 45° through-cutting forceps or a punch to nibble it away to its superior attachment. If there are small or no significant agger nasi air cells, then a 45° scope can be used to inspect the area medial to the ethmoid bulla and lateral to the middle turbinate. It is sometimes possible to see the anterior ethmoid artery in this area. If it is not visible there, then the ethmoid bulla can be removed to reveal the suprabullar recess that extends up into a supraorbital cell: the artery normally lies in the next undulation behind this. Once again the 45° scope is invaluable in visualizing this area.

The unipolar suction diathermy device is ideally shaped to cauterize the artery (Fig. 14.**24 a**, **b**). If a clip is used, it should be applied gently because this is one of the thinner areas of the skull base and it is possible to inadvertently transect the ethmoid artery or go into the skull base. Normally, no packing is required.

### Alternative Surgical Techniques

The external approach is best done using a "seagull-shaped" incision to reduce the likelihood of the scar webbing. Having found and diathermied the angular vein and dissecting down on to the periosteum, the anterior lacrimal crest should be found and then a subperiosteal dissection done posteriorly, staying on the bone of the medial part of the orbit. This will stop orbital fat prolapsing and getting in the way, so it is important to stay in the right plane. It is often surprising to those who are not familiar with the procedure how far back the anterior ethmoid artery is. It can be seen approximately 2.4 cm from the anterior lacrimal crest as what looks like a firm attachment of the orbital periosteum, but in fact it is simply where the anterior ethmoidal artery is going through the periosteum, tenting it as it goes into the anterior ethmoid foramen. The periosteum is mobilized to expose enough of the artery to allow it to be clipped or diathermied.

### Useful Instruments

- The 45° endoscope is ideal to help visualize the skull base and anterior ethmoid artery.
- Bipolar suction diathermy forceps, unipolar suction device.
- Ligaclip applicator and clips.

## ■ Median Frontal Sinus Drainage Procedure

### Terminology and Classification

This procedure consists of opening the frontal recesses to create a central drainage channel by removing the top of the septum, the frontal intersinus septum, and the anterior beak of the frontal bone (Draf et al., 1995) (Fig. 14.**25 a–e**).  *DVD*  9, 10

### Indications

1  Stenosis of the frontal recess secondary to previous surgery.
2  Collapse of the lateral wall of the frontal recess. This is usually secondary to an external frontoethmoidectomy, but it can occur because a mucocele or other pathology has eroded bone.
3  Specific midline tumors (see Chapter 15, Skull Base Surgery).

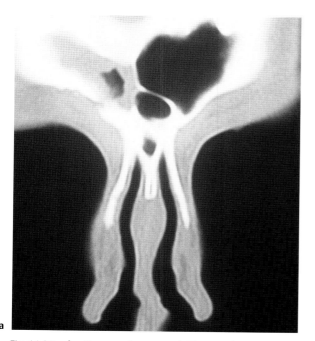

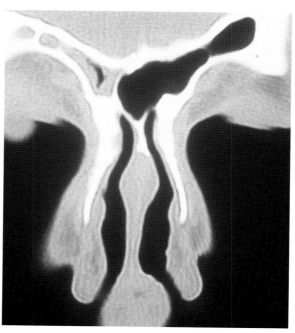

a
b

Fig. 14.**25 a**, **b**   Preoperative coronal CT scans showing postsurgical frontonasal stenosis right side.    Fig. 14.**25 c–e**  ▷

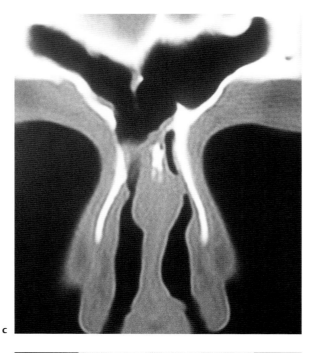

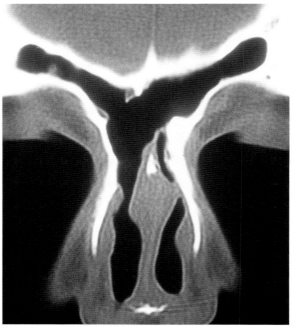

c

d

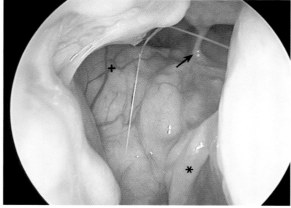

e

Fig. 14.**25 c–e**   A postoperative median drainage channel has been made; (∗) stump of the middle turbinate; (+) right frontal sinus and intersinus septal window to the left side (arrow).

## Contraindications

1   If there has been a previous external approach, then a loss of bony support and scar tissue can cause a lateral loculation and these may not be accessible by a median drainage procedure.
2   Beware that frontal pain, particularly after the patient has had surgery, is often attributed to sinusitis. All too often it is due to tension-type headache or neuropathic pain following previous surgery.

## Surgical Anatomy

The nasal process of the frontal bone is thick and forms a "beak" that restricts both the anterior access to and drainage of the frontal sinus (Fig. 14.**26 a**, **b**). The frontal intersinus septum varies greatly in its position. The extent and direction of pneumatization vary more than in any other area of the paranasal sinuses. The frontal sinus often has more than one drainage channel. Pneumatized cells can travel up into the frontal bone in all directions; anteriorly these form high agger

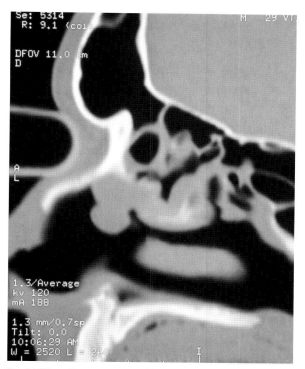

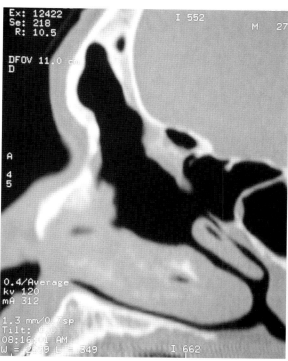

Fig. 14.**26**  **a** Preoperative and **b** postoperative sagittal CT scans show the thick nasal beak of the anterior wall that has been removed to create a large median drainage channel.

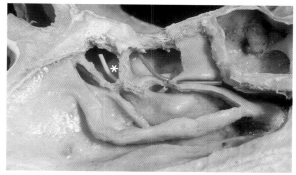

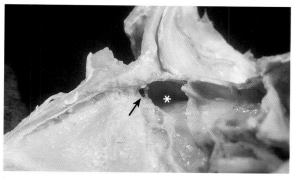

Fig. 14.**27**  **a** View of the right lateral nasal wall: red in the frontal sinus; yellow in the suprabullar recess (∗) and below into the retrobullar recess; and orange in a posterior ethmoid cell.

**b** Shows how the supraorbital cell (∗), an extension of the suprabullar recess, can be mistaken for the frontal sinus. Access to the frontal sinus can be seen as a small anterior dark hole (arrow).

nasi air cells, otherwise known as bulla frontalis, whereas if they extend above the septum they are called intersinus septal cells, and behind the frontal recess they form supraorbital cells (Fig. 14.**27 a**, **b**).

The main concern in this procedure is the cribriform plate that is positioned behind the coronal plane that connects the frontal recesses. Laterally lie the lamina papyracea of the ethmoid bone, the anterior ethmoid air cells, and part of the orbital component of the frontal bone. Not infrequently the me-

dian drainage procedure is indicated because the lateral support has been removed in an external procedure, allowing collapse of the orbital contents medially (Fig. 14.**28**). The anterior boundary of the frontal recess is made of very thick bone, but this is a safe area to operate in as it is away from both the cribriform plate and the anterior ethmoid artery (Simmen, 1997).

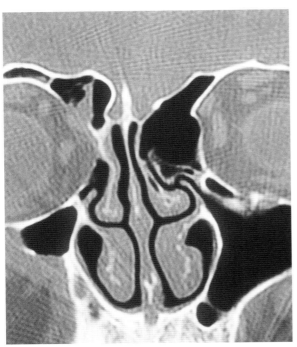

Fig. 14.**28**   Right frontal stenosis following a previous external ethmoidectomy.

## Surgical Technique

The frontal recesses are identified. The frontal recess is positioned adjacent to the middle turbinate and its size depends on the position and size of agger nasi/bulla frontalis/supraorbital cells that "push" the frontal recess medially and relatively anteriorly or posteriorly depending on the relative side of these different groups of cells. It is more anterior if the agger nasi cells are small; it is more posterior if they are large. The degrees of pneumatization of the anterior and posterior cells tend to go together, so that a well-pneumatized system pushes the frontal recess into a narrow "chink" next to the middle turbinate, whereas a poorly pneumatized system leaves the frontal recess readily accessible. A small ball probe can be placed between these cells and the middle turbinate to help locate the frontal recess (see the section on frontoethmoidectomy in Chapter 5, p. 69).

The operator can get an indication whether they are in the frontal recess by placing an angled instrument, such as a ball probe , a Kuhn–Bolger curette, or an olive-ended sucker, in the area they believe to be the frontal sinus and then noting both the angle and length of the probe as it passes the maxillary spine. The instrument is then pinched next to the spine and then removed and placed on the external surface of the nose at the same angle and length from the spine.

If the end of the probe lies well above the supraorbital rim, then it is likely to be in the frontal sinus unless there is a large bulla frontalis or supraorbital cell when the probe is angled laterally as well. These cells can be seen on a CT scan but they are only found by comparing adjacent sections and reconstructing them in the mind's eye. The ability to reconstruct sagittal sections from a spiral CT scan helps in doing this. If the probe lies at the level of the medial canthus or just above it, it is probably in an agger nasi air cell.

It is all too easy to perforate the skull base when operating in this area, especially where the lateral lamella joins the cribriform plate in the region of the anterior ethmoid artery. No pressure should be used when placing any probe or seeker in this area to locate the frontal recess (Fig. 14.29 a–d). If there has been previous surgery or there is scarring and it is very stenosed, then a trephine of the frontal sinus with dye placed within the frontal sinus may help to locate the frontal recess. Image-guided equipment can also help locate its position, but the definition is often not good enough to be relied upon and its main use is to help the surgeon by *confirming* the position. As the anterior ethmoid artery is often dehiscent, it is wise not to grasp mucosa in this area if you are unable to identify the anatomy clearly. In severe polyposis the frontal recess is often open and expanded by the polyps; this makes opening the area easier, but it is important not to avulse these polyps and denude the frontal recess of mucosa.

The anterior upper part of the septum can then be removed with a powered instrument or through-cutters, being sure to stay anterior to the coronal plane between the frontal recesses. It is important not to go posteriorly and risk entering the skull base. The removal of the top of the nasal septum is a bloody procedure and it helps to have a device to irrigate the end of the endoscope. This process is continued superiorly to remove the intersinus septum. It is safe to remove the beak (Fig. 14.30 a–d) or the thick bone that forms the anterior boundary, and this is easier once the intersinus septum has been removed. Unlike in other procedures in the frontal recess, it is not possible to preserve mucosa. The bone of the beak is thick and it takes time to reduce it; again, this area bleeds a lot. The coarse diamond burr combines the advantages of removing bone efficiently while producing relatively little bleeding. At least 3 hours should be put aside for this procedure. After most of the beak has been taken down, it should be possible to examine the frontal sinus more laterally.

When there are no anatomical landmarks because of severe stenosis, adhesions and loss of the middle turbinate, there are two ways of finding the frontal sinus. The first is to remove the anterosuperior part of

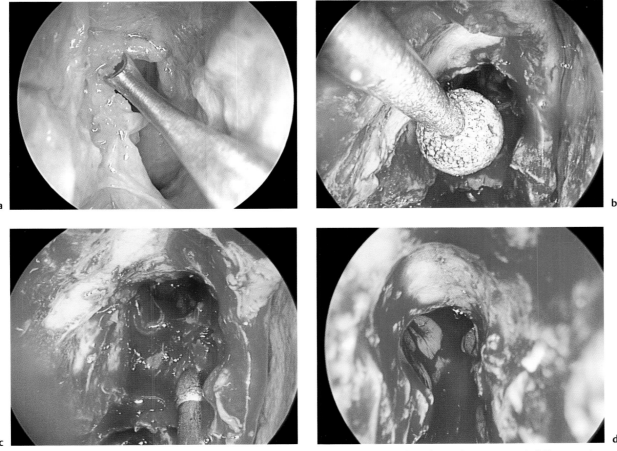

Fig. 14.**29**　**a** A Kuhn–Bolger curette in a cadaver being introduced into the frontal sinus before the anterior cell remnants are curetted. **b** A coarse diamond burr is used to remove the beak of the frontal bone. **c** Right frontal recess exposed with the top of the middle turbinate being retained. **d** Close-up view of the bare bone of the beak with more to be removed. Note the intact mucosa elsewhere.

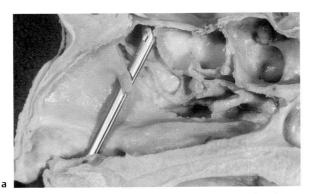

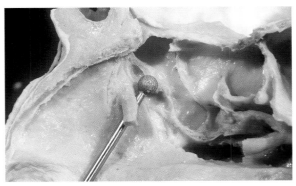

Fig. 14.**30**　**a** Access to the frontal sinus is limited by the attachment of the middle turbinate and the beak of the frontal sinus. **b** A drill has to be used to remove the remains of the most anterior agger nasi cells and beak to gain access to the frontal sinus.

Fig. 14.**30 c, d**　▷

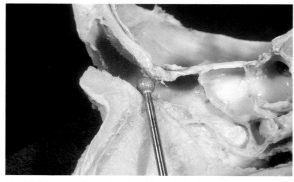

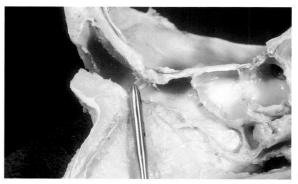

c                                                                                 d

Fig. 14.**30**   **c** Drilling the shoulder of the beak. **d** A straight instrument can now be introduced into the frontal sinus.

the septum, staying as far forward as possible. The second is to define the lacrimal sac as for a DCR and follow it upward as this leads directly to the anterior aspect of the frontal recess (Fig. 14.**31**).

There is no need for a stent (Figs. 14.**32 a–g**, 14.**33 a–f**, 14.**34 a–d**).

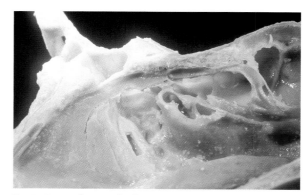

Fig. 14.**31**   Following the lacrimal sac leads up to the area of the frontal recess and the anterior wall of the bulla, which lies posterior to the recess. This is a useful way of finding the frontal sinus when all other landmarks have been lost.

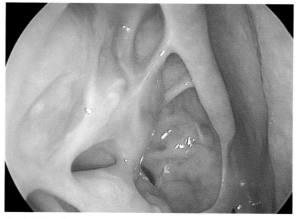

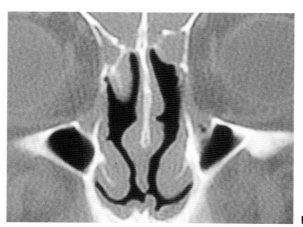

a                                                                                        b

Fig. 14.**32 a**, **b**   Stenosis of left frontal recess after several endonasal and external procedures.

Fig. 14.**32 c–g**  ▷

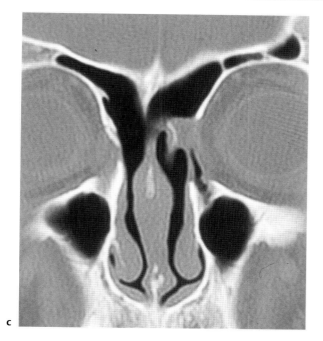

c

Fig. 14.**32** **c** Postoperative coronal CT scan after a median drainage procedure. **d** Postoperative endoscopic view on the left after a median drainage procedure. **e** Closer view over the top of the septum. **f** Postoperative endoscopic view on the right. **g** View looking into the frontal sinus with the remains of the frontal intersinus septum (∗).

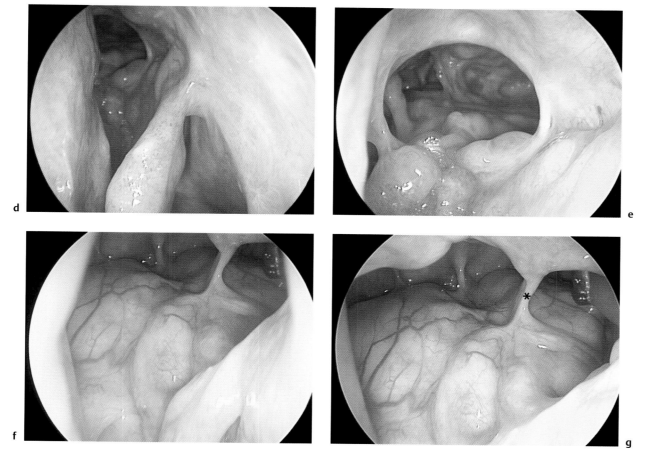

d

e

f

g

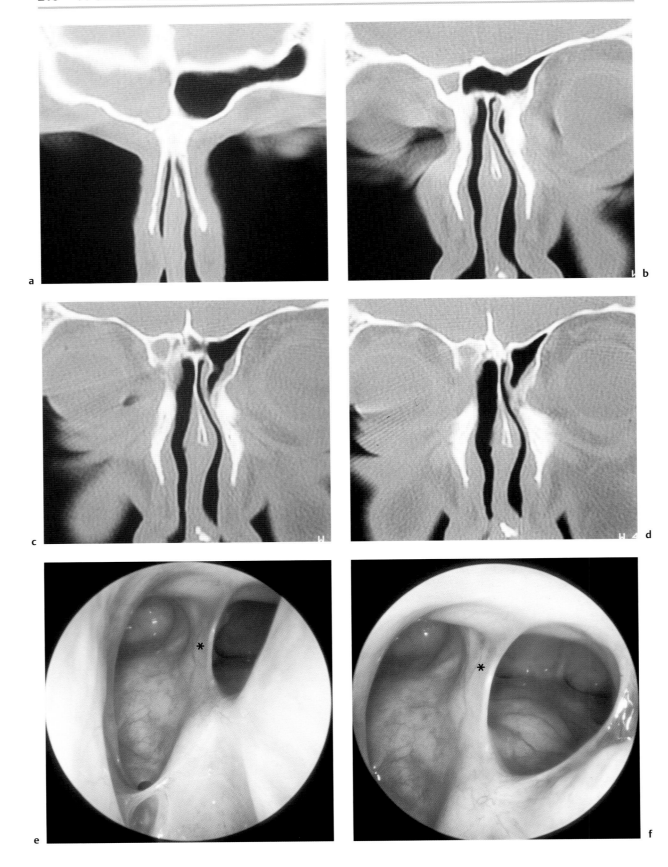

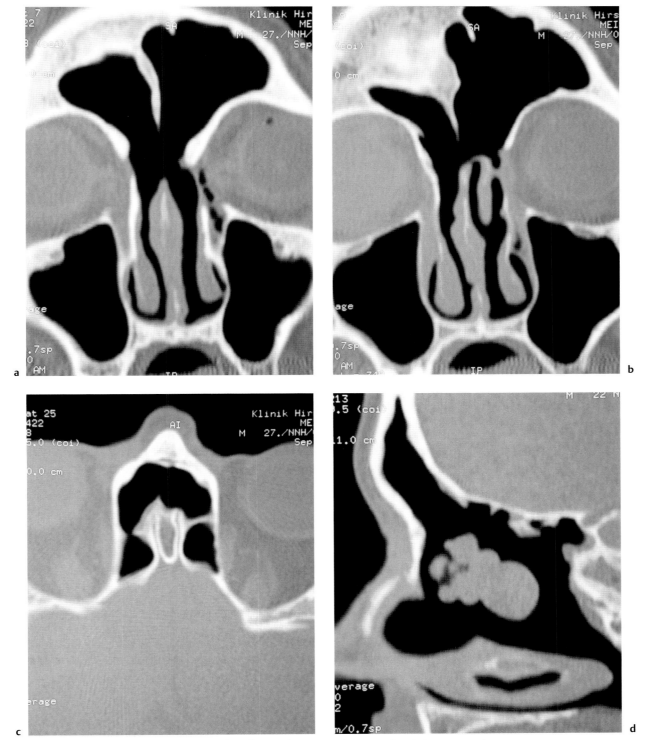

Fig. 14.**34 a–d**    Postoperative coronal, axial, and sagittal CT scans after a median drainage procedure.

◁ Fig. 14.**33 a–d**    Coronal CT scans showing right frontal stenosis as a result of endoscopic sinus surgery. **e, f** Postoperative
view from the right, looking up at the remains of the frontal intersinus septum (∗).

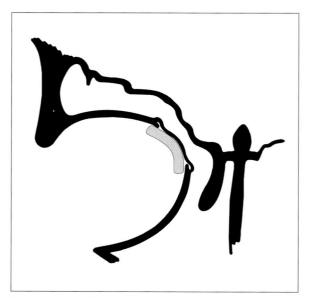

Fig. 14.**35** Line diagram showing how a septal graft can be placed to reduce lateral collapse.

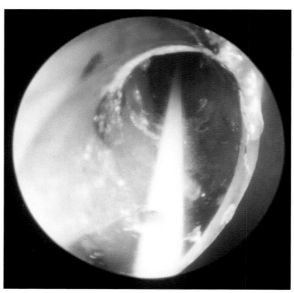

Fig. 14.**36** A stent in the frontal sinus with ongoing infection. The authors do not recommend stents as they appear to stimulate granulation tissue and fibroblast activity.

## Alternative Surgical Techniques

Instead of creating a central drainage channel, it is possible to support and reconstruct the lateral wall of the frontal recess if collapse of that area is the primary problem (Fig. 14.**35**). This particularly applies when an external ethmoidectomy has led to a loss of bone lateral to the frontal recess. There is often a great deal of fibrosis in the area of the frontal recess when it has stenosed after an external ethmoidectomy. The old idea of using as large a stent as possible in the belief that "the larger the stent the greater the chance the recess will have of not stenosing down completely when the stent is removed" is wrong. The pressure necrosis that the large stent causes induces a lot of fibroblast activity (Fig. 14.**36**). An alternative technique is to replace the fibrosed mucosa with new mucosa.

It is rarely possible to reflect a septal flap that extends into this area; a free turbinate graft works well. A free cartilage graft from the septum or conchal bowl is sutured in position with mucosa over it and a loose stent is placed to hold it open. The stent is loose in order to avoid any pressure necrosis on the graft. This will provide lateral support and reduce the chance of further stenosis. Two weeks after surgery, endoscopy will show that the stent is loose and surrounded by healthy mucosa in the frontal recess. This technique is successful in approximately 80 % of patients after 5 years in our hands.

Another alternative is obliteration of the frontal sinuses. This is a large procedure, particularly if the

sinuses are well pneumatized, as is often the case in these patients (Fig. 14.**37** a–d). A coronal flap is done after a plain occipitofrontal radiograph has been taken to work out a template of the extent of the frontal sinuses. It is worth dissecting the periosteum off the frontal bone down to the supraorbital margin. This differs from conventional descriptions of the anterior wall as being hinged on a flap of periosteum inferiorly. This is rarely possible without having tatters of periosteum between areas where bone has been divided along its inferior margin. To add to this, the mucosa of the entire frontal sinus needs to be removed, not only from the posterior wall but the anterior flap, and this is difficult to do thoroughly while it is still attached to the periosteum. It is important to remove all the mucosa from the whole of the frontal sinus because if any is left a mucocele will form. The template is used to estimate the outline of the frontal sinus and an initial hole is made into the sinus in its lateral third. A blunt-ended hook can be used to check the outline of the extent of the frontal sinus, and if it is rotated it to where its end reaches the limit of the frontal sinus it can be followed around with a fissure burr (Murphy and Jones, 2004).

An alternative technique is to place an endoscope into the frontal sinus; its light will illuminate the exact extent of the anterior wall and this will help exact removal. In addition, the surgeon can see where the end of the drill is by looking at the endoscopic view on the screen. This reduces the degree of overhang left after the anterior wall is removed and makes removal of the mucosa easier. It is unwise to make an entry hole high

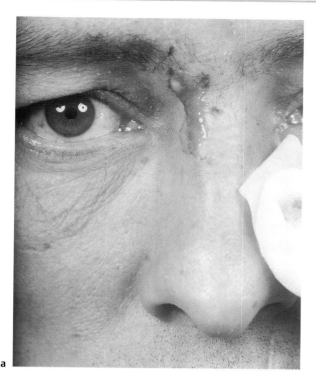

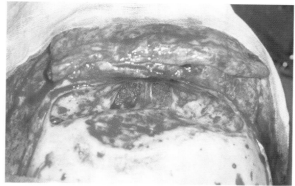

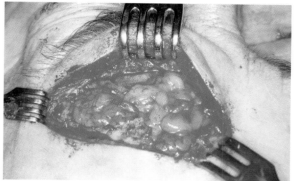

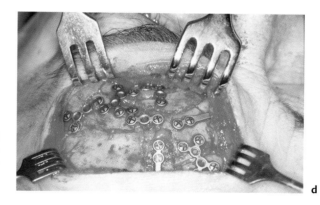

Fig. 14.**37** **a** Pus discharging from a fistula due to an infected implant that had been placed in the sinus. **b** Drill-out of the sinus, with careful removal of every piece of mucosa. **c** Fat obliteration of the frontal sinus. **d** Reconstruction of the anterior wall with split calvarial bone.

in the midline where the venous sinuses are large as entry there can cause torrential bleeding. Before the whole anterior plate is removed, it is worth fixing miniplates onto the anterior wall (these will be removed subsequently) and making burr holes into the cranium to match these plates; this will make replacement of the plate at the end of the procedure not only more accurate but quicker. There are invaginations of mucosa that follow veins into the posterior wall of the frontal sinus and it is important that the posterior wall is drilled to reduce the chance of remnants of mucosa being left behind. The sinus is best obliterated with fat and the frontal recess should be blocked with fascia; both can be obtained from the thigh or abdomen. The

anterior bone flap is susceptible to infection and prophylactic antibiotic cover should be given.

A further technique that can be used when there is osteomyelitis or a loss of much of the anterior wall of the frontal sinus is to remove the whole anterior wall and the mucosal lining, and smooth the supraorbital rims—Riedel's procedure (Fig. 14.**38 a–d**) (Raghavan and Jones, 2004).

### Useful Instruments

1 In a midline drainage procedure, a 45° endoscope, ball probes, and a Kuhn–Bolger frontal sinus curette are helpful.

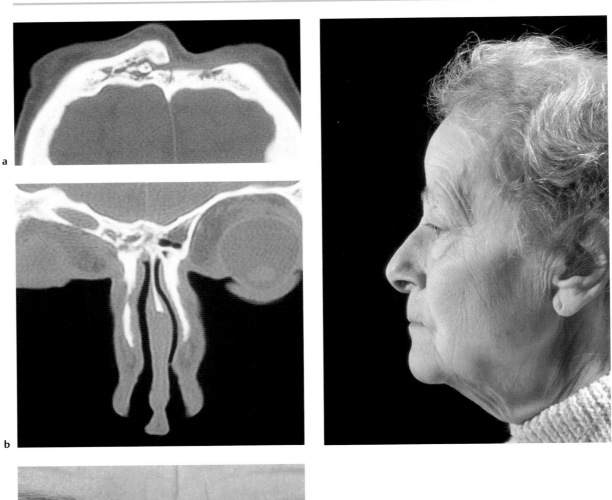

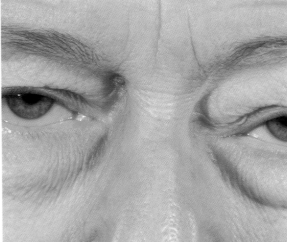

Fig. 14.**38 a**, **b**   Axial and coronal CT scans showing osteomyelitis of the frontal bone. **c**, **d** Preoperative discharging fistula and postoperative appearance after Riedel's procedure.

2  A long-shanked drill with a coarse diamond burr helps in reducing the "beak" of the frontal bone.
3  Image-guided instrumentation.

## Orbital Decompression

### Terminology and Classification

Removing one or more of the bony walls that make up its surrounding can decompress the contents of the orbit. The largest potential amount of decompression is obtained by removing the medial wall of the orbit, next its floor, and then its lateral wall. Decompression can be achieved externally, although the amount of dissection that can take place toward the orbital apex is limited because of reduced visibility and pressure on the orbital contents (Fig. 14.**39**). Many techniques have been described for decompressing the orbit transantrally, or via a subconjunctival or subciliary incision.

### Indications

The primary indication for this procedure is dysthyroid eye disease, either for cosmetic reasons or when vision is deteriorating and steroids and radiotherapy have not controlled this (Fig. 14.**40 a**, **b**). An endoscopic approach can decompress both the medial and inferior aspects of the eye. In experienced hands, it is possible to obtain better access to the orbital apex and even to decompress the optic nerve endoscopically (Gormley et al., 1997) (Fig. 14.**41 a**–**d**). Benign bony tumors can also threaten the viability of the optic nerve and justify removal.

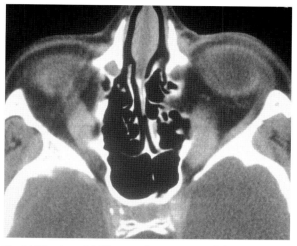

Fig. 14.**39**   An axial CT scan after an external decompression showing poor decompression, in part due to limited posterior access.

### Surgical Anatomy

The medial wall of the orbit is made up of the lamina papyracea of the ethmoid bone, the palatine bone, and more posteriorly the thicker bone of the sphenoid that makes up the apex of the orbit. The degree of pneumatization of the sphenoid sinus determines whether the optic nerve indents, or is even dehiscent in, its lateral wall. The same applies to the posterior ethmoid sinuses, which can envelop the optic nerve before it reaches the sphenoid sinus if there is a sphenoethmoid cell. The inferior-medial strut is made of the maxillary bone, and this is often thick (Fig. 14.**42**). The

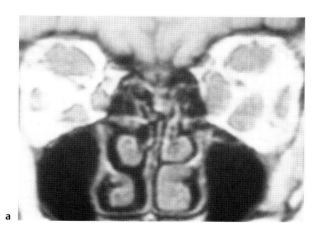

a

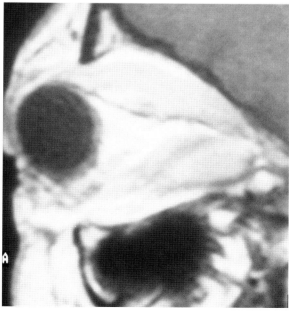

b

Fig. 14.**40**   **a** Coronal and **b** sagittal MR images, showing the hypertrophied muscles and proptosis of dysthyroid eye disease.

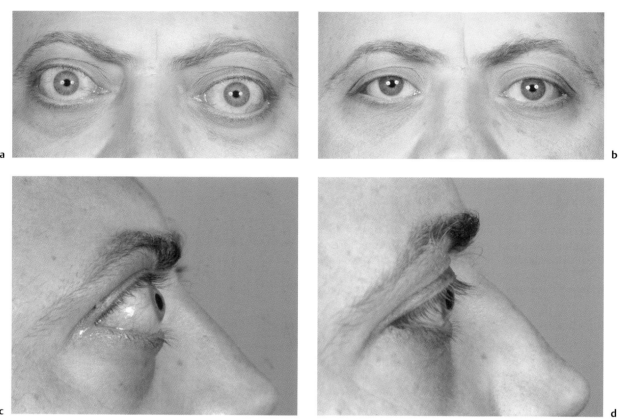

Fig. 14.**41 a–d**    Preoperative (**a**, **c**) and postoperative (**b**, **d**) appearance after bilateral endoscopic decompression for dysthyroid eye disease.

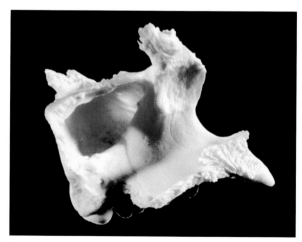

Fig. 14.**42**    The medial aspect of the left disarticulated maxillary bone showing the thick strut that makes up the inferomedial part of the orbit. Do not remove too much as this will cause diplopia.

next area of bony condensation is around the infraorbital nerve in the floor of the orbit and lateral to this the bone is thicker and more difficult to remove (Fig. 14.**43**).

## Surgical Technique

A type III maxillary sinusotomy is undertaken initially and a thorough ethmoidectomy is done to expose the lamina papyracea. The lamina papyracea is readily incised in an oblique direction with a Freer's elevator (Fig. 14.**44 a**, **b**). Through-cutting forceps can be used to remove it sequentially inferiorly, superiorly, and posteriorly. During this procedure the assistant examines the eye to see that it does not move and ballottes it repeatedly to allow the surgeon to see how much of the lateral nasal wall is dehiscent. A thick strut of bone forms the junction between the medial wall and the floor of the orbit, and this is not readily removed. It is advisable to leave this strut because its removal increases the likelihood of diplopia as this is more likely to alter the axis of the globe in spite of the suspensory ligament of the eye not being directly af-

fected. Even if this is done on both sides, it is not easy
to control the axis of the globe where this strut of bone
is removed. The lamina papyracea can be removed
more anteriorly using a back-biter, but it is important
not to come so far forward so that the bone is firm, because it is here that the lacrimal sac is most at risk. The
lamina papyracea can best be removed by dissecting
between it and the orbital periostium with a Freer elevator.

Only when the orbit has been completely decompressed should the orbital periosteum be incised
(Fig. 14.45 a, b). It helps a great deal if the blade is extremely sharp and if only superficial posterior horizontal cuts in the periosteum are done initially:
deeper cuts run the risk of damaging the medial rectus. Multiple rows should be made, and then these
should be followed by vertical cross-hatching incisions, again starting posteriorly. If the first incisions in
the periosteum are anterior, this will limit posterior
access as the fat will prolapse and block the view. It is
helpful to ballotte the eye with the eyelids closed in
order to help the fat prolapse into the nasal airway at
this stage. It also helps put tension on the periosteum
and means that this can be incised more superficially
without entering the contents of the orbit. Once multiple cross-hatching has been done, the orbit can be
pushed inward to break any remaining strands of orbital periosteum. This will encourage the orbital fat to
prolapse medially through the lateral nasal wall. The
degree of proptosis should then be reassessed to ensure that decompression has been adequate. This will
often encourage the surgeon to undertake more cross-
hatching and be more meticulous about the removal of

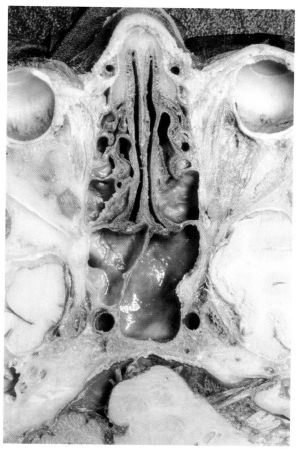

Fig. 14.**43**   Axial section showing the relationship of the medial rectus to the lamina papyracea and the optic nerve in the
sphenoid sinus.

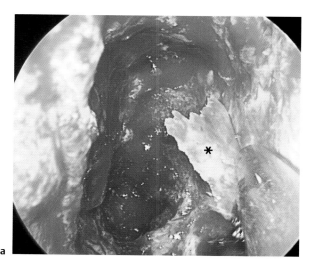

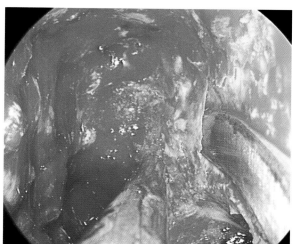

Fig. 14.**44 a**, **b**   Removing the lamina papyracea ( ∗ ) of the left lateral nasal wall.

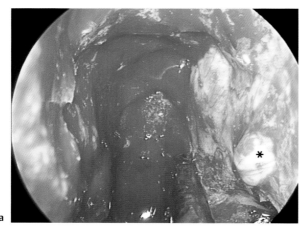

a

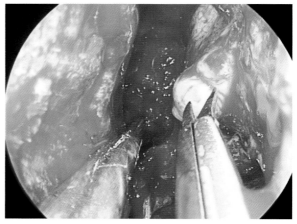

b

Fig. 14.**45 a, b**   The lamina papyracea has been removed and a little fat (∗) can be seen protruding through a small defect of the periorbital layer. Bellucci scissors are then used to carefully divide the periorbital layer.

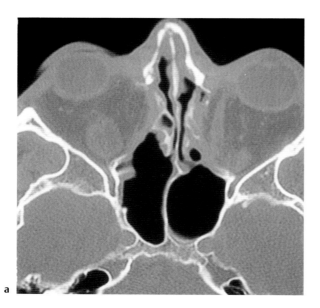

a

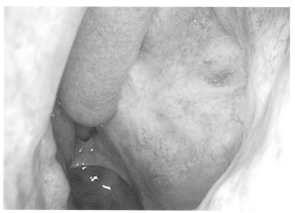

b

Fig. 14.**46**   **a** Postoperative axial CT scan and **b** left endoscopic view to show healed mucosa over the decompressed orbital contents.

any remaining fragments of lamina papyracea or orbital periosteum (Figs. 14.**46 a, b**, 14.**47**).

At the orbital apex, the bone of the sphenoid becomes extremely thick and a coarse diamond burr is needed to reduce the bone here. It is important that this is well irrigated in order to avoid generation of heat and the possibility of this being transmitted to the optic nerve. A thorough orbital decompression means that bone is removed to this area. It is best to assess the thinness of the bone after drilling it using a Freer's elevator and then using a hand curette in order to remove the slithers of bone that remain over the optic nerve. In the lower third of the lateral wall of the sphenoid sinus, it is more common for the maxillary branch of the trigeminal to be seen as a prominence. It is possible to mistakenly decompress this instead of the optic nerve. The optic nerve, in the 20% of patients where it does produce a bulge in the lateral wall of the sphenoid, is usually at the junction of the upper third and lower two-thirds of the lateral wall of the sphenoid.

Look out for periorbital cellulitis that would cause progressive pain and swelling as this is a potential complication. It is interesting that the dehiscent orbital fat is quickly covered by healthy mucosa.

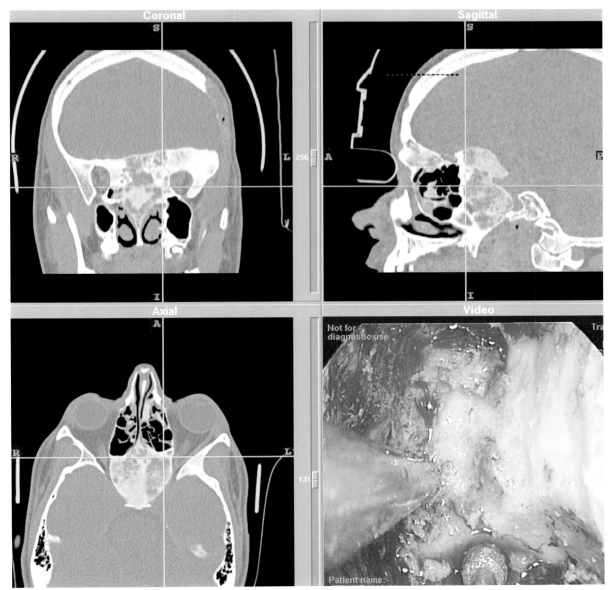

Fig. 14.**47**   Computer-guided images during the removal of fibrous dysplasia to decompress the orbit because of deteriorating vision.

## Useful instruments

1   A long-shanked drill with a coarse diamond burr and a good irrigation system to keep the bone cool.
2   Image guided surgery.

## ■ Optic Nerve Decompression

### Terminology and Classification

Optic nerve decompression is an extension of orbital decompression when the optic nerve in the lateral wall of the sphenoid is decompressed.

### Indications

The indications for this are limited. All too often, damage to the optic nerve is recognized days after the trauma that caused it. The type of head injury that leads to optic nerve damage is usually associated with significant brain damage, whose management takes precedence. The clinical picture is normally clouded by the overall neurological status of the patient. Assessing the optic afferent pathway in these circumstances is not easy, as the patient often requires ventilation and is paralyzed. Under these circumstances, it may be inappropriate for the patient to undergo

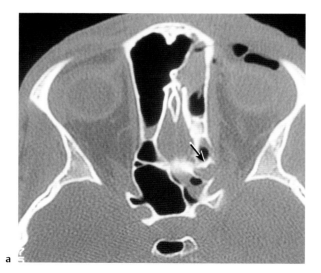

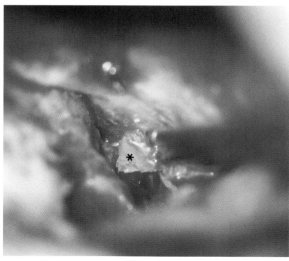

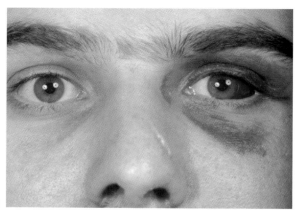

Fig. 14.**48**   **a** Axial CT scan showing a posttraumatic fragment of bone pressing on the optic nerve (arrow). **b** Peroperative endoscopic view showing removal of the bony fragment (∗) responsible 4 hours after accident. **c** Partial loss of vision returned following removal of the bony fragment and decompression of the orbit.

surgery, particularly if they have a Glasgow coma scale score of less than 8 (Jones et al., 1997b). If there is a skull base fracture included in the sphenoid and there is evidence of an afferent defect, then further investigations, including visual evoked potentials (Jones, 1997) or usually a swinging light test (Mason et al., 1998a), should be done. If these are abnormal, then the question remains when it is appropriate to decompress the optic nerve. Several studies suggest that with retro-orbital hemorrhage, decompression of the orbit needs to be done in less than one hour (Mason et al., 1998a). However, where there is no hemorrhage, it is less clear under what circumstances it is beneficial to decompress the nerve pathway.

High-dose steroids are the primary treatment of choice in traumatic optic neuropathy (Sofferman, 1995). However, if the optic nerve function is deteriorating in spite of these it would seem reasonable to intervene (Jiang et al., 2001). If there is an anatomical constriction on CT scans affecting the course of the optic nerve and the patient is fit for anesthesia, then it seems reasonable to remove the bone pressing on the nerve (Fig. 14.48a–c). While the results of optic nerve decompression have been encouraging, the assessment of these patients, the state of the afferent pathway, and knowledge of the ability of the optic nerve to improve without any intervention are too limited to allow clear guidelines at present.

### Surgical Anatomy

See the section above on Orbital Decompression.

### Surgical Technique

First of all, an orbital decompression of the medial wall is done without incising any periosteum at this stage. The optic nerve can often be decompressed in the lateral wall of the sphenoid, but extreme care is needed to avoid heating the bone over it. There has

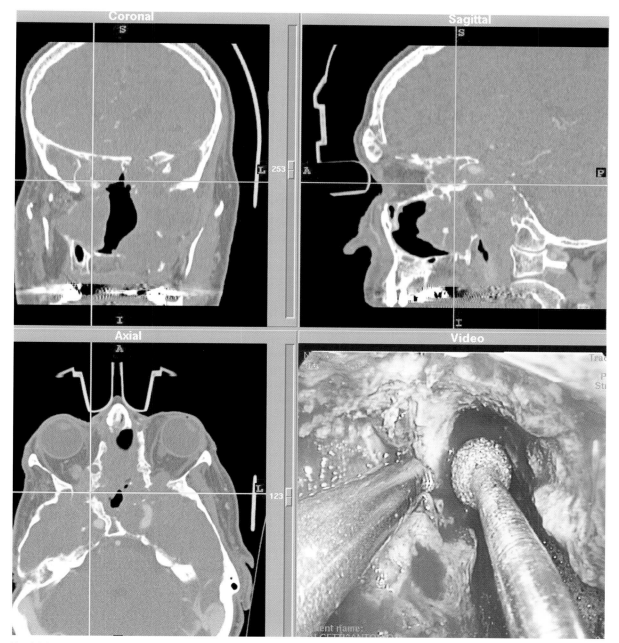

Fig. 14.**49**   Peroperative computer-guided images during the removal of a chordoma pressing on the orbital apex.

been debate whether the sheath of the optic nerve should be incised or not. There is insufficient evidence in favor of this (Jiang et al., 2001). Incising the sheath not only runs the risk of producing a CSF leak but could compromise some of the vascular supply of the optic nerve (Fig. 14.**49**).

Postoperatively it is vital to monitor the vision quarter-hourly for one hour, and then hourly for 4 hours, although decompression is rarely associated with any deterioration in vision. In fact, the immediate

or early results of decompression are frequently extremely gratifying. The patient should be instructed not to blow their nose or stifle sneezes for 4 days in order to avoid surgical emphysema (Fig. 14.**50**).

## Useful Instruments

See the section above on Orbital Decompression.

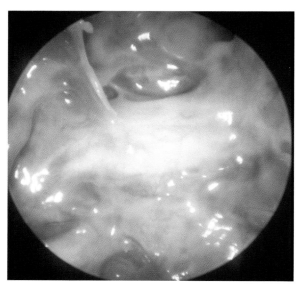

Fig. 14.**50**   View of the left optic nerve 6 months after an optic nerve decompression done for trauma associated with partial loss of vision, which returned.

## ■ Choanal Atresia Surgery

### Terminology and Classification

Choanal atresia is secondary to the unilateral or bilateral persistence of the buccopharyngeal membrane. It can be membranous or bony. It is important to define how thick any bony stenosis is and study the anatomy of neighboring structures such as the carotid artery.

### Indications

A newborn infant relies on its nasal airway. It is particularly compromised during suckling. It is not possible to leave bilateral choanal atresia untreated. Rapid assessment and correction are needed to provide a nasal airway, and an oropharyngeal airway has to be held in place in the meantime. Bilateral choanal atresia is often associated with other congenital abnormalities (the CHARGE syndrome in particular) that also need to be investigated.

First of all an attempt to pass a fine nasogastric tube into the nasopharynx should be made to help confirm the diagnosis. An axial CT should be done, but only after decongesting the mucosa and sucking any mucus (this avoids mucus producing the false appearance of a mucosal obstruction). A unilateral atresia often presents later in the early teens when the patient realizes that they cannot breathe through one side. They can also present with a unilateral mucoid discharge.

### Surgical Anatomy

A persistent membrane or bony plate separates the nasopharynx from the nasal airway. Not only does the thickness of any bony obstruction need to be assessed but also its lateral and medial intrusion into the airway. There may be no complete bony partition, but thick lateral bone that protrudes medially and narrows the airway will need a lot of bony work in order to widen it.

### Surgical Technique

#### Bilateral Atresia

If the obstruction is due to soft tissue then it is possible to palpate it and see with an endoscope where it should be perforated and opened up. If there is a complete bony plate, it is important not to lose your way, and most surgeons initially find it safer to place their finger in the nasopharynx and aim the drill at it. It is now possible to visualize the posterior aspect of the septum and the back of the inferior turbinate and use these landmarks to drill through the atretic plate under endoscopic control. Having made an opening by whatever means, it can then be widened endoscopically in a controlled way (Fig. 14.**51** a, **b**). The primary goals of surgery are to provide a wide airway with as little collateral mucosal damage as possible (Fig. 14.**52** a–c). Conventionally, a wide stent has been inserted, but this causes pressure necrosis of any viable mucosa and it appears to encourage fibrosis and stenosis once the stent is removed. A loose stent is better, and the strut joining the two cylindrical stents should not press on the columella. An endotracheal tube that has a section cut out of it to leave one flat connecting piece between the two tubes can lightly rest on the columella with a loose circumferential tie placed through the tubes and around the nasopharynx to retain it.

#### Unilateral Atresia

In unilateral choanal atresia a simple technique that allows aeration and restoration of mucociliary clearance of the blocked airway relies on removing the vomer. This can be done endoscopically by incising through all layers just behind the quadrilateral cartilage and then removing all layers of the vomer with through-cutting forceps (Cumberworth et al., 1995). The septal branch of the sphenopalatine artery usually needs to be cauterized. No stent is required (Fig. 14.**53** a–c).

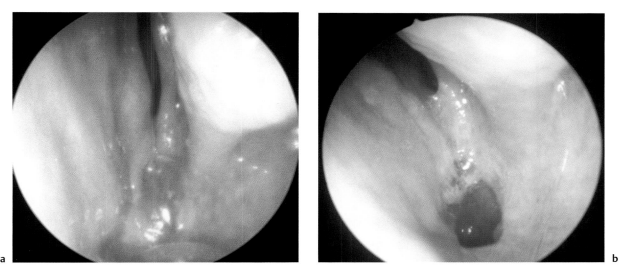

Fig. 14.**51** **a** Preoperative and **b** postoperative views of left choanal atresia in a neonate. The changes were the same on both sides.

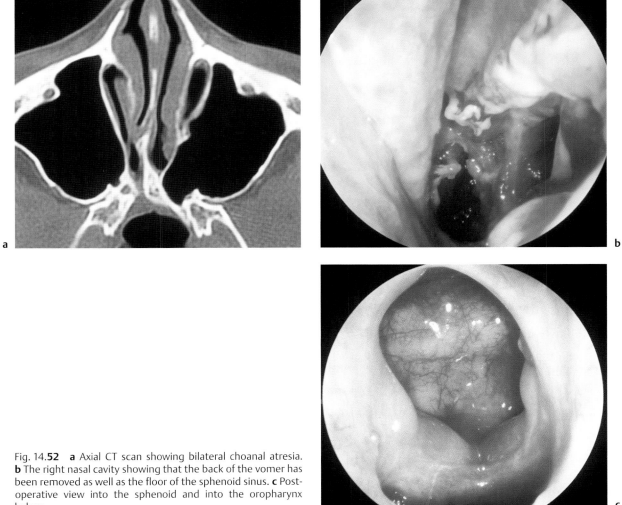

Fig. 14.**52** **a** Axial CT scan showing bilateral choanal atresia. **b** The right nasal cavity showing that the back of the vomer has been removed as well as the floor of the sphenoid sinus. **c** Postoperative view into the sphenoid and into the oropharynx below.

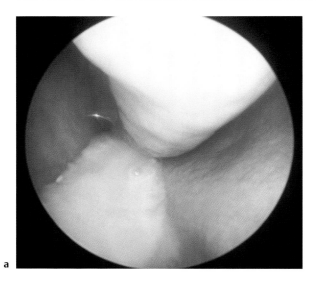

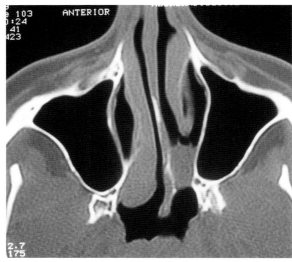

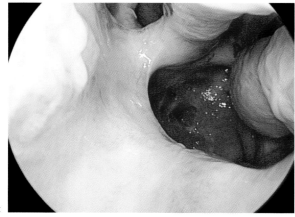

Fig. 14.**53**  **a** Mucus stagnation in unilateral choanal atresia. **b** Axial CT scan showing a left unilateral membranous choanal atresia. **c** Postoperative endoscopic view showing a patent posterior choana 8 years later.

### Alternative Surgical Techniques

Transpalatal techniques allow direct exposure but cause more disruption and fibrosis of the palatal muscles.

### Useful Instruments

1  A long-shanked drill with irrigation and a coarse diamond burr.
2  An image guided system.
3  A 120° endoscope to visualize the nasopharynx while drilling is being done.

### ■ Medial Maxillectomy

### Terminology and Classification

Medial maxillectomy entails total resection of the lateral nasal wall (ethmoidectomy) including the anterior and posterior fontanelles, the inferior turbinate, and tissue from the pyriform aperture as well as the posterior wall of the maxillary sinus (Kraft et al., 2003). **DVD** 14

### Indications

Indications are extensive inverted papilloma affecting the lateral nasal wall and involving the maxillary sinus (Fig. 14.**54** a, **b**) and benign tumors of the medial wall of the maxilla.

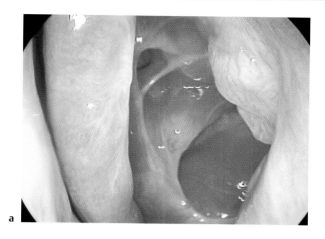

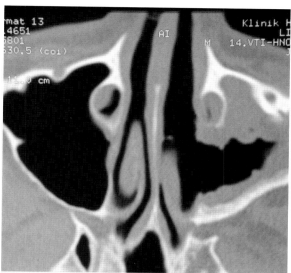

Fig. 14.**54**  **a** Endoscopic view and **b** axial CT scan showing recurrent inverted papilloma involving the anterior wall of the left maxilla.

## Surgical Anatomy

The bony medial surface of the maxilla is wide open (see Fig. 14.**42**). The medial wall of the maxillary sinus is made up of the inferior turbinate, the uncinate bone, part of the ethmoid complex, and the palatine bone (Fig. 14.**55**). The remaining wall that separates the maxillary sinus from the nasal airway is made up of the mucus membrane of both the maxillary sinus and the lateral nasal wall, and the areas that have no intermediate bone form the anterior and posterior fontanelle (Fig. 14.**56 a–c**).

## Surgical Technique

First of all, a type III maxillary sinusotomy is fashioned with its posterior limit extending level with the posterior wall of the maxillary sinus. This often means that the anterior branch of the sphenopalatine artery needs cauterizing. An anteriorly based mucosal flap over the frontal process of the maxilla and the anterior lacrimal crest is elevated to expose the anterior lacrimal crest. The anterior lacrimal crest is removed along its whole length using a Hajek–Kofler punch, and toward the top a coarse diamond burr is used to remove it up to its superior limit. The sac is resected up to its upper third. Bone is removed down to the level of the nasal floor using the side-biting antrum punch forceps. Any remaining bone around the lacrimal fossa, the bony ridge along the anterior rim of the maxilla, and the ridge of bone remaining inferiorly between it and the floor of the nose is drilled down level to the anterior wall and floor of the maxillary sinus (Fig. 14.**57 a–d**). A

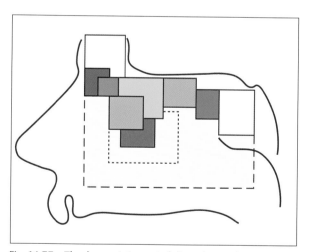

Fig. 14.**55**  The heavy interrupted line shows the extent of bone that needs to be removed in a medial maxillectomy.

3 mm chisel can be used to remove the thicker bone of the anteroinferior margin that makes up the rim of the pyriform aperture. This now allows you to visualize the entire maxillary sinus, although a 70° endoscope may be needed to see its anterior wall. Any exposed orbital periosteum is left intact (Fig. 14.**58 a–d**). The margins of the opening that expose the maxillary sinus will then be smooth and leave no crest (Fig. 14.**59 a, b**).

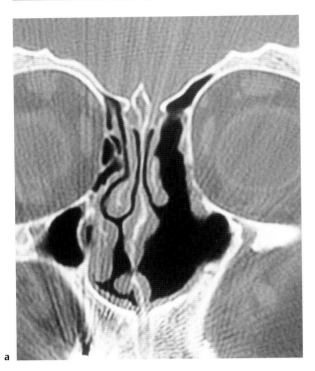

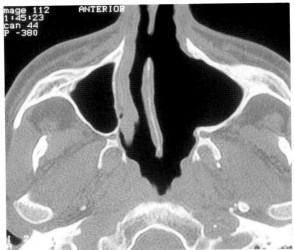

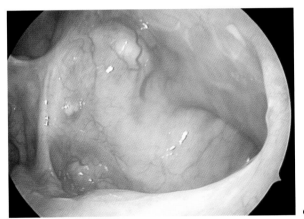

Fig. 14.**56**   **a** Coronal and **b** axial CT scans along with **c** the endoscopic appearance after a left medial maxillectomy.

This procedure is usually combined with an anterior ethmoidectomy. In the radical removal of a tumor, the middle turbinate may also need to be resected (Fig. 14.**60**).

### Alternative Techniques

Lateral rhinotomy or midfacial degloving provide good access and visibility to the maxillary sinus and lateral nasal wall. An external scar is the main disadvantage of a lateral rhinotomy (Fig. 14.**61 a–d**). In the hands of an experienced endoscopic surgeon, the visibility is the same. Some endoscopic sinus surgeons do a Caldwell–Luc procedure at the same time as their endoscopic surgery in order to help visualize the maxillary sinus.

### Useful Instruments

1  Stammberger side-biting antrum punch forceps.
2  Hajek–Kofler punch.
3  A long-shanked drill with a coarse diamond to remove the bone at the top of the lacrimal crest and the rim of the medial surface of the maxillary sinus where it is too thick to be removed by a punch.

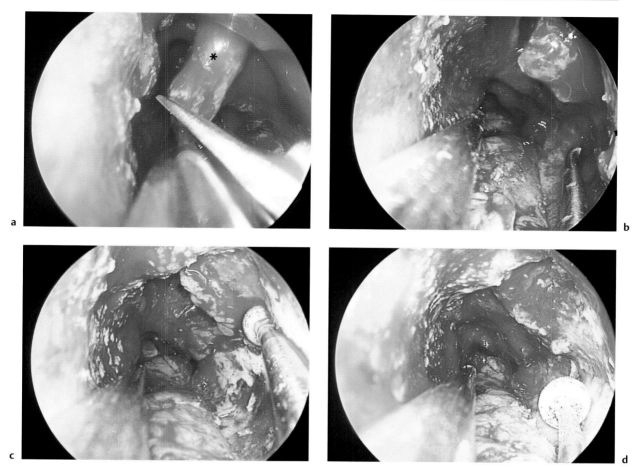

Fig. 14.**57**    **a** Dividing the exposed left lacrimal sac ( ∗ ). **b** Dissecting the mucosa off the margins of the left maxillary sinus.

**c** Further drilling the shoulder of the left lacrimal crest. **d** Leveling the ridge dividing the maxilla from the floor of the nose.

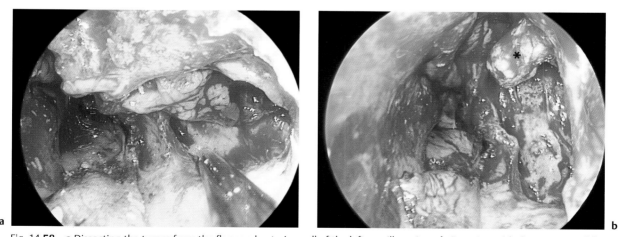

Fig. 14.**58**    **a** Dissecting the tumor from the floor and anterior wall of the left maxillary sinus. **b** Overview with the remnant of the left lacrimal sac ( ∗ ).

Fig. 14.**58**   **c, d**   ▷

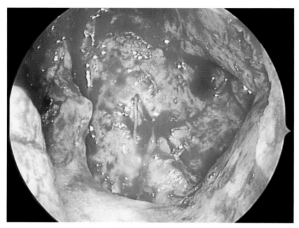
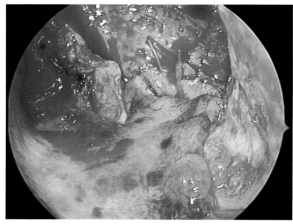

c

d

Fig. 14.**58**   **c** Before and **d** after folding the medially based flap of mucosa over the floor of the nose and maxilla.

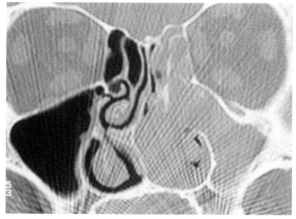

a

Fig. 14.**59**   **a** Preoperative coronal CT scan and **b** postoperative endoscopic appearance of inverted papilloma involving the maxillary sinus.

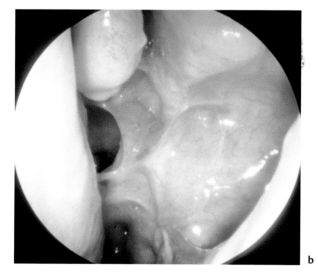

b

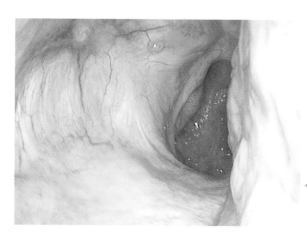

◁ Fig. 14.**60**   Often the medial wall of the maxillary sinus medializes and fills in to give this appearance. This is the view 3 years after the endoscopic resection of a low-grade adenocarcinoma on the right side.

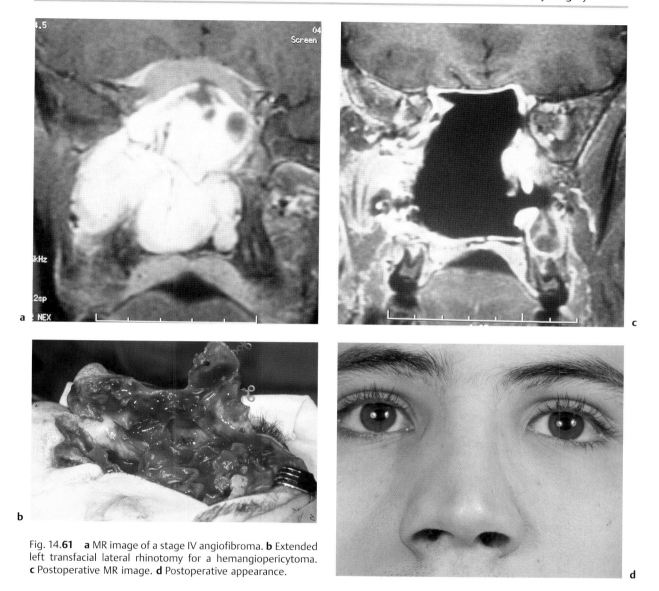

Fig. 14.**61** **a** MR image of a stage IV angiofibroma. **b** Extended left transfacial lateral rhinotomy for a hemangiopericytoma. **c** Postoperative MR image. **d** Postoperative appearance.

## ▪ Pituitary Surgery

### Terminology and Classification

The pituitary can be approached in several ways, which include:

- Transseptal, transsphenoidal
- Transnasal
- Via an external ethmoidectomy approach
- Through the upper buccal sulcus of the mouth and then transseptal, transsphenoidal
- Via a craniotomy, e.g., an anterolateral approach, or a frontal approach

### Indications

Pituitary tumors occur in 9 in 100 000 people and comprise 10 % of intracranial tumors. The commonest pituitary tumors in patients under 35 years secrete prolactin and adrenocorticotropin, whereas after 35–50 years they generally secrete growth hormone. After that, nonsecreting tumors are more common. Symptoms can be caused by pressure on the anterior pituitary and hypopituitarism, or by an extrasellar growth that can produce headaches, pressure on the optic chiasm, or brain. The dopamine receptor agonists inhibit prolactin and shrink many of the prolactin-secreting

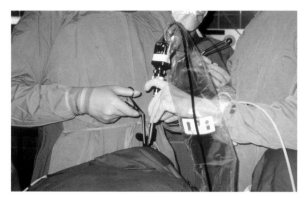

Fig. 14.**62**    The neurosurgeon working with the rhinologist.

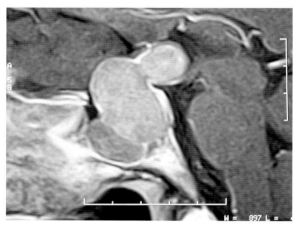

Fig. 14.**63**    Sagittal reconstruction of a macroadenoma of the pituitary gland.

tumors. Somatostatin analogues have a variable degree of success in reducing the secretion and size of growth hormone-secreting tumors. Dopamine receptors also occur in a proportion of nonfunctioning tumors, but long-term treatment provides sustained improvement in only a small proportion of this group. Surgery is the first-line treatment in acromegaly, where up to 90% of microadenomas are cured, although the results are not so good in larger tumors.

Surgery for pituitary disease must be based on an assessment of the patient by a multidisciplinary team (Fig. 14.**62**). The medical management of many pituitary tumors has reduced the frequency of the need for surgery in many patients. Medical management is rarely of use in tumors that extend into the suprasellar area and extend above the diaphragma sellae. Hourglass tumors cannot readily be dealt with using an inferior approach alone unless only partial debulking of the tumor and/or a biopsy is required.

Whatever approach is used to the sphenoid sinus and pituitary fossa, the endoscope gives excellent visibility within the sphenoid sinus, and with a 45° endo-

scope it is possible to see more detail within the pituitary fossa than with the microscope. The advantages of the transnasal, transseptal, or lower buccal approach is that it avoids an external scar, and by removing the posterior part of the septum, vomer, and anterior wall of the sphenoid this approach allows wide access. In the transnasal technique, mucosal preservation is an added advantage. All these techniques allow the surgeon to work bimanually if necessary. This is valuable in the occasional case when there is moderate or severe bleeding as this situation is then controlled more readily. It is difficult to deal with bleeding if the only access has been endoscopically through a unilateral sphenoidotomy, even if two experienced endoscopists are working together with one holding the endoscope to allow the other surgeon the use of both hands. An external ethmoidectomy approach produces a scar and has the potential to cause stenosis of the frontal recess.

## Surgical Anatomy

The vomer consistently joins the sphenoid in the midline and this is a very reliable landmark. The sphenoid intersinus septum is often asymmetric (> 75%) and the preoperative CT scans should be studied before operating. The degree of pneumatization of the sphenoid also varies a great deal (Lang, 1989). Axial cuts complement coronal sections and sagittal reconstruction helps (Fig. 14.**63**). The natural sphenoid ostium is relatively high in the posterior wall of the sphenoid and is often placed at the level of the superior turbinate. It may be readily visible after gentle lateralization of the middle turbinate. The bony anterior wall of the sphenoid sinus is often thin or deficient 1–1.5 cm above the posterior choana. The lateral wall of the sphenoid has indentations from various structures:

1  In its upper third the optic nerve can indent its surface.
2  In its middle third the maxillary nerve can form an almost horizontal, semicircular intrusion that may be mistaken for the optic nerve.
3  The degree of pneumatization of the sinus varies and influences how prominent structures are in its lateral wall. Pneumatization can extend to the clivus, the lesser wing, and the root of the pterygoid process. Agenesis of the sphenoid sinus occurs in 0.7% of patients. It is small and confined to the anterior aspect of the sphenoid (a conchal sinus) in 5% of cases. In 28%, it extends to the coronal plane level with the anterior wall of the sphenoid (a presellar sinus). And in 67% it is both presellar and postsellar.
4  The carotid artery bulges into its lower lateral wall and it can be dehiscent in up to 30% of patients,
5  The vidian nerve can bulge into its floor.

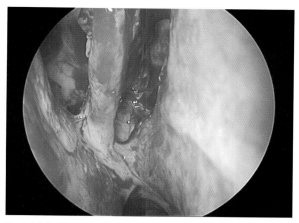

Fig. 14.**64**   Transnasal approach to enlarge one sphenoidotomy before removing the back of the vomer retrogradely.

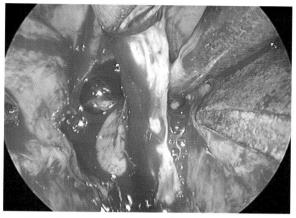

Fig. 14.**65**   The transseptal approach, removing the back of the vomer to access the sphenoid sinus in the midline.

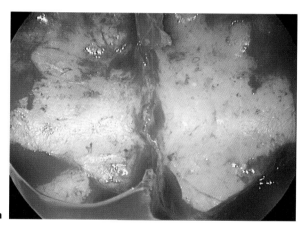

a

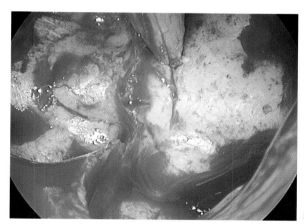

b

Fig. 14.**66 a, b**   The back of the sphenoid intersinus septum with the mucosa removed and an osteotome being used very carefully to remove the thin bone over the pituitary.

## Surgical Technique

A transnasal endoscopic approach starts by making a sphenoidotomy on the side of the tumor or, when it is in the midline opening, the side where the sinus is larger. The sphenoidotomy is opened up to the level of the skull base using a sphenoid punch. Suction diathermy will be needed to stop bleeding from the posterior branch of the sphenopalatine artery when opening the sphenoidotomy inferiorly (Fig. 14.**64**). Any vomerine spur should be removed. After carefully examining the CT scan and endoscopically inspecting the sphenoid sinus to check on the proximity of the lateral structures, the lateral aspect of its anterior wall can be removed if necessary. A Kerrison antrum punch is good for doing this as its small diameter means that the bone can be removed in small pieces with good visibility. If more space is needed across the midline,

the vomer can be fractured across or it can be incised 1 cm in front of the sphenoid and removed. As the vomer joins the sphenoid it can be very thick, but it rarely needs drilling (Fig. 14.**65**). The pituitary often bulges into the roof of the sphenoid and the bone may be very thin (Fig. 14.**66 a, b**). If the bone is thick, a coarse diamond burr should be used to thin it. This is better than a tungsten burr, which can catch and skid away and potentially damage other structures. A diathermy point is useful to open the dura by making a cross-shaped incision through it. A 45° endoscope gives excellent visibility and helps to avoid going through the diaphragm sellae. A Hajek punch helps to remove the bone over the pituitary (Fig. 14.**67 a, b**).

The tumor is often gray in color, but occasionally it can be vascular and ooze moderately. The pituitary fossa can be closed at the end of the procedure with

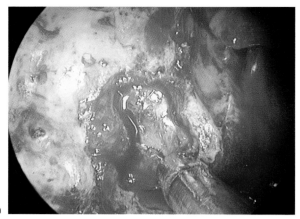
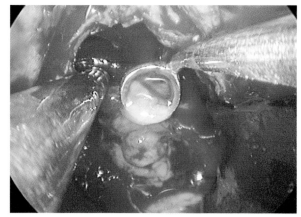

a

b

Fig. 14.**67**   **a** The roof of the sphenoid sinus is removed to expose the floor of the pituitary. **b** A ring curette is used to remove the pituitary tumor.

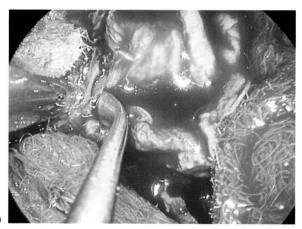
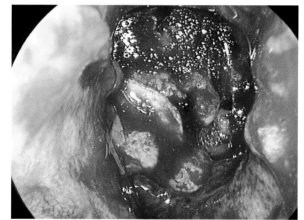

a

b

Fig. 14.**68 a, b**   If there is a CSF leak, fascia is first placed and then it is supported by fat.

septal bone placed in the bony defect. If there is a CSF leak, fascia and fat may also be needed in order to stop it (Fig. 14.**68 a, b**).

It is possible to approach the pituitary via a limited sphenoidotomy, although this reduces access and visibility. As well as providing an approach that is not centred on the midline and will increase the possibility of damaging lateral structures.   **DVD** 17

### Alternative Surgical Techniques

#### Transbuccal-Septal-Sphenoid Approach

In this approach, there is no external scar, the approach is at an angle that is directed toward the roof of the sphenoid, and it gives good visibility of the pituitary. This approach involves a longer distance or tun-

nel to work through than other approaches. Much of the nasal septum is removed to allow access, but it is vital to preserve the anterior 0.5 cm from where the septum is attached to the spine in order to avoid loss of tip support. It is wise to electively remove the necessary segment of cartilage intact so that it can readily be reinserted at the end of the procedure to minimize the risk of a perforation, as septal tears often occur during the procedure. Replacing the cartilage as well as suturing any tears will minimize the possibility of creating a perforation.

#### External Transethmoidectomy Approach

This allows the microscope to be used and the sphenoid can be opened in a plane that approaches it directly along the axis of the nose onto the anterior wall of the sphenoid. However, with this method the axis of approach to visualize the pituitary is not ideal, there is an external scar, and there is the possibility of producing stenosis of the frontal recess.

### A Craniotomy (e.g., an Anterolateral Approach), or a Frontal Approach

This is for lesions where there is a significant suprasellar extension and these techniques lie outside the remit of this book.

### Useful Instruments

1   A Hajek–Kofler punch to remove thick bone. The rotating sleeve allows its jaws to be pointed in any direction and for the handle to be in a comfortable position for the operator.
2   A Kerrison punch allows fine controlled removal of small segments of bone and the slight reversed angle of its jaws helps to remove the back of the vomer.
3   A long-shanked drill with a coarse diamond to remove any bone in the roof of the sphenoid bone in a controlled way.
4   A computer-guided system.

# 15 Skull Base Surgery

We are not advocating that the majority of lesions in and around the skull base should be resected endonasally, but we believe that the endoscope can provide improved access and visibility in specific circumstances without compromising tumor resection. The following circumstances are discussed in this chapter:

- Cerebrospinal fluid (CSF) leaks
- Encephaloceles
- Benign tumors
  - Mucoceles
  - Inverted papilloma
  - Osteoma
  - Hemangioma
  - Angiofibroma
  - Schwannoma
  - Chordoma
  - Chondroma
  - Langerhans cell histiocytosis
  - Pleomorphic adenoma
- Malignant tumors
  - Olfactory neuroblastoma
  - Malignant melanoma
  - Plasmacytoma

The management of tumors of the skull base should be done as part of a multidisciplinary team and the surgeon should be able to undertake an external approach and know how to deal with the majority of possible complications. This includes being able to change to an external approach if necessary. The following principles apply to the planning of endoscopic procedures at the skull base:

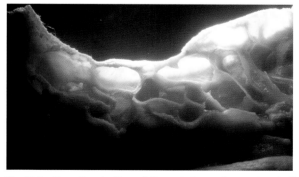

Fig. 15.**1** Transillumination of the anterior and posterior skull base showing how thin the bone can be.

- An understanding of the pathology of any lesion at the skull base is essential in its management.
- Peers from other relevant disciplines should be involved in making a treatment plan.
- An extended range of equipment is needed to do this type of surgery.
- Imaging should be done to define the extent of any tumor and angiography with or without embolization may be necessary.
- Preoperative counseling is very important.

## ■ Management of Skull Base Lesions with a CSF Leak

### Terminology and Classification

A CSF leak results from a breach in the dura, which may be spontaneous, secondary to a fracture, related to surgical trauma, or associated with pathology of the skull base and/or secondary to a high-pressure system (Fig. 15.**1**).

### Indications

The primary reason for repairing a CSF leak is that it is associated with a 10% risk per year of developing meningitis (Eljamel, 1993). There is debate whether a CSF leak resulting from a fracture of the anterior skull base always needs repairing, as a proportion stop spontaneously within 6 weeks (other than those of the posterior wall of the frontal sinus or a large defect, which are unlikely to stop). Those who have a leak repaired electively still have a slightly increased risk of developing meningitis in the future, but this is less than in those whose leak stops spontaneously. In other words, active leaks should probably be repaired at any stage.

### Surgical Anatomy

The skull base is made up anteriorly of the posterior wall of the frontal sinus, which is thick frontal bone that extends posteriorly to form the roof of the ethmoid sinuses (fovea ethmoidalis) on either side of the cribriform plate that comprises part of the ethmoid bone (Fig. 15.**2**). The cribriform plate joins the fovea through the lateral lamella and this can be almost non-

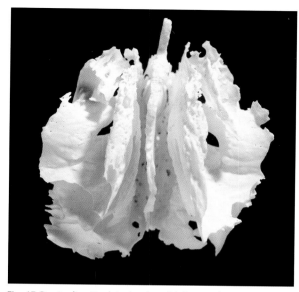

Fig. 15.**2** A disarticulated ethmoid bone showing the cribriform plate with the crista galli above and the vertical plate of the ethmoid below.

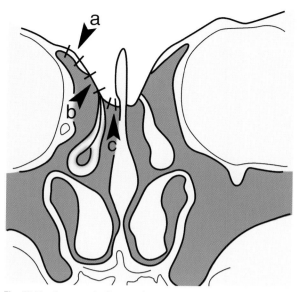

Fig. 15.**3** Arrow **a** indicates the roof of the ethmoid sinuses; arrow **b** indicates the lateral lamella, and arrow **c** indicates the medial aspect of the cribriform plate.

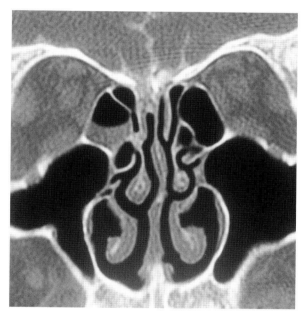

Fig. 15.**4** CSF leak due to a small encephalocele of the right cribriform plate.

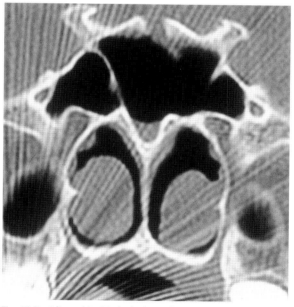

Fig. 15.**5** Idiopathic CSF leak through the posterior wall of the sphenoid sinus near the midline.

existent when the cribriform plate and fovea ethmoidalis are on the same plane, or it can form the thin vertical bone connecting them, depending on how far the cribriform plate dips into the nose (Fig. 15.**3**). Posteriorly, the sphenoid sinus and posterior ethmoidal air cells form the inferior relationship of the skull base.

The commonest site of a spontaneous CSF leak is the area of the cribriform plate where dura around the olfactory nerves appears to have extended through the cribriform plate and ruptured (Fig. 15.**4**). The next most common leak is from a very well-pneumatized sphenoid sinus (Fig. 15.**5**). A high-pressure system may be a contributing factor in these cases and a shunt or ventriculostomy may be required.

CSF leaks complicating intranasal surgery are often found around the lamina lateralis (the vertical

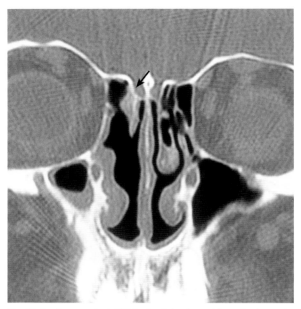

Fig. 15.**6** Postsurgical CSF leak of the lateral lamella (arrow).

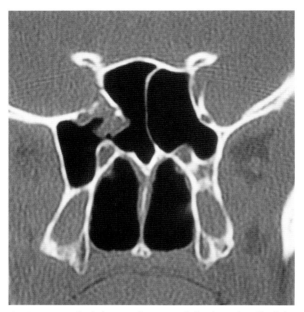

Fig. 15.**7** CSF leak from a fracture of the lateral wall of the sphenoid sinus.

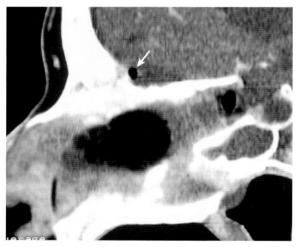

Fig. 15.**8** Sagittal CT scan showing a pneumocephalus (arrow) due to a CSF leak from the posterior wall of the sphenoid sinus after pituitary surgery.

thin bone joining the cribriform plate to the fovea ethmoidalis) near the anterior ethmoid artery (Fig. 15.**6**).

Posttraumatic CSF leaks commonly originate from the cribriform plate, the fovea ethmoidalis, and the posterior wall of the frontal sinus or sphenoid sinus (Fig. 15.**7**). Leaks of the anterior and middle cranial fossa occurring after neurosurgical procedures most commonly follow pituitary surgery (Fig. 15.**8**). Post-

neurosurgical leaks also come from the posterior wall of the frontal sinus when it has not been cranialized, and they are more likely if a pericranial flap has not been used to repair any dural defect.

## Diagnosis

- It is vital to localize the site of a leak (Marshall et al., 2001 a).
- Any fluid should be tested for immunofixation of beta-2-transferrin (Fig. 15.**9 a**, **b**).
- Consider whether there is an underlying high-pressure system.
- Successful closure depends on defining the exact site of any defect.
- No single technique works in all situations.

The glucose oxidase test has a poor predictive value and gives too many false-positive results to be useful in making or excluding this important diagnosis (Bateman and Jones, 2000); it is therefore obsolete. It is very important to confirm the diagnosis with immunofixation of beta-2-transferrin as this is an extremely specific and sensitive test. Unilateral autonomic rhinitis is unusual but it can feign CSF rhinorrhea and this is another reason for confirming the diagnosis as described.

Next, the site of any defect should be defined using high-resolution coronal CT (Lloyd et al., 1994; Simmen et al., 1997). Remember that CT images are made up of an averaging effect and therefore a defect seen on two

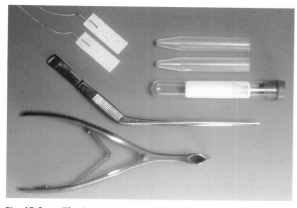

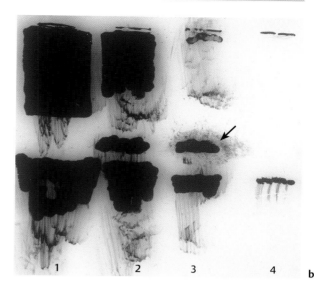

Fig. 15.**9**   **a** The instruments used to collect CSF if none can be collected by the patient. **b** Silver-stained immunofixation of beta-2-transferrin: column 1, the patient's serum; column 2, CSF; column 3, right nostril, positive to beta-2-transferrin (arrow); column 4, left nostril, no beta-2-transferrin.

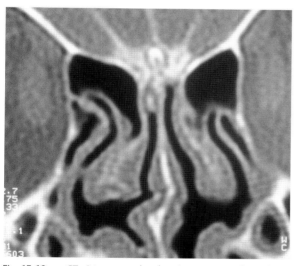

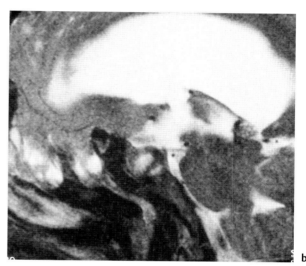

Fig. 15.**10**   **a** CT cisternography showing contrast through the medial aspect of the right cribriform plate. **b** Sagittal MR image showing a CSF leak into the sphenoid sinus.

2 mm slices is likely to be at least 6 mm wide. If CT fails to define the site of the defect, T2-weighted MRI may help (Stafford Johnson et al., 1996). This has superseded CT cisternography (Fig. 15.**10a**, **b**). In a small proportion of patients, the site of the leak is uncertain, or after trauma it could be that there is more than one leak. Under these circumstances, a diagnostic or preoperative fluorescein lumbar puncture will help define the source of the leak (Fig. 15.**11**). The use of a polymedic 24-gauge "pencil point" needle is associated with fewer headaches than the use of standard beveled needles (Bateman et al., 1999) (Fig. 15.**12**). It is vital to ensure that there is a free flow

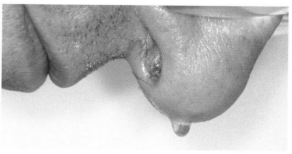

Fig. 15.**11**   Fluorescein stained CSF. This can be used as a diagnostic test to confirm that there is a genuine CSF leak as well as to help localize the site of the leak.

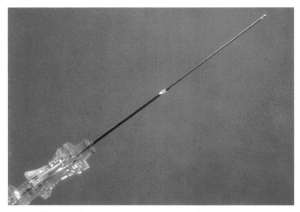

Fig. 15.**12**   A 24 gauge polymedic "pencil point" needle.

of CSF before proceeding to inject any fluorescein. This minimizes the chance of entering the surrounding space and causing arachnoiditis. It is important to aspirate 10 ml of CSF and dilute the fluorescein with it before the fluid is slowly reinjected. Only 0.25–0.5 ml of 5% sodium fluorescein specifically for intrathecal use should be diluted with the CSF before it is reinjected. The ideal time for the fluorescein to be injected is one hour beforehand or alternatively after induction, but time should be allowed for the fluorescein to reach the site of the defect. If the patient is placed in a 10° head-down position this will help. The fluid will appear bright yellow, unless a blue filter is used when it appears fluorescent green (Fig. 15.**13 a–d**).

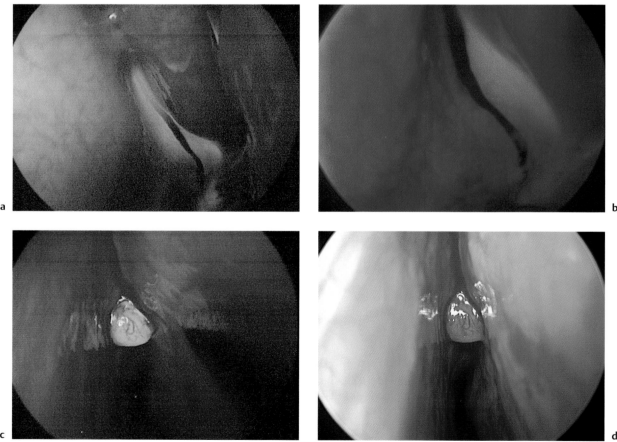

Fig. 15.**13**   **a** The fluorescein tracking down between the middle turbinate and septum. **b** With a blue filter. **c** This was followed upward to reveal a small encephalocele with brightly fluorescein-stained CSF within it. **d** Without filter.

## Surgical Technique

### Graft Materials

Fascia can be harvested from the temporalis muscle, but this is not very thick and it is limited in size. The rectus abdominis provides thicker fascia via a 2 cm incision adjacent to the umbilicus, and fat can also be collected at the same time. Fascia lata is very thick and a large sheet can be harvested along with fat. This can cause a great deal of local discomfort, but it is necessary if there is a large defect. Fascia is preferably used as an underlay, but this is not always possible. Fat is useful to support a graft in position. It can act like glue to hold fascia in place, and it makes fibrin glue unnecessary. It is always wise to harvest a little more than you think you will need. If there is a defect larger then 2 cm, it may be desirable to reinforce the repair with cartilage or bone. Cartilage may be available from the septum. If not, a postauricular approach to the conchal bowl will obtain a good quantity. Bone can be taken from the vomer or the inferior turbinate, but the quality and amount of the latter vary. For a very large defect, a cortical bone graft may be necessary. A good free thick mucosal graft is obtained from a generous inferior turbinectomy and this can be dissected off its underlying bone, but this has to be done with care using nontoothed forceps (Fig. 15.**14**). **DVD** 15

The method used to close a leak is largely determined by the site of the leak.

### A Cribriform Plate Defect

Once the site of the defect has been defined, the mucosa should be gently dissected away, freshening the edges to define the size of the defect. This often reveals a larger bony defect than appeared on CT scans. Most defects in this area can be repaired by fascia or a free nasal mucosal graft from the turbinate (Simmen and Bischoff, 1998) (Fig. 15.**15**). Defects larger then 2 cm can be supported by conchal cartilage overlaid with fascia or mucosa. Some surgeons advocate an "underlay" technique, placing any rigid graft above the bony defect, and placing any mucosal graft under the surrounding mucosa (Fig. 15.**16 a, b**). It is wise not to poke any material intracranially, to minimize the chance of causing hemorrhage.

### Lamella Lateralis

The hardest area to repair is around the lamella lateralis because it is adjacent to the anterior ethmoid artery and the surrounding bone is so thin that any instrumentation in this area often makes the defect bigger. Having freshened the mucosa around the defect, we use an overlay of fascia or turbinate mucosa supported by fat or oxidized cellulose. Another option is to

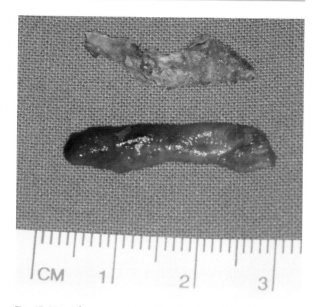

Fig. 15.**14**  A free mucosal graft and slither of bone from an inferior turbinate.

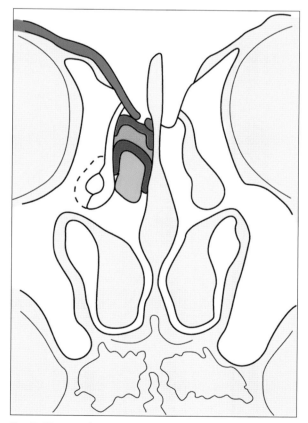

Fig. 15.**15**  Line diagram to show a fascia overlay with free mucosal graft that was secured with oxidized cellulose to close a defect in the cribriform plate.

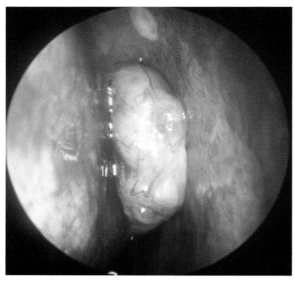
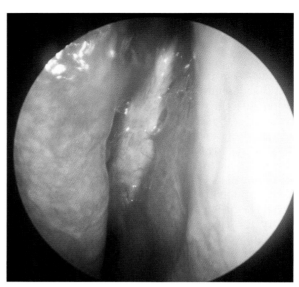

a                                                                                                    b

Fig. 15.**16**   **a** An encephalocele of the medial aspect of the cribriform plate. **b** Two years postoperatively, where a free bone and mucosal graft have been used to seal the leak.

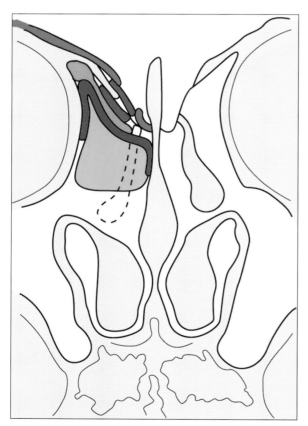

Fig. 15.**17**   A line diagram to show a free mucosal flap used to overlay fascia that has been placed on either side of the defect. The mucosa from the medial part of the middle turbinate can be used to provide a vascularized flap over any repair.

carefully remove part of the middle turbinate having dissected the mucosa off it so that it remains attached medially and then to swing the mucosa laterally over the defect (Figs. 15.**17**, 15.**18 a–c**).

### Ethmoid Roof

Repairing defects in this area is easier because the bone is thicker and the dura is well formed. The principles are the same as for the cribriform plate. It is often easier to insert an underlay graft here because the bone is thick and stable around the defect (Figs. 15.**19 a–d**, 15.**20 a–d**).

### Frontal Sinus

The endoscopic repair of frontal sinus CSF leaks is rarely possible because of reduced access and visibility. Only small defects of the area that can be seen bulging anteriorly when the frontal recess has been opened can be dealt with endoscopically. If there is a lateral defect in the posterior wall of the frontal sinus, this can be dealt with via an extradural approach, minimizing the risk of intracranial complications (Fig. 15.**21 a–d**). Usually a coronal flap with removal of the anterior wall of the frontal sinus allows access to the defect. The pericranium is best preserved and replaced over the bone, which is reattached with miniplates, as trying to swing a bone flap down on attached periosteum usually results in tearing it and it is then of little use. The site of the defect can then be defined and repaired with fascia and fat to hold the graft

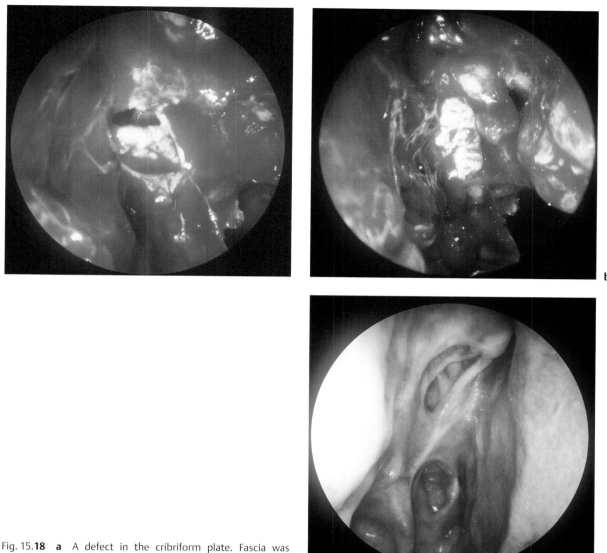

Fig. 15.**18**  **a**  A defect in the cribriform plate. Fascia was placed above it. **b** Fascia overlay over the defect. **c** Endoscopic appearance of the CSF leak repair at 3 years.

in position. If there is severe disruption of the frontal recess, then the frontal sinus is obliterated with fat (it is imperative to remove all underlying sinus mucosa and to drill the bone that is covered by mucosa with a diamond drill in order to avoid leaving any residual mucosa that could lead to the formation of a mucocele) (Weber et al., 1999).

### Sphenoid Sinus

Within the sphenoid sinus most surgeons use fascia supported by fat (Fig. 15.**22 a–c**). The repair is most difficult when the sinus is extremely pneumatized later-

ally into the pterygoid plates; defining its edges is then not easy. In these cases it helps to remove the root of the medial pterygoid plate. In order to do this, the sphenopalatine artery has to be exposed and diathermied. It is important to freshen the edges of any defect before placing a graft, as this seems to be an important part in initiating the repair process.

### Packing and Aftercare

Whatever graft is used, it is normally supported by fat or oxidized cellulose; some surgeons use an antiseptic pack to support this. An overnight stay in hospital is

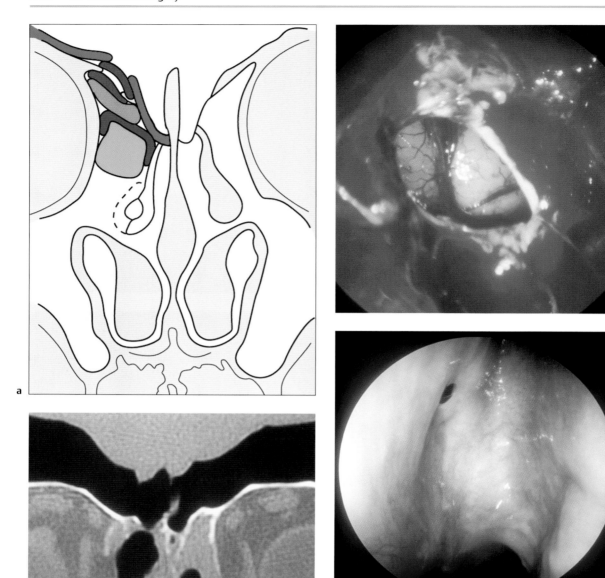

Fig. 15.**19    a**   Line diagram of fascia underlay/overlay covered by a free mucosal graft. **b** Defect in the roof of the right ethmoid sinuses. **c** CT scan of the defect in the roof of the right ethmoid sinuses with pneumocephalus. **d** Postoperative appearance after repair of the CSF leak at 2 years.

required following the procedure and the only morbidity experienced by the patient is if a nasal pack is left in situ. A broad-spectrum antibiotic such as co-amoxiclav is given for 10 days postoperatively. We do not routinely use lumbar drains following transnasal endoscopic repair of CSF leaks. The patients are advised to avoid straining, to sneeze with their mouth open, and not to stifle sneezes, so as to avoid any abrupt increases in intranasal pressure, for one month following repair.   **DVD** 15

## Comment

It appears that most endoscopic techniques produce a success rate of approximately 90% after one attempt, which compares favorably with the transcranial tech-

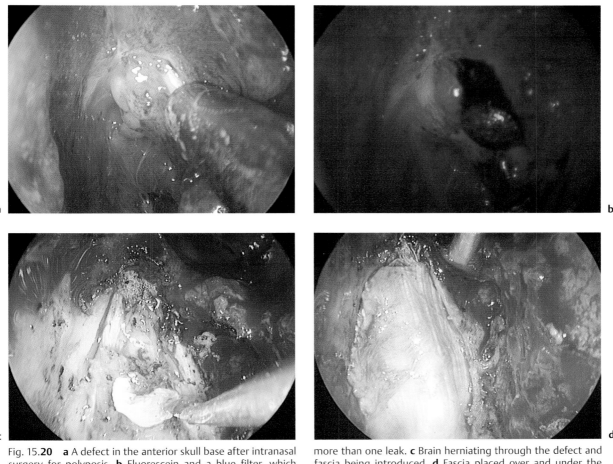

Fig. 15.**20**   **a** A defect in the anterior skull base after intranasal surgery for polyposis. **b** Fluorescein and a blue filter, which helped to define the extent of the leak and show that there was more than one leak. **c** Brain herniating through the defect and fascia being introduced. **d** Fascia placed over and under the skull base defect.

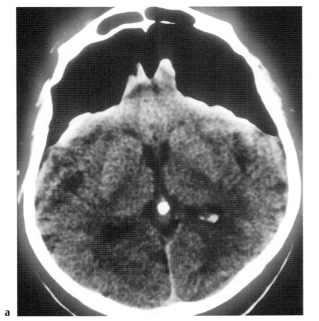

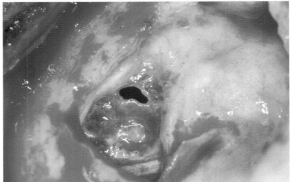

Fig. 15.**21**   **a** Extensive pneumocephalus due to a fracture involving the posterior wall of the frontal sinus. **b** Transfrontal osteoplastic approach to define the defect in the posterior wall of the frontal sinus.

Fig. 15.**21**   **c**, **d**   ▷

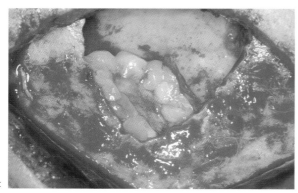

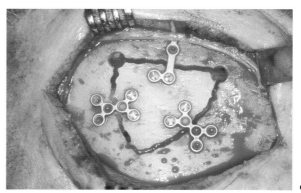

c

d

Fig. 15.**21**   **c** Fascia and fat overlay grafts. Note that the incision was done through a forehead crease in an elderly man. **d** Plating of the osteoplastic flap.

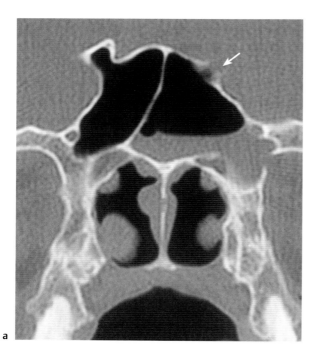

a

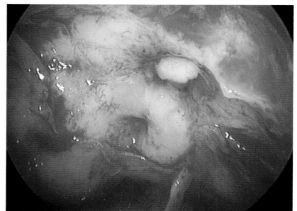

b

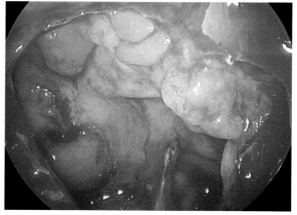

c

Fig. 15.**22**   **a** Coronal CT scan with a defect in the sphenoid sinus (arrow). **b** Fascia plug into the defect between the optic nerve and carotid artery. **c** Fascia and fat overlay in the lateral wall of the sphenoid sinus.

niques that have a success rate of approximately 75 % (Jones, 2001 b; Simmen et al., 1998). The endoscopic repair of anterior and sphenoid CSF leaks or encephaloceles is now the treatment of choice in most of these lesions. A recent meta-analysis (Hegazy et al., 2000) confirms this view. It reduces the significant morbidity and mortality associated with a transcranial approach (loss of sense of smell, length of inpatient stay, epilepsy, cerebral edema, frontal lobe dysfunction, osteomyelitis of the frontal bone flap and rarely, but importantly, postoperative intracranial hemorrhage). An extradural approach is often needed for defects of the posterior wall of the frontal sinus as these may not be accessible endoscopically. Defects larger

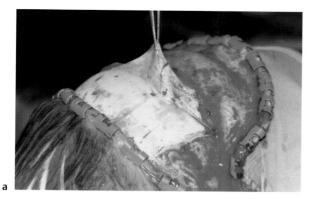

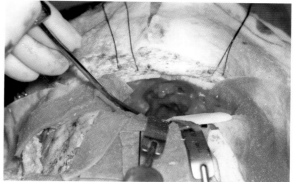

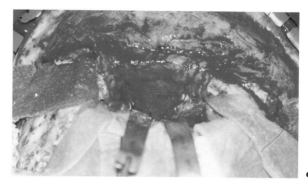

Fig. 15.**23**   **a** Raising a pericranial flap. **b** Cranialization of the frontal sinus in an anterior skull base tumor. Note that the posterior wall of the frontal sinus and *all* the frontal sinus mucosa have been removed. **c** The pericranial flap in position.

than 5 cm cannot readily be managed endoscopically (Fig. 15.23 a–c). If there is an associated malignancy or an extensive cosmetic deformity, then craniofacial surgery needs to be done in conjunction with repair of a leak. The majority of other CSF leaks are highly amenable to an endoscopic repair.

## Modifications and Alternatives

If a CSF leak occurs in conjunction with a tumor of the skull base or a severe skull base fracture, a craniotomy and removal of the posterior wall of the frontal sinus and its lining, along with reconstruction of the anterior wall of the frontal sinus with split calvarial bone, is indicated (Donald, 1982). The use of a pericranial flap to cover any dural defect reduces the incidence of postoperative CSF leaks.

## ◼ Encephaloceles

## Terminology and Classification

An encephalocele is a herniation of a part of the intracranial contents through a defect in the skull. Encephaloceles may present as obvious malformations or they may be occult and only come to light following a complication. Basal encephaloceles can be classified on the basis of their location into: transethmoidal (Fig. 15.24 a, b), sphenoethmoidal, transsphenoidal, frontosphenoidal, or rarely basioccipital-nasopharyngeal. Encephaloceles may be congenital in origin and represent a primary anomaly of the neural tube and its skeletal cover. Acquired encephaloceles may be posttraumatic (Fig. 15.25 a, b) or follow neurosurgery or sinonasal surgery.

## Indications

People with encephaloceles have an increased risk of developing meningitis, particularly if there is an active CSF leak. From the anterior skull base, the encephalocele can be large enough to cause nasal obstruction. Encephaloceles can be associated with craniofacial abnormalities requiring surgery in their own right.

## Surgical Anatomy

The neck of the encephalocele may be small (Fig. 15.26) with a large sac whose content may vary in extent, but any brain tissue within it is likely to be nonfunctioning unless the sac is sessile and very broad based.

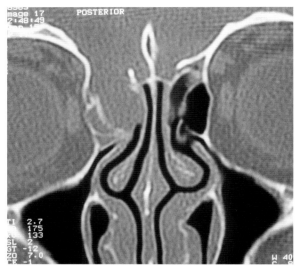

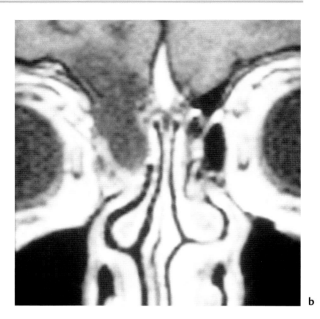

Fig. 15.**24** **a** CT and **b** MR images showing an encephalocele of the roof of the right ethmoid sinuses.

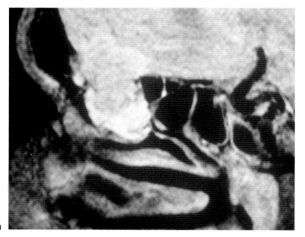

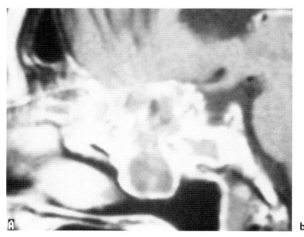

Fig. 15.**25** **a** Sagittal MR image of a posttraumatic frontoethmoidal encephalocele. **b** Sagittal MR image of a sphenoethmoid encephalocele 20 years after skull base radiotherapy.

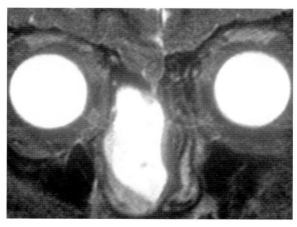

◁ Fig. 15.**26** Sagittal MR image of an encephalocele in a child successfully closed endoscopically.

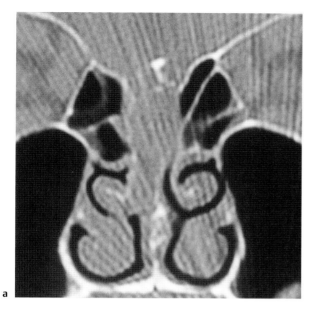
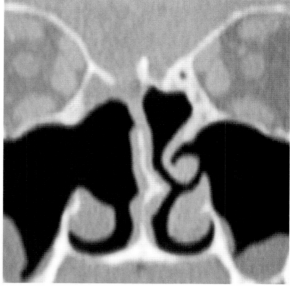
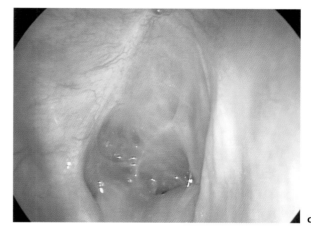

Fig. 15.**27 a**, **b**  Coronal CT scans of a right ethmoid roof encephalocele preoperatively (**a**) and postoperatively (**b**) with the defect having been repaired with an underlay and overlay fascia graft. **c** The endoscopic view following the repair at 3 years.

## Surgical Technique

Outpatient nasendoscopy and a high-resolution coronal CT scan can help define the site and size of any bony defect. MRI is of particular benefit in defining the contents of the sac and the vascularity of its contents.

The surgical technique is similar to that described previously for the treatment of CSF rhinorrhea. The neck of the encephalocele is identified and any overlying mucosa is removed, although the sac has usually become so distended that the mucosa is not distinguishable from the dura. If the size of the sac limits access to define its neck, the sac can be incised and thereby deflated. It is then possible to resect the sac up to the site of the defect. The encephalocele is then excised and the edges of the bony defect are freshened.

The encephalocele should be excised as the neural tissue within it is redundant, and by reducing it intracranially the possibility of a septic focus is introduced (Marshall et al., 2001 b). The remaining dural defect is then repaired exactly as described in repairing a CSF leak (Fig. 15.**27 a–c**).

## Alternative Surgical Techniques

There is a role for extracranial techniques where there is an extensive defect, further cosmetic craniofacial reconstruction is needed, or it is not possible to visualize the defect.

Where there is a large defect or multiple defects of the skull base, an external transethmoidal approach

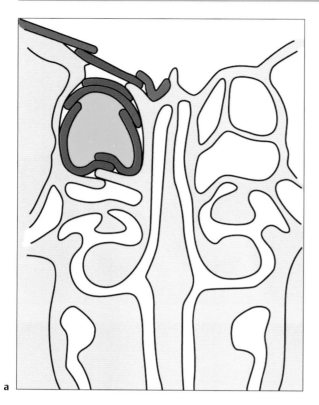

a

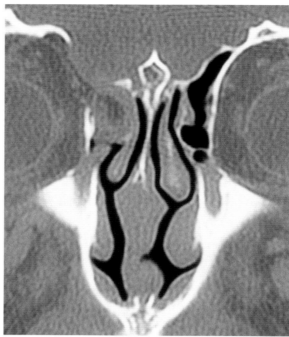

b

Fig. 15.**28** **a** Line diagram of a transfrontoethmoid partial fat obliteration for extensive defects with preservation of the olfactory mucosa. **b** Postoperative CT scan.

followed by peeling down the mucosa from around the defect, be it the septum or the middle turbinate, exposes the defect, which is then covered by fascia and fat before the unpeeled mucosa is replaced (Simmen et al., 1998) (Figs. 15.**28**a, b, 15.**29**a–c).

Traditionally, encephaloceles have been treated neurosurgically via a transcranial approach, which is associated with significant morbidity: a loss of sense of smell, postoperative intracerebral hemorrhage, cerebral edema, epilepsy, frontal lobe dysfunction with memory and concentration deficits, and potential osteomyelitis of the frontal bone flap. In addition to these risks, repair by this technique requires 5–7 days in hospital, hair loss along the incision line, and a period off driving postoperatively.

A transcranial approach remains the method of choice in combination with an extracranial approach for large congenital lesions over 5 cm in diameter and when cosmetic craniofacial reconstruction is needed.

A transpalatal or a sublabial transseptal approach can be used to repair transsphenoidal encephaloceles. The morbidity of these techniques is less than in an intracranial approach, but they are associated with a longer hospital stay of several days, more soft-tissue trauma and discomfort, and the risk of a septal perforation or disruption to palatal muscles.

## ■ The Role of Endonasal Surgery in Benign Tumors

### General Principles

- Be sure that you are certain about the pathology of the lesion (particularly if surgery has the potential to cause any significant morbidity).
- Beware of other pathology that can simulate benign and malignant neoplasms, for example, inflammatory polyps, fungal infection, Wegener granulomatosis, sarcoid, and rhinoscleroma (Jones, 1999 b).
- Excision depends on a thorough knowledge of the surgical anatomy:
  - Ensure adequate access and visibility.
  - Ensure that you do not damage surrounding vital structures.
  - If it is a vascular lesion, make sure that bleeding can be controlled.
- Be able to convert to an open approach if necessary.
- The fact that a lesion is benign does not mean that it should not be completely resected, with few exceptions: e.g., where resection would lead to unacceptable morbidity or risk mortality such as in fibrous dysplasia of the skull base, where complete

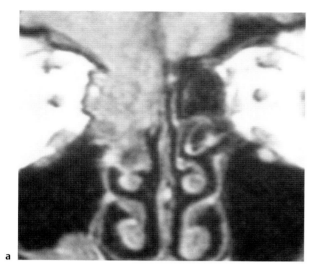

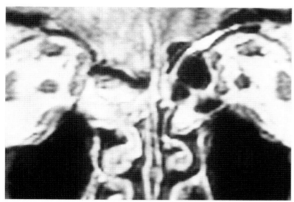

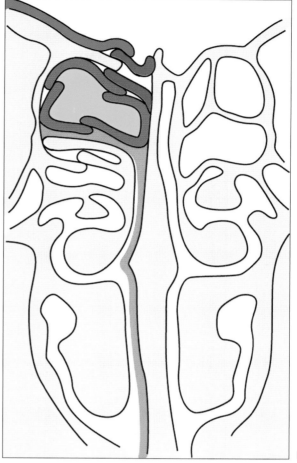

Fig. 15.**29**   **a** Coronal MR image of right ethmoid encephalocele. **b** Line diagram of transfrontoethmoid partial fat obliteration for large defects without preservation of olfactory mucosa.

**c** Postoperative coronal MR image showing fat that was used to support the repair of the skull base defect.

resection is often not possible without causing damage to one or more cranial nerves or major vessels.

- Weigh the pros and cons of intervening: for example, mild cosmetic asymmetry in many patients with fibrous dysplasia, against the morbidity of surgery.
- Have good preoperative imaging (this includes angiography in most vascular lesions).
- Endoscopy often has the potential to reduce the morbidity of surgery, but it may not necessarily be the best approach if it compromises the margin of resection.
- Surgery for most benign lesions depends on its anatomical site; sites can broadly be grouped into the following areas:
  - Cribriform plate and fovea ethmoidalis
  - Frontal sinus
  - Ethmoid complex and orbit
  - Maxillary sinus, lateral nasal wall
  - Pterygopalatine fossa
  - Sphenoid sinus, clivus, and cavernous sinus

## Specific Conditions

### Mucoceles

The majority of mucoceles can be marsupialized endoscopically with minimal morbidity and with long-term results that are as good as, if not better than, those done by a conventional external approach. Concerns that the marsupialization of mucoceles may not halt their expansion have been found to be unwarranted. Mucoceles accessible with the endoscope should be opened as widely as possible using through-cutting forceps in order to minimize the amount of scar tissue that forms around the edges, and which might lead to a recurrence (Fig. 15.**30 a–d**). The wider a mucocele is marsupialized, the better (Fig. 15.**31 a**, **b**).

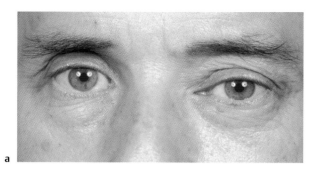

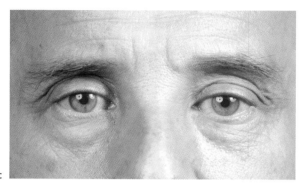

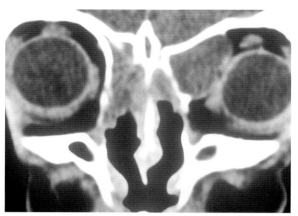

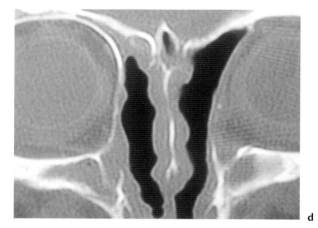

Fig. 15.**30**   **a** Displacement of the left orbit due to a mucocele. **b** Coronal CT scan—note typical lateralized remnant of the middle turbinate after previous surgery for polyposis. **c** Postoperative view after endoscopic marsupialization of the mucocele. **d** Postoperative CT scan following endoscopic drainage of the mucocele.

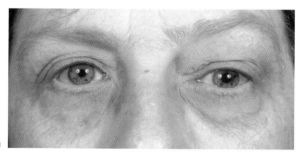

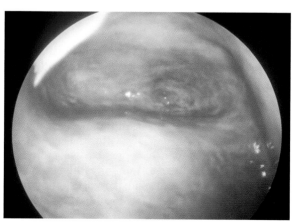

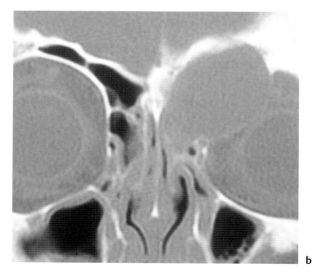

Fig. 15.**31**   **a** Displaced left eye due to a frontoethmoidal mucocele. **b** Coronal CT scan of a left frontoethmoid mucocele. **c** Endoscopic view into the marsupialized mucocele once its contents have been aspirated.

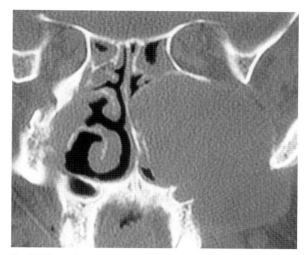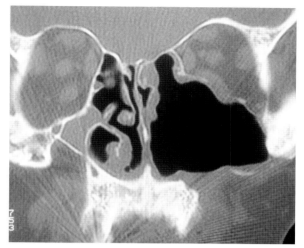

Fig. 15.**32** **a** Preoperative and **b** postoperative coronal CT scans of a left maxillary sinus mucocele.

Maxillary sinus mucoceles are less common. Most mucoceles can be marsupialized well with the endoscope except for those lying in the lateral aspect of the frontal sinus (Figs. 15.**32 a**, **b**; 15.**33**), those that are secondary to malignancy (which will require an en bloc resection and a craniofacial resection), and those that are secondary to pathology such as Paget disease or fibrous dysplasia that makes an endoscopic approach technically difficult or puts the eye or dura at an increased risk (Beasley and Jones, 1995 b). Once a frontal and/or ethmoidal mucocele has been marsupialized, the expanded "shell" of bone that remains can often be pushed manually in order to correct any bony swelling that may cause a cosmetic defect or displacement of the orbit. Some posteriorly placed mucoceles leave the orbit displaced even after marsupialization, and then the orbit will need to be decompressed by removing its lateral wall as in an orbital decompression (Conboy and Jones, 2003). **DVD** 10

Accordingly, mucoceles that are unsuitable for an endoscopic approach include:

- Hypertrophic bone in the area of the frontal recess.
- Revision surgery where the previous operation was an external fronto-ethmoidectomy, and if the recurrence is located lateral to the area that is accessible even via a median drainage procedure.
- A laterally placed frontal mucocele.
- Malignancy associated with a mucocele.

### Inverted Papilloma

It is important to exclude any coexisting malignancy or atypia present at diagnosis as these occur in 8–15% of cases on presentation, and these justify an en bloc resection with possible radiotherapy, depending on the histology and degree of invasion (Fig. 15.**34 a**, **b**). It is

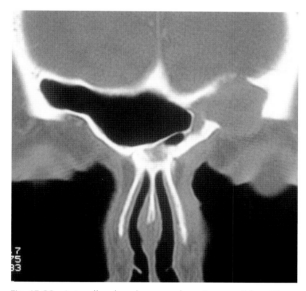

Fig. 15.**33** Laterally placed mucocele not accessible with an endoscope.

important that all macroscopically diseased tissue is examined in order to avoid malignancy being missed (Fig. 15.**35 a–d**).

The management of lesions without malignancy or atypia is more contentious, as the orthodox view has been that wide excision leads to reduced recurrence rates and a reduced risk of malignant transformation. A review of the world literature shows that, while malignant transformation does occur, it is very unusual (Jones, 1998 b).

The main determinant of the endonasal approach in benign lesions is the extent of disease and whether it

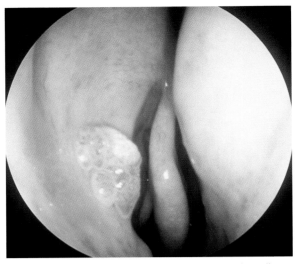
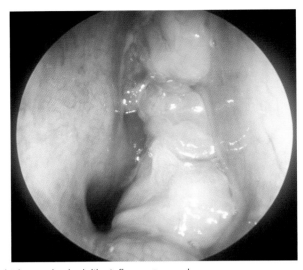

Fig. 15.**34 a**, **b** Endoscopic appearance of inverted papilloma, which can also look like inflammatory polyps.

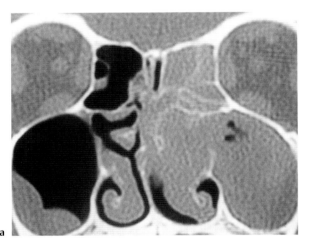
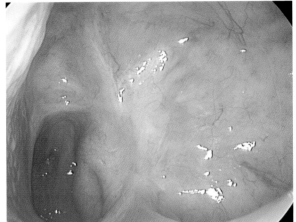

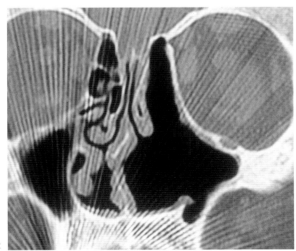
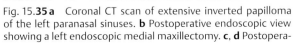
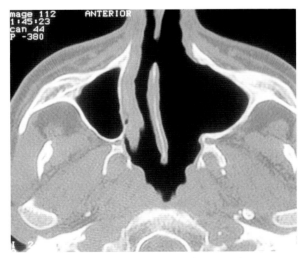

Fig. 15.**35 a** Coronal CT scan of extensive inverted papilloma of the left paranasal sinuses. **b** Postoperative endoscopic view showing a left endoscopic medial maxillectomy. **c**, **d** Postopera- tive coronal (**c**) and axial (**d**) CT scans after an endoscopic me- dial maxillectomy.

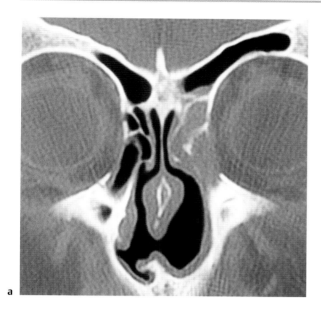

a

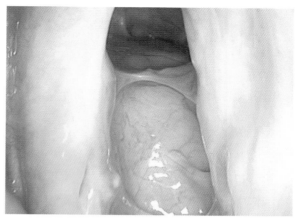

b

Fig. 15.**36** **a** Preoperative CT scan and **b** postoperative endo-scopic view of an inverted papilloma of the left ethmoid sinuses and frontal recess.

is possible to remove all macroscopic disease. This is one circumstance when the edict that mucosa should be preserved at all costs does not apply, and success is influenced by the ability to remove all the diseased mucosa. It is now recognized that when there is *no* malignancy it is purely a mucosal disease and that the likelihood of cure depends not only on the removal of all macroscopically diseased tissue but also on host immunity and resistance. It is associated with human papilloma viruses 16 and 11; these probably alter the mucosa's genome and they may also be present in some tissue that has yet to show macroscopic evidence of disease.

The authors have operated on patients with very extensive disease (many previous procedures involving all sinuses bilaterally, and the septum) and, in spite of thorough attempts to remove all diseased tissue, have felt that they had not been successful. However, some of these patients have then been disease free while others have had very limited residual disease reappear, but surprisingly not affecting a number of areas where a reappearance of disease was anticipated. This has led us to believe that there is also an immunological aspect to this disease that affects prognosis. Perhaps a reduction in tumor antigen load in these patients after surgery may help eradicate any residual disease. Smaller lesions may not only be more readily excised but may represent better host immunity.

Recurrence rates are often quoted as being over 30 % and this of course represents residual disease. The most difficult areas for excision are the frontal sinus

(Fig. 15.36 a, b), the anterior wall of the maxilla, and the nasolacrimal system.

There are now several series that show similar results from both endoscopic and more radical surgery (Waitz and Wigand, 1992; Tufano et al., 1999; Chee and Sethi, 1999), although others have shown better results with more radical surgery (Mansell and Bates, 2000). Endoscopic surveillance is needed after excision, allowing any recurrence to be excised early in order to limit its spread (Fig. 15.37 a, b). The authors have never seen a recurrence when endoscopy has been clear for 3 years and we have 90 % who are disease free after a mean of 10 years following endoscopic medial maxillectomy (Kraft et al., 2003). There are many reports of disease appearing long after excision, but these come from the pre-endoscopic era. **DVD** 14

### Osteoma

Approximately 3 % of people have paranasal sinus osteomas according to Earwacker (1993). In his series of 1500 CT scans, only two patients were symptomatic. This is the authors' experience. Many osteomas are found incidentally and are blamed for causing headaches or excision is recommended before they cause symptoms (Hehar and Jones, 1997). In practice, osteomas rarely cause any problems other than cosmetic. If they do cause symptoms by obstructing the frontal recess, their history should include symptoms that are worse after upper respiratory tract infections and there should be endoscopic and CT scan signs of mucosal disease (Fig. 15.38 a–c). All too often tension-

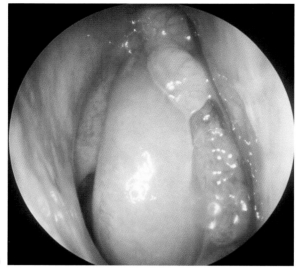

a

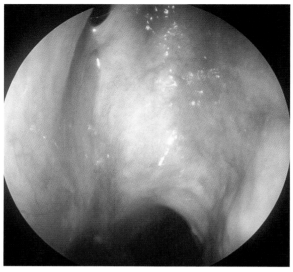

b

Fig. 15.**37**   **a** Inverted papilloma in the olfactory cleft and **b** appearance 7 years later after resection. The mucosa was removed and the CSF leak created was repaired with a fascia overlay graft.

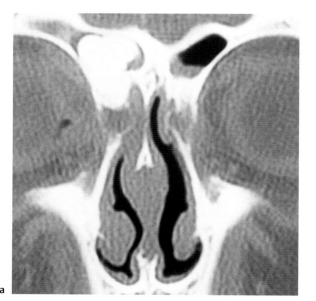

a

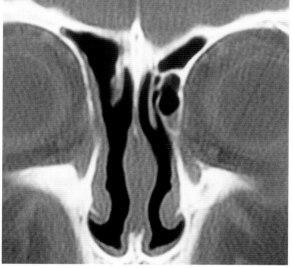

b

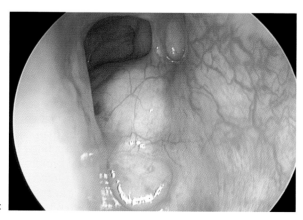

c

Fig. 15.**38**   **a** Osteoma obstructing the right frontal recess; note whether there is evidence of other paranasal sinus pathology, otherwise reconsider the need to operate. **b** Postoperative CT scan and **c** endoscopic view.

type headaches are blamed on an osteoma that is coincidental.

The removal of osteomas depends on how accessible they are (Schick et al., 2001) (Fig. 15.**39**). The endoscope can be used to shell out the osteoma and then its walls can be removed or fractured inwards. As the most symptomatic ones are in the frontal recess, it is important to reconstruct the mucosal lining with a septal flap or a free mucosal graft or to combine their removal with a median drainage procedure.

### Hemangioma

Most hemangiomas that appear in childhood involute spontaneously and no intervention is required. Occasionally they can enlarge, endangering vital structures, and then steroids or interferon alfa-2 have a role (Ezekowitz et al., 1992). Later in life, smaller capillary, venous, or cavernous hemangiomas can present, often with epistaxis. They can originate from the septum or the turbinates and alarm the patient and primary care physician, who may suspect malignancy. They can emulate pyogenic granulomas (granuloma gravidarum, which is due to a florid reaction as a result of local trauma, typically in the third trimester of pregnancy) (Fig. 15.**40 a–d**). Outpatient endoscopic examination along with gentle palpation with a round-ended probe will help make the diagnosis as this will help define its base and differentiate it from a hemorrhagic tumor originating from the skull base or lateral nasal wall (Fig. 15.**41 a–c**). All these lesions are readily removed endoscopically after infiltration and by taking a margin of tissue around the lesion. More ex-

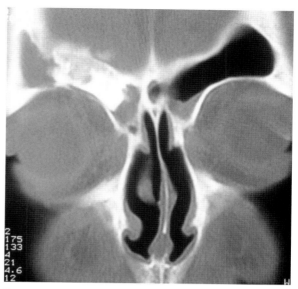

Fig. 15.**39**  Laterally placed osteoma not accessible endoscopically. Note that there is disease present, otherwise surgery would rarely be justified.

tensive hemangioma should not be removed surgically unless imaging, including angiography, has shown that resection and vascular control are possible. These lesions often require major surgery, sometimes with preoperative embolization, and they are not suitable for endoscopic excision. Their blood vessels do not contract and the bleeding that can occur with their removal can be life-threatening. (Fig. 15.**42 a–d**).

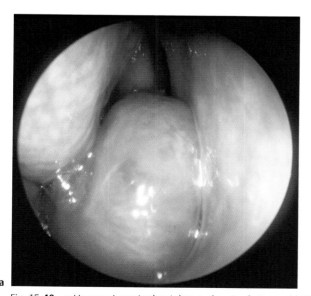

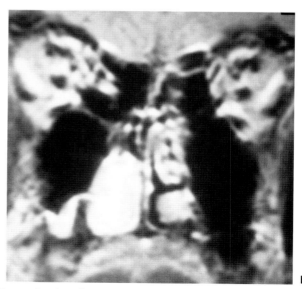

Fig. 15.**40**  **a** Hemangioma in the right nasal cavity. **b** Coronal MR image showing a hemangioma coming from the sphenopalatine artery.

Fig. 15.**40**  **c, d**  ▷

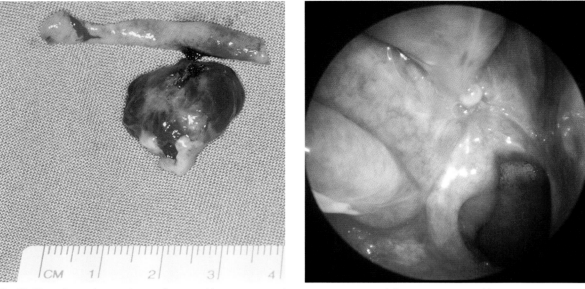

Fig. 15.**40** **c** Operative specimen of resected hemangioma. **d** Postoperative cavity following resection of hemangioma.

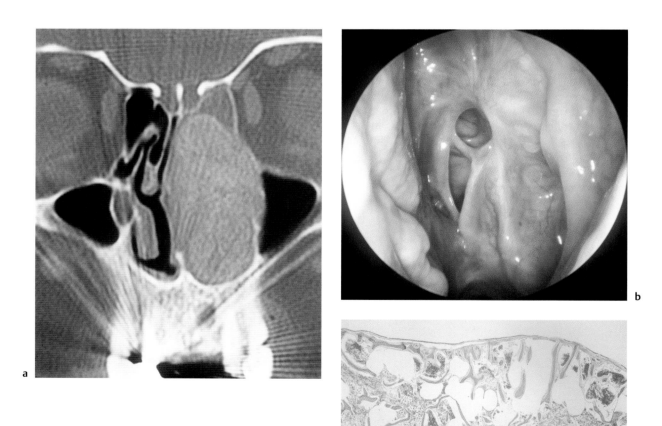

Fig. 15.**41** **a** Coronal CT scan of a left cavernous hemangio-osteoma. **b** Postoperative cavity after resection of cavernous hemangio-osteoma. **c** Histology showing a hemangio-osteoma.

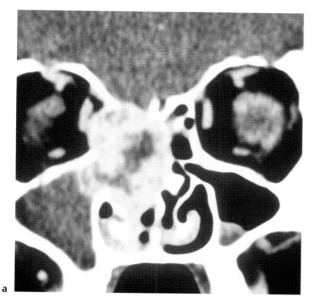

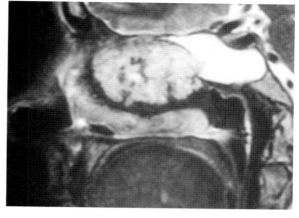

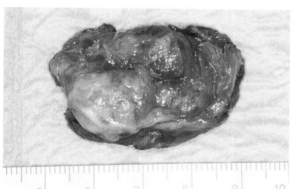

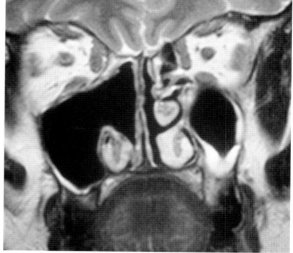

Fig. 15.**42** **a** Coronal CT scan of giant pyogenic granuloma that has eroded the skull base. **b** Sagittal MR image showing sizable vessels within the pyogenic granuloma. **c** Operative specimen of pyogenic granuloma. **d** Postoperative coronal MR image scan following resection of pyogenic granuloma.

## Angiofibroma

Angiofibromas originate from the sphenopalatine foramen at the junction of the sphenoid process of the palatine bone and the pterygoid process of the sphenoid. Whether endoscopic excision of an angiofibroma is possible depends on its size, on knowledge of its blood supply, and on whether it can be embolized safely (Fig. 15.**43 a–e**). It is not possible to excise them endoscopically without preoperative embolization. Total removal depends on accessibility and control of their blood supply. The conventional approaches are via a lateral rhinotomy and medial maxillectomy, midfacial degloving (Price et al., 1988) or transpalatally (Sessions et al., 1993). Larger lesions require the addition of a lateral infratemporal approach.

Angiofibromas at stage Ia, IIa or IIb according to Fisch may be suitable for endoscopic excision (Ene-pekides, 2004). These lesions comprise only a fifth of all angiofibromas (Newlands et al., 1999). It is important that any surgeon embarking on an endoscopic resection should be able to convert to an open approach as bleeding can necessitate this. It is also important to have blood saved and at least six units of blood cross-matched and to have access to fresh frozen plasma.

Endoscopic resection consists of a type III maxillary sinusotomy, an ethmoidectomy, and removal of the posterior wall of the maxillary sinus in order to define and clip the terminal branches of the maxillary artery and its sphenopalatine branches. The sphenoid is opened if access is possible and then the lesion is removed. The aim is to remove the whole lesion in one piece, but it is often removed in several pieces. It is often necessary to pack and apply pressure to the area

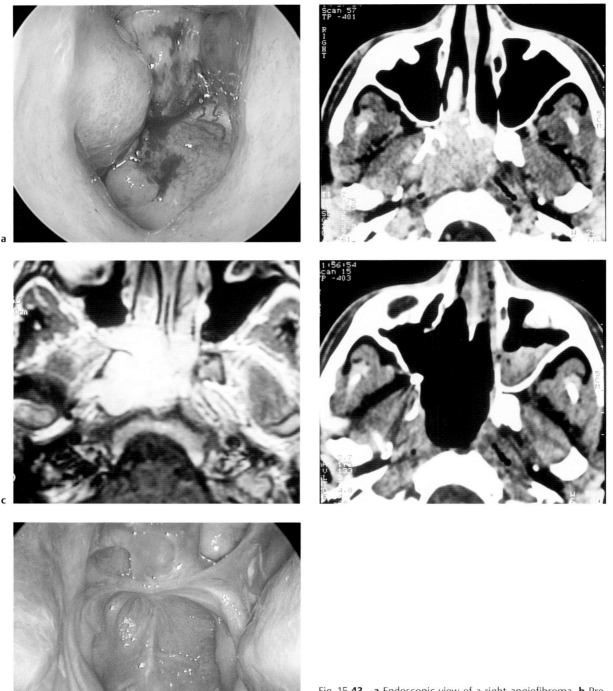

Fig. 15.**43**    **a** Endoscopic view of a right angiofibroma. **b** Preoperative axial CT scan with contrast. **c** Preoperative MR image and **d** postoperative axial CT scans. **e** Endoscopic view at 3 years after resection of angiofibroma.

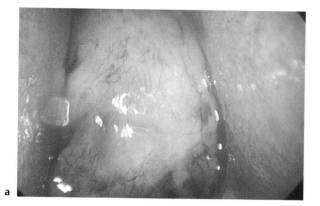

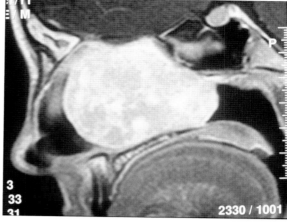

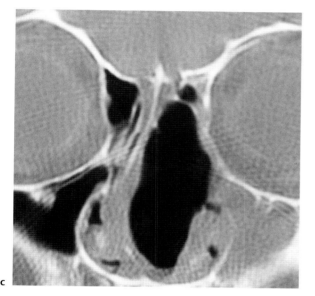

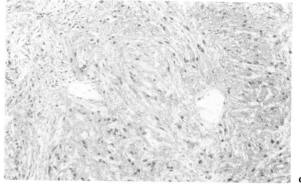

Fig. 15.**44    a** Left schwannoma based on the sphenoethmoid recess. **b** Sagittal MR image of schwannoma. **c** Postoperative coronal CT scan. A septoplasty was needed to help get around the lesion. **d** Histology, showing a schwannoma.

temporarily in order to reduce bleeding before the next attempt is made to remove any remnant. Large suckers are needed to remove enough blood quickly and allow the lateral wall to be visualized. A suction catheter passed through the other nostril into the nasopharynx also reduces the reservoir of blood in the nasopharynx and helps visibility. The main problem area is removing disease that goes behind and lateral to the pterygoid plates and clivus. The 45° endoscope helps visualize this area, but bleeding often limits this. This is one of the areas where it helps to have one surgeon holding the endoscope while the other has two hands free.

Concern has been expressed that preoperative embolization can lead to a higher recurrence rate by reducing bleeding from the tumor, which often has no defined capsule, and this makes it more likely that a remnant will be left behind (McCoombe et al., 1990). It is rarely possible to resect an angiofibroma endoscopi-

cally without pre-embolization, and we recommend that it is done.

### Schwannoma

Unusual isolated lesions can occasionally be resected endoscopically, but their suitability for this approach depends on their extent and site (Fig. 15.**44**a–d).

### Chordoma

Chordomas often present late with neurological or ophthalmological symptoms, but occasionally they present earlier with nasal symptoms of obstruction or epistaxis. CT scanning and MRI are important in assessing their extent. Biopsy must differentiate it from a chondrosarcoma. Large lesions often require a transfacial approach, access via a Le Fort I osteotomy, or lower lesions by a mandibular split. Some anterior le-

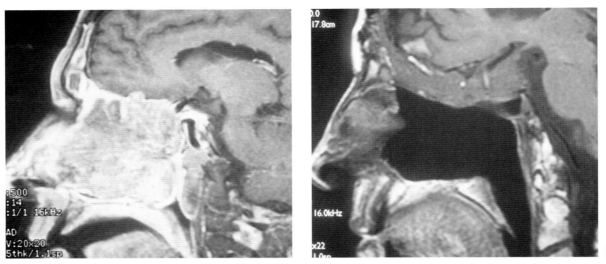

Fig. 15.**45**  **a** Preoperative and **b** postoperative sagittal MRI views of a chordoma subtotally removed endoscopically.

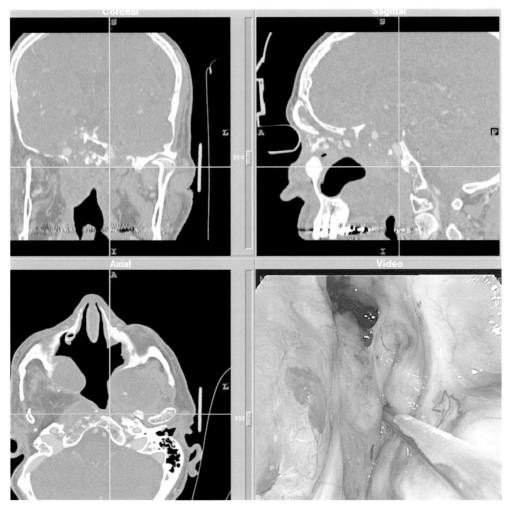

Fig. 15.**46**  Peroperative view using computer-aided surgery in a recurrent chordoma removed because of deteriorating vision. Note its faint yellow color.

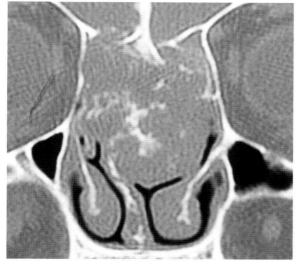

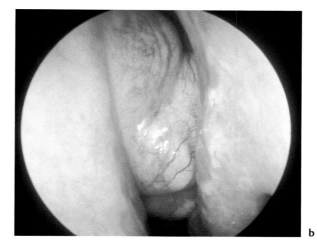

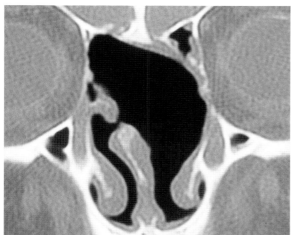

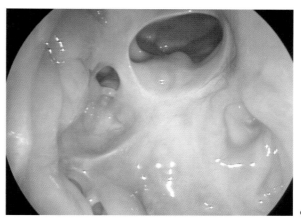

Fig. 15.**47**  **a** Coronal CT scan of an anterior skull base chondroma. **b** Endoscopic appearance of a chordoma. **c** Postoperative coronal CT scan and **d** endoscopic appearance after resection of chordoma.

sions based on the anterior aspect of the sphenoid can largely be removed endoscopically (Fig. 15.**45 a**, **b**), although it is relatively unusual to be able to excise them completely (Fig. 15.**46**). This approach normally involves a bilateral sphenoid sinusotomy type III when the sphenoidotomy is extended to the floor of the sinus and laterally to the vital structures. The carotid arteries and optic nerves can almost be skeletonized using a long-shanked drill and a well-irrigated coarse diamond burr.

Chordomas are moderately radiosensitive and radiotherapy is often done in conjunction with surgery. Cure is rare as recurrence is common, and while the long-term prognosis is poor they often grow slowly and patients can live for several years.

### Chondroma

Chondromas can be localized to the ethmoid sinuses, maxilla, or septum and can be amenable to endoscopic removal (Fig. 15.**47 a–d**). If they are large and spread outside the paranasal sinuses, they may need to be excised via a lateral rhinotomy or midfacial degloving.

### Langerhans Cell Histiocytosis

These lesions are rare in the paranasal sinuses and in adults they are normally self-limiting. Intralesional steroids can be used but are rarely necessary. In children under 2 years, it is an unpleasant multisystem disorder that requires chemotherapeutic agents.

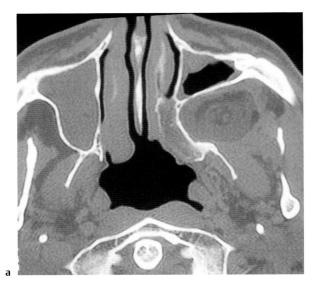

a

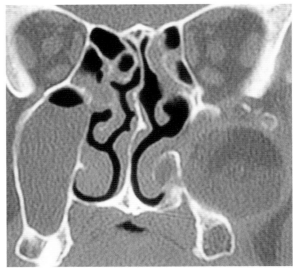

b

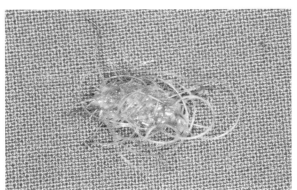

c

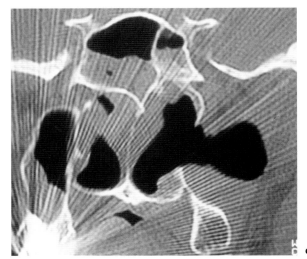

d

Fig. 15.**48**   **a** Axial and **b** coronal CT scans of a left pterygo-palatine fossa teratoma. **c** Operative specimen and **d** post-operative coronal CT scan after resection of pterygopalatine fossa teratoma.

### Pleomorphic Adenoma

When pleomorphic adenomas occur they can be found in the septum and can be excised endoscopically with a small but macroscopically clear margin to leave a perforation. This can be inspected for recurrence and reconstructed after a disease-free interval. When removing one of these lesions, it is particularly important to have a clear margin and remove it in one piece, otherwise recurrence is likely.

### Other Benign Pathological Lesions

Almost every type of benign lesion has been reported in the paranasal sinuses (Harrison and Lund, 1993).

Apart from the lesions mentioned, surgical management usually depends on the anatomical site (Fig. 15.**48** a–d). **DVD** 16

## Surgical Approaches for Benign Paranasal and Skull Base Lesions

### Lesions of the Cribriform Plate and Fovea Ethmoidalis

Preoperative imaging to define the extent of the disease and in particular the extent of any intracranial involvement is vital. Surgery to resect lesions in this area should be done where there are the expertise and the facilities to do a craniotomy if necessary or to deal

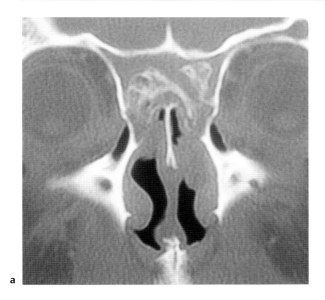

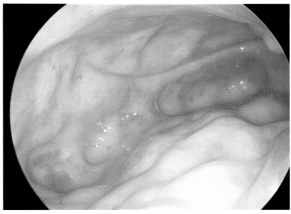

Fig. 15.**49**  **a** Preoperative coronal CT scan showing extensive inverted papilloma in the frontal sinus and characteristic calcification within it. **b** Postoperative endoscopic view of the frontal sinuses 3 years after a median drainage procedure.

with any intracranial complications, although these should be rare.

Otologists are familiar with the dura, both operating next to it and dealing with it when it is damaged. Rhinologists may be less comfortable dealing with exactly the same problems, but tears to the dura are readily dealt with (see section on the management of CSF leaks in Chapter 15, p. 240). The main surgical principles are:

- Define the extent of the lesion (this in part relies on radiology).
- Establish a preoperative plan that will enable the lesion to be removed safely, but also anticipate what problems may be faced and how they might be dealt with. For example, an anterior skull base defect may be created that is larger than might have been desired. Ideally patient consent should be obtained in such a way that they have been warned of this possibility. A graft of fascia or chondral or septal cartilage may be needed to close any defect.
- Gain surgical control by defining the margins of the lesion.
- Do not grab and twist any bone attached to the anterior skull base—including the lesion—as this may fracture the skull base unpredictably.
- Reconstruct any defect (see the sections Management of Skull Base Lesions with a CSF Leak and Encephaloceles, Chapter 15).
- Bleeding and reduced visibility are the main causes of poor surgical technique. It is worth taking time and using topical vasoconstrictors such as 1 : 10 000 epinephrine on a neurosurgical patte or 1 cm ribbon gauze. Sections of the cribriform plate or fovea ethmoidalis can be removed, and it is best if the dura is preserved. It is important to use a fenestrated sucker and not to apply anything but minimal suction to brain tissue if it is exposed. Careful dissection, avoiding trauma that might produce intracranial bleeding, and respecting the dura will allow the resection of tumors that involve the skull base if their removal is indicated.
- Patients having surgery of this type should give fully informed consent.

### Frontal Sinus

Most benign lesions that involve the frontal sinus are best managed by an external approach (Beasley and Jones, 1995 a). After their removal, most lesions in this area result in a loss of lateral support, which produces stenosis of the frontal recess, although this may take years to develop. While a median drainage procedure can be done to overcome this (Fig. 15.**49** a, b), it is not easy, and an external incision with reconstruction of the lateral wall and the mucosa of the frontal recess gives good access and results. A lesion in the lateral part of the frontal recess usually escapes removal using the endoscope. An external incision, preserving as much healthy mucosa as possible to minimize the chance of loculations forming, with reconstruction of its wall works well. If there is marked disruption of the frontal sinus, then obliteration may be necessary.

Few benign frontal lesions are amenable to endoscopic resection. These are normally in the midline and are removed after gaining control by removing all the air cells around them and opening the frontal recesses. Image-guided surgery can help in this area.

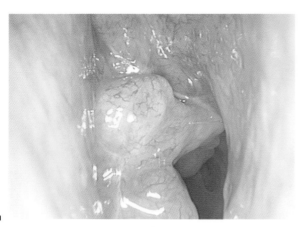
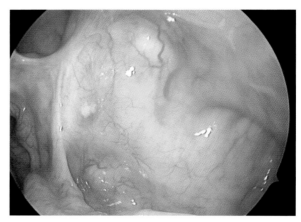

a                                                                                                                                                                              b

Fig. 15.**50**   **a** Preoperative and **b** postoperative endoscopic views of recurrent inverted papilloma in the left maxillary sinus extending around the floor and anterior wall.

### Ethmoid Complex, Lateral Nasal Wall, and Orbit

It is rarely possible to remove a lesion in this area in one piece unless it is small. In order to remove the whole lesion, it may be necessary to remove the lamina papyracea, which can be done with minimum morbidity. The periosteum should not be cut if possible, as orbital fat will prolapse into the operating field and make further surgery more difficult. The same principles should be followed as for a frontoethmoidectomy. It is best to start with a maxillary sinusotomy in order to establish a good landmark and create the space to make further work on the ethmoid sinuses easier.

### Maxillary Sinus

The medial and posterior walls of the maxillary sinus are readily accessible after a type III sinusotomy. The medial wall can be resected endoscopically by doing a medial maxillectomy (Fig. 15.**50 a**, **b**). This sounds like a major procedure because historically it was associated with doing a lateral rhinotomy incision (although now a midfacial degloving approach would often be a better alternative). However, an endoscopic medial maxillectomy is not a very difficult procedure (see Chapter 14), and the main surgical problem is controlling any potential bleeding from the branches of the sphenopalatine artery that run over the posterior fontanelle and through the inferior turbinate. These are best controlled by initially identifying the branches of the sphenopalatine artery and cauterizing them with suction diathermy. The resection can then proceed with relative ease.

The anterior wall and floor are more difficult to visualize. In lesions such as inverted papilloma it may be possible to do this by making a type III sinusotomy and using a 70° endoscope, or after an endoscopic medial maxillectomy.

### Pterygopalatine Fossa

The main pathological lesion in this area is the angiofibroma and its resection has been described earlier in this chapter. Other lesions in this area need the same approach, with control of the terminal branches of the maxillary artery being obtained by doing a type III maxillary sinusotomy, removing its posterior wall, and defining, and coagulating the artery. A long-shanked drill with a coarse diamond burr helps remove the bone here as this can often be very thick (Fig. 15.**51 a–c**).

### Sphenoid Sinus, Clivus, and Cavernous Sinus

It is essential to know the pathology, to have detailed imaging, and to have weighed the pros and cons in removing benign lesions in this area (Fig 15.**52 a**, **b**). They often present late when there are cranial nerve or eye signs and they are often not completely resectable. The benefit of debulking many of these lesions, whose troublesome margins are producing the symptoms, is not always clear. It is often the edges of these lesions that are spreading through the skull base that cannot be resected. The main strategy is to do bilateral sphenoid type III sinusotomies and extend them down to the floor of the sinus and then laterally to the vital structures. The carotid arteries and maxillary and optic nerves can be skeletonized if necessary using a well-irrigated coarse diamond burr. The surgeon must possess the expertise to convert to an open approach (Le Fort I osteotomy/mandibular split) if necessary. In open approaches, the endoscope can help visualize this area. The 45° endoscope can aid access to areas that evade the operating microscope.

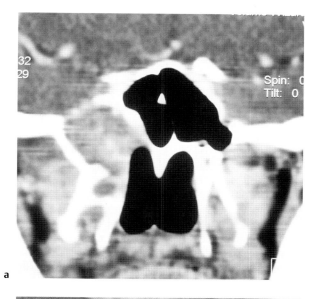

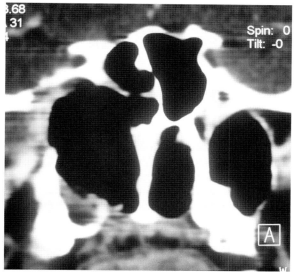

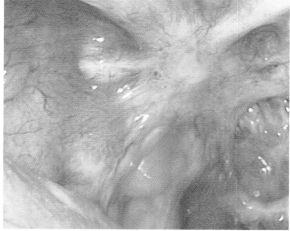

Fig. 15.**51**   **a** Preoperative and **b** postoperative coronal CT scans of a hemangiopericytoma of the pterygopalatine fossa. Note that the lateral wing of the pterygoid and part of the floor of the sphenoid were removed. **c** Endoscopic view 6 years after surgery.

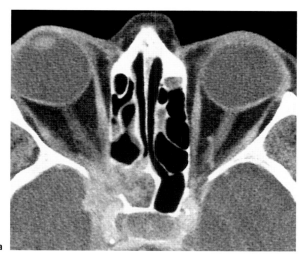

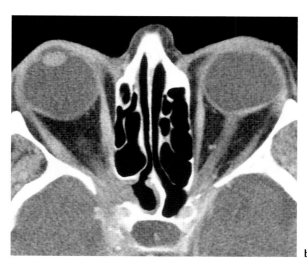

Fig. 15.**52**   **a** An axial CT scan showing a lesion at the orbital apex going into the cavernous sinus, associated with blindness thought to be due to malignancy. A biopsy showed that this was aspergillosis. **b** This CT scan shows some resolution after 6 months on itraconazole. The patient is well 1 year after completing a 2-year course of intraconazole.

### Access for Biopsies

It is important that all tissue, whether it looks harmless or not, is sent for histological examination. We found that 1 % of 2021 nasal polyps had pathology that differed significantly from the clinician's diagnosis, and this then altered management (Diamantopopolous and Jones, 2000). Endoscopic biopsy can reduce morbidity (Trimas and Stringer, 1994) as well as preserving oncological barriers so that an en bloc resection can potentially be carried out without compromising oncological resection as well as increasing the rate of histological diagnosis. Biopsy should ideally be done after imaging so that the artifacts that occur after surgery do not complicate image interpretation (Myers and Carrau, 1993).

### Postoperative Monitoring

The endoscope offers excellent visibility of the lateral nasal wall or postoperative craniofacial cavity, whether the initial resection was done endoscopically or not (Homer et al., 1997). *DVD* 14, 16, 17

### ■ The Role of Endonasal Surgery in the Resection of Malignant Tumors

While the endoscope has the potential to help visualize the paranasal sinuses and reduce the morbidity associated with the resection of lesions in this area, it is vital that the surgical resection and its margins are *not compromised* by the use of these techniques. An understanding of the pathology of lesions in this area and formulation of a treatment plan with an oncological team are important.

- If the endoscope is used in the removal of a malignant lesion, its use should *not compromise the extent of the resection.*
- The management of all malignant lesions should be done in conjunction with a multidisciplinary team.
- The en bloc resection of malignant tumors is usually the surgeon's main goal. However, this is not always possible and in some circumstances (tumor abutting the internal carotid, the optic nerve, or cavernous sinus) removal without a clear margin, or incomplete removal, will occur. Under these circumstances, additional treatment such as radiotherapy or chemotherapy is often given, depending on the pathology, the patient's condition, and the relative benefit compared to the morbidity these may produce.
- In studies of malignant disease of the paranasal sinuses, only a small minority of cases are suitable for endoscopic resection (Tufano et al., 1999).

- The endoscope can be used to assist in defining the intranasal extent of a tumor in conjunction with a craniofacial resection (Thaler et al., 1999).
- The expertise must be available to do a craniotomy if it becomes apparent that this is needed to resect the tumor or deal with a complication.
- It is important to recognize when resection is not in the patient's interest, for example, tumor into the frontal lobes, through prevertebral fascia, or affecting both optic nerves (Sissons et al., 1989). While more recent techniques have extended what can be resected, such as lesions involving the cavernous sinus, there is no evidence that these increase life expectancy or reduce morbidity (Janecka et al., 1994).
- Longer-term follow-up than is currently available, and comparative trials, are needed before the endoscopic resection of malignant tumors can be advocated.

### Surgical Technique

#### Combined Craniofacial and Endoscopic Resection

The main use of the endoscope is to help obtain a clear inferior margin (Fig. 15.**53 a–e**). Before operating, the radiographs and the endoscopic appearance need to be studied to estimate the extent of the lesion. When the margin of the tumor is not clear, it is helpful to take endoscopic biopsies at the start of the procedure and send these for frozen section. The craniofacial resection can then proceed, and the wait for the pathologist's reply will not prolong the procedure.

A thorough frontosphenoethmoidectomy can be done away from the tumor margin, if possible to add to the margin of the resection. The septum can be divided endoscopically to help the specimen be delivered en bloc via the craniotomy. If the tumor extends to involve the medial wall of the orbit, this can be removed via the craniotomy, and the endoscope can help in ensuring that its inferior margins are cleared.

#### The Endoscopic Resection of Malignant Anterior Skull Base Tumors

This is controversial at present. No evidence exists, as yet, that supports the endoscopic "debulking" of tumors followed by radiotherapy. Craniofacial en bloc resection remains the gold standard that has increased life expectancy in skull base tumors (Howard and Lund, 1993). The integrity of the dura is critical in the management of this condition. A tumor invading the dura is associated with a poor prognosis, but thankfully the dura often forms a good barrier.

The endoscopic resection of malignant skull base lesions may have a role in small tumors, where a margin of resection is possible (Fig. 15.**54 a–c**).

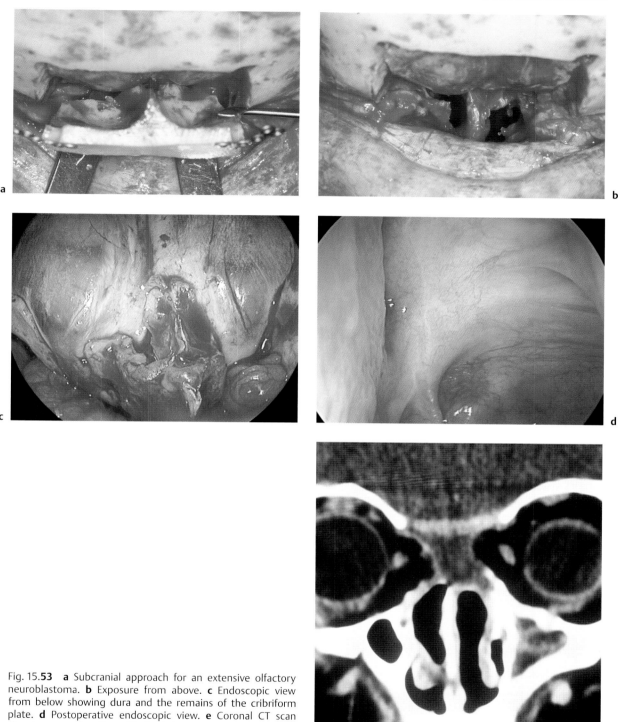

Fig. 15.**53** **a** Subcranial approach for an extensive olfactory neuroblastoma. **b** Exposure from above. **c** Endoscopic view from below showing dura and the remains of the cribriform plate. **d** Postoperative endoscopic view. **e** Coronal CT scan showing reconstruction with fascia lata.

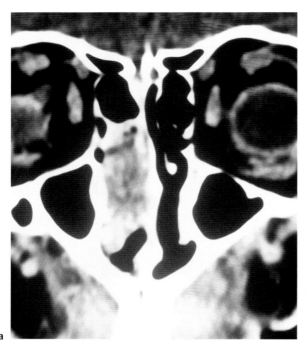

a

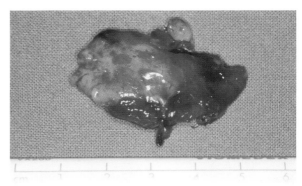

b

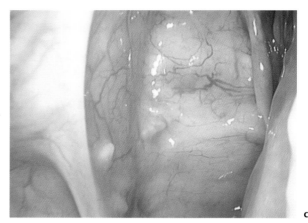

c

Fig. 15.**54**  **a** Preoperative coronal CT scan of an adenocarcinoma. **b** Operative specimen of resected adenocarcinoma with a surrounding cuff of bone and soft tissue. **c** Postoperative endoscopic appearance showing the reconstructed skull base 5 years after surgery.

The same technique should be used as has been described above (in the section Surgical Approaches for Benign Paranasal and Skull Base Lesions, p. 268) except that every attempt should be made to remove the tumor and its bony base in one piece. However, it is often necessary to debulk a tumor hanging into the airway in order to improve the visibility of its margins and the roof of the sinuses. Powered instrumentation helps, but all material must be collected in a trap, in series with the suction tube, for histological examination.

## Specific Malignant Conditions

### Olfactory Neuroblastoma

Endoscopic resection has been advocated for tumors of Kadish stage A or B (no evidence of intracranial extension). Endoscopically, it is possible to resect the cribriform plate, the crista galli, the olfactory bulbs, and their surrounding dura along with the top of the septum and the middle turbinates where they are attached to the skull base (Casiano et al., 2000) (Fig. 15.**55 a–d**). The question is whether this approach enables an adequate margin of resection and, if not, whether this matters—particularly if postoperative

radiotherapy is given. Series have been small, and with limited follow-up, and do not provide enough evidence that this method is better than a craniofacial approach at present (Bradley et al., 2003). It can be argued that the primary determining factor affecting prognosis is the degree of differentiation (if staging is controlled for). It can also be argued that poorly differentiated tumors may have already metastasized, and that it is best to minimize surgical morbidity and mortality by endoscopic resection, as craniofacial resections have a complication rate of almost 1 in 4 (Levine et al., 1999). However, the series reporting endoscopic resection are few and limited. Tumors resected in conjunction with radiotherapy have not shown an increase in local recurrence rates, but larger numbers, ideally controlled for stage and differentiation and with a longer follow-up, are required before these techniques can be advocated.

### Malignant Melanoma

The management of malignant melanoma suggests that an initial en bloc resection with radiotherapy is associated with a lower local recurrence and metastatic rate in spite of its relatively low radiosensitivity.

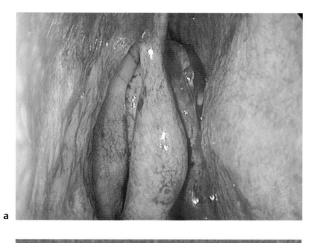

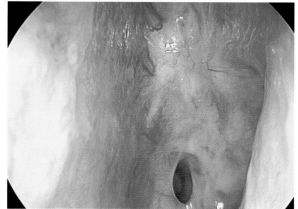

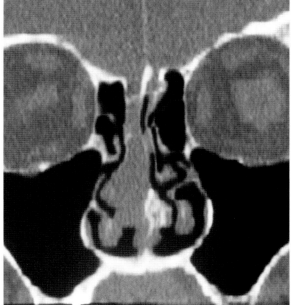

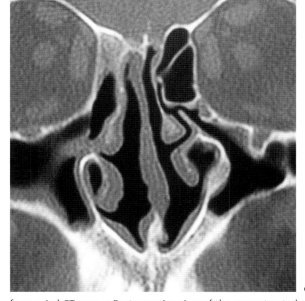

Fig. 15.**55**    **a** A right hemorrhagic polyp in the olfactory cleft—an olfactory neuroblastoma. **b** Reconstructed coronal CT scan from spiral CT scan. **c** Postoperative view of the reconstructed skull base. **d** Postoperative CT scan.

However, the prognosis is poor, with approximately only 1 in 4 surviving 5 years. The endoscope is useful for examining the nasal lining for evidence of satellite lesions, although about a one-third are amelanotic. The endoscope has the potential to reduce morbidity in dealing with *recurrent* disease and there is no evidence that doing a wider resection when it has recurred gives a better result than piecemeal resection (Fig. 15.**56** a, **b**).

### Plasmacytoma

The management of these lesions depends on an understanding of their pathology, since their behavior and management differ. Granuloma, pseudolymphoma, reactive plasmacytic hyperplasia, olfactory neuroblastoma, lymphoma, anaplastic carcinoma, and metastatic tumors can all have a very similar appearance (Fig. 15.**57**). Biopsy is essential, as in every lesion of this type. The diagnostic classification of plasma cell neoplastic disorders includes:

1   Solitary plasmacytoma of bone
2   Extramedullary plasmacytoma
3   Myelomatosis
4   Plasma cell leukemia

Solitary plasmacytoma of bone commonly presents as a single large osteolytic lesion, often with multicystic areas of rarefaction. However, almost 50% of solitary plasmacytomas will convert to multiple myeloma

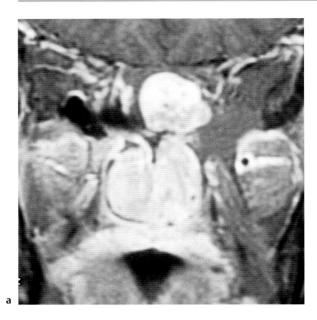

a

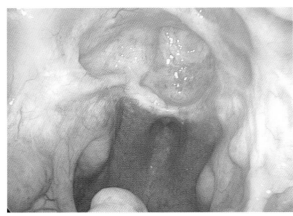

b

Fig. 15.**56**  **a** Preoperative coronal MR image showing extensive malignant melanoma in the posterior nasopharynx—much of it was polypoid. **b** Postoperative appearance 3 years after endoscopic removal of the mucosa on the septum, floor of the sphenoid, and bilateral sphenoethmoid recesses.

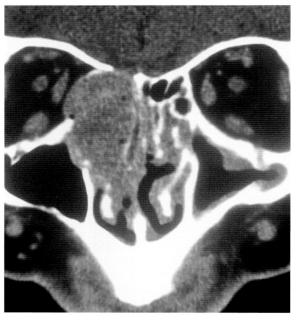

Fig. 15.**57**  CT scan of a plasmacytoma involving the right frontoethmoid sinuses.

(Majumdar et al., 2002). It is important to look for evidence of systemic involvement and the presence of paraprotein. Extramedullary plasmacytomas present as sessile, pedunculated, or polypoid masses with a pale yellow hue, and fewer patients convert to multiple myeloma.

Solitary lesions can be excised but, as they are highly radiosensitive, they should only be removed if this can be done with minimum morbidity. Radiotherapy is the treatment of choice. Adjuvant chemotherapy is sometimes indicated in an attempt to delay conversion to myeloma.

### Other Malignant Skull Base Tumors

There is, at present, little evidence that the endoscope is of benefit in resecting other malignant tumors affecting the skull base or paranasal sinuses, for example, adenocarcinoma (Fig. 15.58 a–f), squamous cell carcinoma (Fig. 15.59 a–c), nasopharyngeal carcinoma, neuroendocrine tumors other than olfactory neuroblastomas, lymphoma (Quraishi et al., 2000), undifferentiated carcinoma (Fig. 15.60 a–d), small-cell carcinoma, adenoid cystic carcinoma, sarcomas, and metastases. However, some malignant tumors can be resected with as wide a margin as can be obtained using other techniques in the hands of an experienced endonasal surgeon. *This should only be done in conjunction with a multidisciplinary team.*

Fig. 15.**58**  **a** Preoperative coronal and **b** axial CT scans of ▷ adenocarcinoma of the posterior skull base. **c** Postoperative coronal and **d** axial CT scans of adenocarcinoma of the posterior skull base—the patient also received radiotherapy. **e** Endoscopic appearance at 5 years of the posterior nasal cavity and **f** close-up view with recess above the pituitary gland (∗).

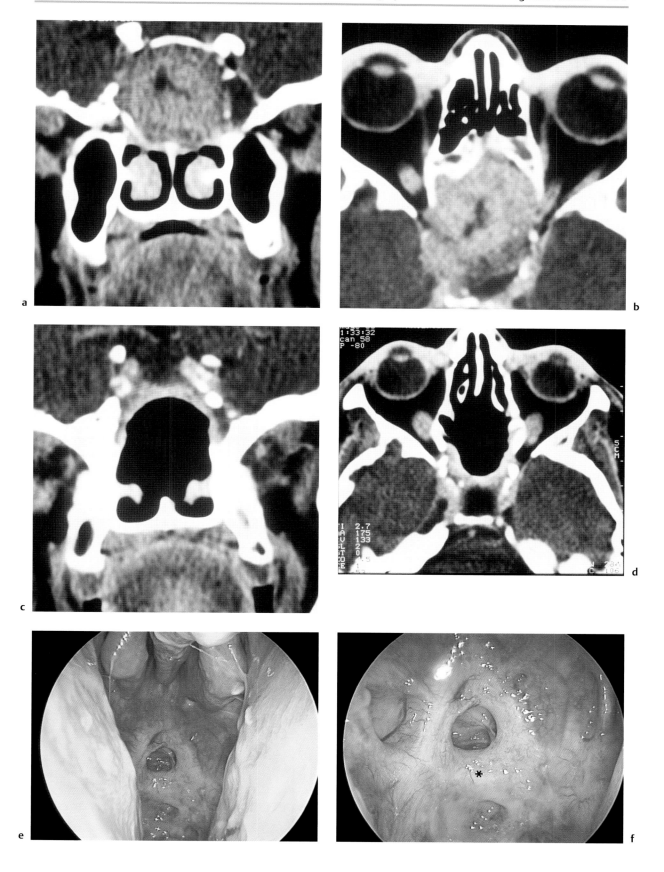

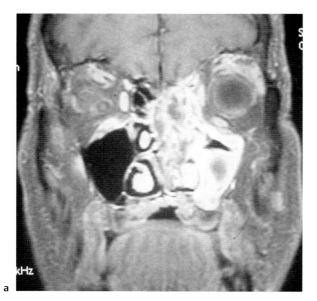

a

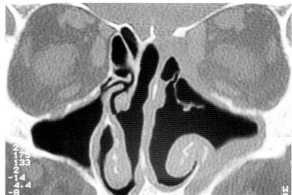

b

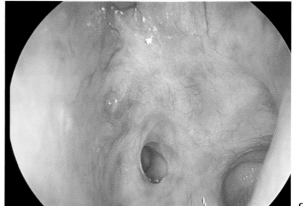

c

Fig. 15.**59** **a** Preoperative MR image and **b** CT scan after endo-scopic resection and radiotherapy in a moderately differen-tiated squamous cell carcinoma of the left paranasal sinuses. **c** Four year follow-up appearance after endoscopic resection and radiotherapy for squamous cell carcinoma.

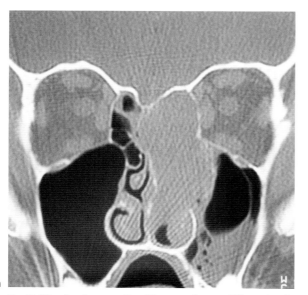

a

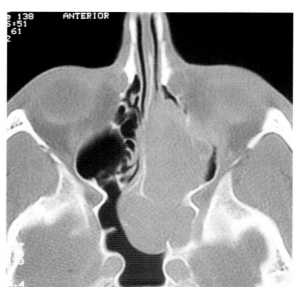

b

Fig. 15.**60 a**, **b**   Preoperative CT scans of an undifferentiated carcinoma involving the paranasal sinuses.        Fig. 15.**60 c**, **d**   ▷

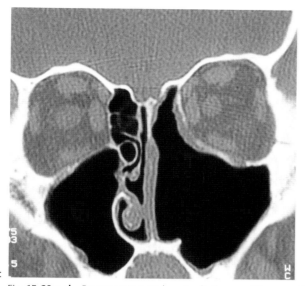
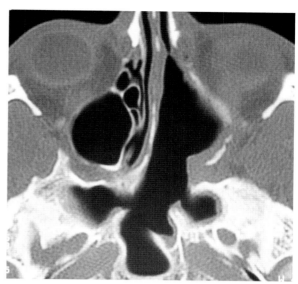

c

d

Fig. 15.**60 c, d**    Postoperative and postradiotherapy CT scans—the patient died of brain metastases 3 years later.

## Recurrent or Residual Malignant Disease

The endoscopic debulking of disease can sometimes help in palliation by providing a nasal airway. The KTP laser is particularly useful in debulking hemorrhagic lesions. The endoscope has little else to offer under these circumstances.

# 16 The Way Forward

## ■ Advances in Medical Management

It is said that to be a good surgeon you also have to be a good physician. Surgical maneuvers cannot cure the majority of patients with noninfective nasal polyps, any more than they can cure allergic rhinitis. Advances in instrumentation, computer-aided surgery, and optics may refine surgical techniques, but it seems likely that the main advances will come through research into the etiology and pathological mechanisms of allergic and idiopathic rhinitis and nasal polyposis, and the development of new medical therapies.

At present, medical management has focused on the treatment of allergy and infection. What is not well understood is the reason for the inflammatory changes that are found in the absence of an infectious agent or allergy—as they are conventionally understood.

### Nasal Polyps

The cause of most inflammatory polyps remains a mystery in spite of extensive work describing their cell morphology, IgE, and cytokine profiles (Kramer et al., 2000), as well as exploring some possible genetic associations (Irving et al., 1997). Why nasal polyps present more than twice as frequently in men is unknown. It is often said that polyps are caused by allergy, although atopy is no more prevalent in patients with nasal polyps than in the whole population (Slavin, 1997). However, a higher proportion of women than men with nasal polyps have asthma (Drake-Lee, 1987). With this in mind, it is important to define the term atopy and not equate it with asthma, as the majority of people with late-onset asthma are nonatopic (i.e., skin-prick test negative and normal serum IgE levels). Nasal polyps from both atopic and nonatopic patients sent for histological examination are invariably reported as "allergic" because of the presence of eosinophils. Raised levels of IL-5 and IgE have been found in both groups (Kramer et al., 2000), so is it possible that there is local "allergy" to inhaled inert antigens, bacterial (Bachert et al., 2001), fungal (Ponikau et al., 1999), or viral (Perelmurrer et al., 1979) antigens.

## Immunoglobulin E, Cytokines, and Chemokines in Rhinitis

Several workers have reported the local production of IgE in patients with a negative skin-prick test (Huggins and Brostoff, 1975), and in a proportion of people who are now classified as having nonallergic or idiopathic rhinitis (Powe et al., 2001, 2003). Several groups have proposed that the nasal mucosa has the ability to produce allergen-specific IgE locally (Huggins and Brostoff, 1975; Kleinjan et al., 2000; Powe et al., 2001). There may be mechanisms other than allergy that can produce eosinophilia. For example, the common cold has been shown to produce a prolonged influx of IgE receptor-bearing eosinophils in patients with allergic rhinitis (Van Benton et al., 2001). Are the mucosal changes the aftermath of an infection that has upregulated cytokines (Kramer et al., 2000), resulted in chemokines such as eotaxin-2 (Jahnsen et al., 1999; Murdoch and Finn, 2000), and altered the genetic expression of mucus (Voynow et al., 1998) or the production of proteoglycans (Lee et al., 2001)? Cytokines and chemokines act as mediators, chemoattractors, and activators of inflammation, but the trigger for their production in the absence of infection or allergy is not known.

## Nitric Oxide

Nitric oxide, a potent biological mediator synthesized from L-arginine by the enzyme NO synthase (NOS), is a small lipophilic molecule that can diffuse rapidly across cell membranes. One form of NOS is neuronal NO synthase found in the nonadrenergic, noncholinergic nerves of the peripheral nervous system; a second is endothelial NO synthase; and the third is inducible NO synthase (Conboy and Jones, 2000). Inducible NO synthase can be induced by inflammation or infection and a range of cell types, by pro-inflammatory cytokines such as IFN-$\gamma$, IL-1$\beta$ and TNF-$\gamma$, by IgE immune complexes, or by bacterial products such as lipopolysaccharide and lipotechoic acid, and by viral infections. In animal models, inducible NO synthase inhibitors reduce the late-phase response after allergen challenge. Inducible NO synthase knockout mice appear to have an enhanced $T_H1$ phenotype with an increase in IFN-$\gamma$ and a decrease in IL-4. Inducible NO synthase inhibitors, therefore, have potential as anti-inflammatory agents in rhinitis.

## Novel Therapeutic Strategies

Therapeutic attempts to reduce the action of cytokines and chemokines offer promise. The chemokine receptor CCR3 is expressed on mast cells, eosinophils, basophils and IL-2-activated T lymphocytes. It appears that activation of these receptor sites can influence the migration of these cells into mucosa (Murdoch and Finn, 2000). Chemokine receptor antagonists have the potential to inhibit eosinophilia in particular. Other chemokine receptor antagonists that offer promise are CXCR1 and 2.

The implementation of monoclonal antibodies in humans has been slow because, when they are created from rat B cells, they are recognized as being foreign. However, hybrid antibodies are now being engineered to block a variety of molecules such as IgE (Adelroth et al., 2000), IL-4 and IL-5, or entire cell lineages such as T$_H$2 cells by adding exotoxins to the antibodies (Leckie et al., 2000) (Fig. 16.**1**).

Another strategy is to block key molecules involved in inflammation. Trials of soluble IL-4 receptors in asthma have already taken place (Borish et al., 2001).

It has been suggested that there is a balance in an individual's helper T-cell response between T$_H$1 cells and T$_H$2 cells (Berger, 2000). T$_H$1 cells produce cytokines that produce the pro-inflammatory responses responsible for killing intracellular parasites and for perpetuating autoimmune responses. T$_H$2 cells produce cytokines associated with the promotion of IgE and eosinophilic responses in atopy (Fig. 16.**2**). It has been suggested that in allergic rhinitis and seasonal asthma, an individual with a genetic predisposition toward a T$_H$2-biased immune system could move away from this bias if exposed to certain environmental stimuli early in life (Openshaw and Walzl, 1999; Openshaw and Hewitt, 2000). Early exposure to microbial agents may be the appropriate stimulus causing the immune system in these individuals to move toward a T$_H$1-dependent system (Strachan et al., 2000). Without this biological programming, the bias would persist and the individual would tend toward a T$_H$2-dependent system—for example, atopy. Ways are now being sought to augment the T$_H$1 response by methods such as recombinant IL-12 or Toll-like receptors that recognize DNA motifs in bacteria and induce IL-12 and other host defenses when activated (Hemmi et al., 2000).

Gene therapy is a broad term for many possible techniques, including neutralizing segments of genes and altering the gene sequence or messenger RNA. Antisense therapy involves using complementary coding sequences and binding these irreversibly to sense RNA, preventing protein translation, or to genomic DNA, thereby blocking transcription. While the potential for these techniques is great, their safe application in humans poses great problems at present.

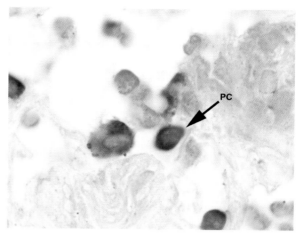

Fig. 16.**1**   A micrograph (×100) showing a mast cell expressing IL-4 in close proximity to a plasma cell (PC).

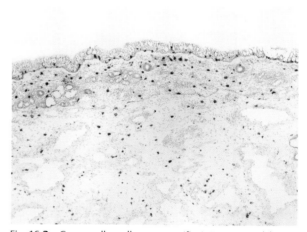

Fig. 16.**2**   Grass pollen allergen-specific IgE is stained brown and is localized to mast cells within the nasal mucosa of this atopic individual with persistant allergic rhinitis.

Phosphodiesterase inhibitors also have potential as anti-inflammatory agents in rhinitis. Cyclic AMP (cAMP) is metabolized by a superfamily of phosphodiesterases and has broad effects in suppressing the immune and inflammatory cell activity. Phosphodiesterase inhibitor-4 is the major cAMP-hydrolyzing isoenzyme in inflammatory and immune cells. Phosphodiesterase inhibitors have activity on a variety of human inflammatory cells (basophils, monoctyes) in vitro. Phosphodiesterase inhibitors can also inhibit the antigen-induced proliferation and cytokine production of peripheral mononuclear cells obtained from atopic individuals. Their development holds promise in the treatment of asthma and rhinitis.

A better understanding of the genetics of mucus production (Voynow et al., 1998) and of mucus rheology (Quraishi et al., 1998) may help those in whom

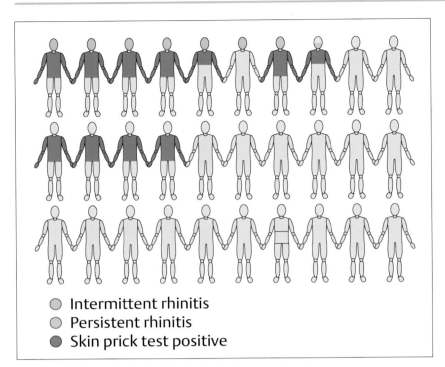

Fig. 16.**3** The distribution of positive skin prick tests in the general population.

○ Intermittent rhinitis
○ Persistent rhinitis
● Skin prick test positive

these appear to be abnormal and improve biorheological matching or the efficiency of mucociliary clearance.

### Immunotherapy

The use of immunotherapy in grass pollen allergic rhinitis has been proven in the short- and long-term (Durham et al., 1999). However, if there is cross-reactivity to a range of inhaled allergens, then immunotherapy directed at one allergen is less effective. Similarly, the evidence to support allergen avoidance is mixed. The results of house dust mite desensitization have been equivocal. Fungal immunotherapy following surgery for allergic fungal sinusitis has helped prevent recurrence and it has been postulated that this may help patients with eosinophilic mucin rhinosinusitis (Ferguson, 2000). The benefits of allergen avoidance are contentious. When there is a marked single allergen, for example, to house dust mite, then going to great lengths to avoid this allergen has been shown to help. However, it is debatable how well these studies can be extrapolated into day-to-day practice, and whether patients are ready to comply with these measures. It appears that half-measures to reduce exposure to such allergens have little effect on the allergen load and are likely to be of little benefit.

### The Markers of Atopy

In allergic rhinitis there is good epidemiological and basic scientific evidence that there is an inherited genetic component that is responsible (Moffat et al., 1994; Jones et al., 1998 b). However, why do 15.5% of asymptomatic people who have a positive skin-prick test not develop any allergic symptoms (Droste et al., 1996) (Fig. 16.**3**), and not all those with a raised IgE have symptoms of rhinitis (Panzani et al., 1993) (Fig. 16.**4**)? In another study of skin-prick tests, 18% of children changed over a 2-year period (Droste et al., 1996). An understanding of the normal course of these processes may help us to influence our immune status and suppress the excessive response to some foreign antigens that leads to the symptoms of allergic rhinitis.

In summary, research on the pathogenesis of all the forms of rhinosinusitis and a better understanding of their etiology and inflammatory mechanisms should lead to advances in the treatment of our patients.

### Radiology

Teleradiology with electronic data transmission and the availability of online consulting between a radiologist and the ENT surgeon may help when a rapid second opinion is needed. Similarly, in this fast-growing field online surgery can be used as part of a distance-learning program.

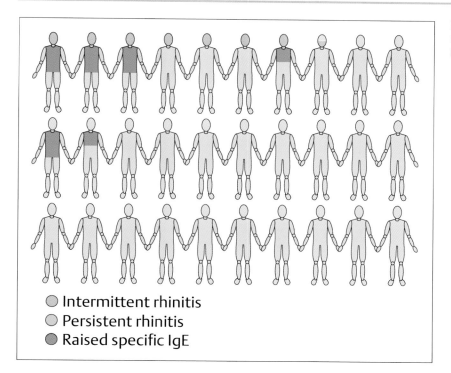

◯ Intermittent rhinitis
◯ Persistent rhinitis
⬤ Raised specific IgE

The objective assessment of olfaction has remained elusive, but recent developments such as functional MRI show more promise than electrophysiological tests (Fig. 16.**5**).

## ■ Surgical Tools

### Optics and Camera Systems in Surgery

Although endoscopic surgery provides an excellent image, it gives a two-dimensional view of three-dimensional structures and some of the depth of perception is lost. Some studies suggest that three-dimensional vision improves performance (Tevaearai et al., 2000). Attempts are being made to place two digital sensors at the end of a rigid light delivery system. The alignment of the sensors' images will be such that when the individual images are fed to the respective eyes this will provide stereoscopic vision. At present, the definition of the images and the fragility of the cameras make this system impractical.

Conventional camera systems are becoming smaller, lighter, more light-sensitive, and with better definition. It is likely that this trend will continue. The technology that allows digital video recording is progressing to enable "averaging" between captured "frames" of information, effectively creating an inter-

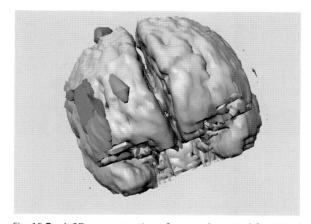

Fig. 16.**5**  A 3D reconstruction of an amalgamated functional MRI/PET study, with the red areas showing activity after stimulation with smell of rose, and green after stimulation with pheromones and smell of rose. (In collaboration with the University Hospital of Zurich.)

mediate image that is then placed between the captured "frames." This gives a better and smoother playback.

It seems difficult to imagine that the optics of modern endoscopes can be improved upon, but only recently the development of the 45° endoscope has significantly improved visibility of the frontal recess. There is some optical distortion and foreshortening in

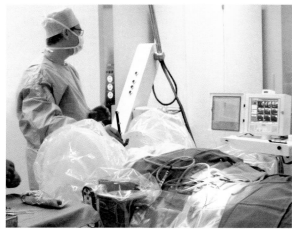

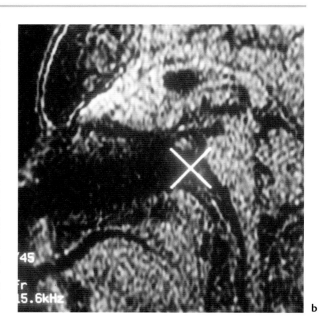

Fig. 16.**6**  **a** Peroperative setup of real-time MRI. The head is between the "doughnuts" of the MRI machine. (Acknowledgement to Dr. R. Bernays, University of Zurich.) **b** Peroperative sagittal MR image showing the position of the end of the endoscope.

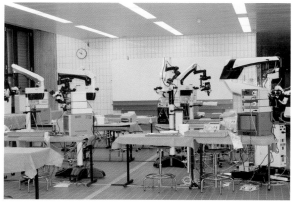

Fig. 16.**7**    Course setup in endoscopic sinus surgery.

the peripheral image of all endoscopes, and this may be improved.

The role of real-time MRI in the operating room with nonferromagnetic instruments is being investigated. It has particular potential where there is brain shift in tumor resection and it accounts for changes that have occurred as the result of surgery. At present it has been shown to help in pituitary and glioma surgery (Fig. 16.**6**a, **b**).

### Surgical Training

The core of surgical training in endoscopic sinus surgery is based on hands-on instructional courses using anatomical specimens (Groscurth et al., 2001)

(Fig. 16.**7**). Good preservation of specimens is important. The bony scaffolding of the paranasal sinuses is the ideal basis for creating a virtual-reality environment that can provide the trainee with experience of a variety of hypothetical surgical situations. Attempts to do this are under way, providing both visual feedback and haptic feedback (a sensation of the force required to undertake a maneuver), in order to simulate different surgical situations (Rudman et al., 1998).

The training of rhinologists should include the holistic management of patients. This should include not only training in how to communicate with patients but the medical management of patients whose disease is not solely confined to the nose (e.g., asthma, immunosuppression, sarcoid, vasculitis, and ciliary dysmotility). Many rhinologists are aware of the psychological aspects of rhinological symptoms (Homer et al., 2000), yet this subject is not well covered in the medical literature or in teaching and research. Many patients who complain bitterly of postnasal drip or catarrh as primary symptoms describe them as having a much greater effect on their life, or ability to function, than might be expected. One pervading theme for the future is that surgeons should not perceive themselves as being the only people who can help their patients and that a team approach (nurse practitioners, asthma and allergy nurses) involving other disciplines (immunologists, respiratory physicians, ophthalmologists, pathologists, radiologists, neurosurgeons, anesthetists) can help everyone (Gawandee, 2001).

# Appendix
# Information for Patients

## ■ Endoscopic Sinus Surgery

### What is Endoscopic Sinus Surgery?

The sinuses are the spaces in the bones of the face above and to either side of the nose, and in the forehead and cheeks. They open into the air passages of the nose through narrow channels. There are several sinuses, which are like rooms that connect to one another and open or drain into the nose. Infection or blockage in the sinuses can block the nose, reduce the sense of smell, and produce infected or discolored mucus down the back of the nose into the throat. When infection and blockage is severe, it can produce pain.

Endoscopic surgery is performed by a surgeon using telescopes to see inside the nose and sinuses. The aim of the operation is to remove part or all of the sinuses so that their drainage channels are opened. This is like plumbing of the sinuses that will help drain any infection. Opening the sinuses will also help sprays or drops to reach the lining of the sinuses. Quite often surgery produces an improvement in breathing as well as the sense of smell. Mucus often becomes less mucky a few weeks after surgery, but this is less predictable; and as normal sinuses produce a cupful of mucus a day, you should expect to be aware of some in spite of surgery.

### What Can I Expect When I Have This Operation?

The operation is performed inside the nose; there is rarely any visible incision or stitching—that is one of the advantages of this type of surgery. After the operation you may have a dressing in the nose, so the nose will feel blocked until the packing is removed. Having endoscopic sinus surgery is not very painful, but you should expect moderate discomfort afterward. If you need nasal packs or dressings, these are uncomfortable for a few seconds when they are removed. Most people go home the day of surgery or the morning after surgery and need a week off work. During that week you can expect the nose to feel blocked up with a blood-stained nasal discharge that lasts a few days.

Irrigation or "douching" of your sinuses is recommended at least three times a day for at least the first two weeks, and if the lining of your nose has been very infected or damaged you may need to continue it for longer. Lots of humidity to the nose (for example, steam inhalations from a bowl or a facial sauna) is often helpful in loosening secretions, but you are advised to blow your nose gently for the first four days. Regular simple painkillers are recommended. After about a week you will have an appointment to come back to clinic to have the sinus cavities checked. The full benefit of the operation may not be experienced until several weeks later, as the surgery produces some swelling inside the nose which takes a while to settle.

### What Complications Can Occur?

Everybody gets some bleeding or blood-stained mucus from the nose for a few days after the operation, and especially after any dressings are removed. A nosebleed usually settles with some pressure placed either side of the lower part of the nose for 20 minutes. It is said that crushed ice cubes or a packet of frozen peas placed over the top of the nose can help, but very occasionally the bleeding can be bad enough to need packing to be placed in the nose or, very rarely, a return to the operating room. Very occasionally some slight bruising from the operation can appear in the eyelids during the week after surgery, but this is not serious and settles on its own.

Rarely, people who had a sense of smell before surgery lose their sense of smell, but this is unusual. It is far more common for your sense of smell to improve if it was poor beforehand—although this cannot be guaranteed. Occasionally the sinuses can get infected after surgery. This would be recognized by an increase in pain around the eye or nose, perhaps with a temperature or a severe headache. If this happens, you need to ring up the hospital and come back to have it checked and treated. It is important to remember, however, that the majority of people having surgery of this type do not experience any complications at all.

## ■ Douching

Some operations in the nose leave the surface raw inside like a graze. But unlike a graze, on the knee for example, you do not get a dry scab with healing underneath. In the nose the "scab" gets very soggy with all the mucus that the nose produces. In between times the mucus can occasionally dry out, and when several layers of mucus do this a crust is formed. Germs can collect within a thick crust and it can become infected and interfere with healing.

In order to keep your sinuses clean and healthy after your surgery it will be helpful to you if you can douche your nose regularly. To start with it is a good idea to do this at least three times a day for the first two weeks and then to reduce it as instructed. Generally this means cutting down on the number of times you douche each day if your nose feels clearer or you are not washing out much mucus or many crusts.

It is usual for you to feel blocked for the first two to three weeks following surgery, until the lining has settled down. Your nose may also run a lot for the first few days with blood-stained mucus. It is also normal to feel some pressure under your nose and forehead and you may need to take some painkillers for the first few days.

There are commercial douching sprays that have the advantage of being sterile and easy to use. These are partially desalinated seawater that has been sterilized and can be delivered under pressure in a jet of water or a spray. They are helpful in getting you used to washing out your nose.

To douche your nose without using a commercial douching spray, make the following mixture: Mix half a teaspoon of salt, half a teaspoon of sugar, and half a teaspoon of sodium bicarbonate in one pint of boiled water that has been left to cool. The problem with this is that it tastes salty and you need to spit it out if it reaches the back of the throat. Put some mixture into a saucer, or the palm of your hand, block off one nostril with one finger and then sniff up the solution into the other nostril. Let it run out afterwards. When you have got used to how this feels, try and sniff up hard so that you can clean out any old blood clot or mucus. Continue until no debris is washed out, and then do the same with the other nostril. If you are advised to use nose drops or sprays, please take them after you have douched.

## ■ Nasal Allergy

### Allergy

This is due to allergens, or substances breathed in that cause the nasal lining to swell, make it produce more fluid, and cause it to become irritated. The allergen that causes this reaction affects the lining of the nose and causes it to release chemicals that cause swelling and obstruction as well as an increase in secretions. The nerves that line the nose are irritated and this produces itching, sneezing, and running.

### What is an Allergen?

An allergen is an irritant particle that produces an allergic reaction. The most common allergens are pollens, molds, house dust mite allergen, and the dried saliva from animals such as cats and dogs.

### Intermittent Allergy

The allergy appears at certain times of year when the pollens are carried by the wind. Examples are tree pollen in the spring such as alder, hazel, oak, elm, and birch; grass pollen in early to mid summer—mainly ryegrass and timothy grass; in autumn weed pollen and mold spores.

### Persistent Allergy

Perennial or "all year round" allergens give persistent symptoms that are similar to the seasonal variety or hay fever but they are there all the time. The most important allergens are the house dust mite and animal dander.

Perennial allergy can also be worse in the hay fever season if the person is also sensitive to pollen.

### Diagnosis

A diagnosis is made on the basis of history and clinical examination. This is helped by investigations such as skin-prick tests that help to find which allergens contribute to the problem. A skin-prick test is a simple test that involves putting these substances on the skin and making a tiny prick that is very superficial and doesn't draw blood.

## Treatment

### Allergen Avoidance

This means making an effort to avoid the allergen or irritant particle that is responsible for the allergy. These measures are most effective if you are only allergic to one substance in particular. For allergy to house dust mite, avoidance means that quite an effort is required, as the use of energy-saving double glazing, along with the use of central heating, have increased the number of house dust mites that live in our homes. These measures appear to be worth doing only if they are done thoroughly.

### House Dust Mite Control Measures

(This is mainly of use if it is the sole allergen causing a problem.)

#### The Bedroom

- Use allergen-impermeable mattress, duvet, and pillow covers, ideally ones that enclose the whole of the contents.
- A weekly hot wash for the sheets.
- Avoid thick pile carpets if possible—wooden or tiled floors are ideal. If you have carpets, these can be sprayed with an anti house dust mite spray that will reduce the numbers of mites for several months.
- Vacuum the floor weekly (this should not be done by the patient).
- Damp dust weekly (this should not be done by the patient)
- Cotton curtains—wash periodically
- Use a filtered vacuum cleaner, but do not use it on the mattress as this will disperse the allergen into the air.

#### Other Rooms

- Remove dust from upholstered furniture.
- Damp dust and vacuum at least twice a week, ideally done by someone other than the patient.
- Furry toys can be washed or placed in the deep-freezer overnight to reduce mites.
- While the rooms are being cleaned, any affected people should be elsewhere.

### Pets

- Wash the pets regularly (the main allergen is the dried salivary proteins on their fur and these are very soluble in water).
- No pets in the bedroom.

### Pollen Avoidance Methods

- Keep windows closed when the pollen count is high, particularly in the late evening.
- Use high-efficiency particulate filter (HEPA) in cars.
- Air conditioners and circulators are now available with pollen filters and can these can cut down the pollen count indoors.

### Medical Treatment

If allergen avoidance does not reduce the patient's symptoms sufficiently then medication can help. If it is possible to anticipate the onset of the symptoms such as in hay fever, then it is better to start the medication before the onset of the symptoms rather than waiting until they have started.

#### Topical Steroid Sprays or Drops

Steroids can be delivered topically (to the surface) using sprays or drops to the nose or they can be taken by mouth. The new generation of topical nasal steroid sprays or drops can be taken to control symptoms for many years as very little is absorbed into the body. Topical nasal steroid sprays are particularly effective at improving the nasal airway, as well as helping to reduce itching, sneezing, and nasal discharge. Occasionally these sprays can produce some dryness or spotting of blood. If the spray is used in the right hand for the left nostril, and vice versa, the bleeding can be minimized because the spray doesn't always hit the same part of the partition down the middle of the nose (the septum).

Steroids in tablet form can provide good relief of symptoms if the problems are severe, but the effects are short-lived and they have to be used sparingly because of concern about side effects.

#### Antihistamines

Histamine is an important chemical released from cells within the nasal lining in response to contact with a nasal allergen. Histamine increases blood flow to the nose, causing itching, sneezing, and a watery discharge.

Antihistamines are usually taken as tablets and work by blocking the effect of the histamine that is released. They are more effective if taken regularly and *before* any symptoms occur. Antihistamines are of some help in reducing the symptoms of itching and sneezing, but they have little effect on reducing nasal blockage.

Side effects are unusual, particularly with the newer antihistamines, but they can occur and can sometimes interact with other medications that you may be taking, so please read the packet and if in any doubt contact your pharmacist or doctor before taking any medication.

Antihistamine nasal sprays are also available. They have minimal side effects but they are not as effective as topical nasal steroids in helping symptoms of blockage.

**Ipratropium Bromide**

Given in spray form ipratropium bromide reduces the watery discharge in "autonomic" rhinitis. This is a condition where the glands secrete more mucus. It is normally found in people over 60 years old and there are few other symptoms except a clear discharge. Ipratropium bromide has little effect on improving nasal blockage, a symptom that is rarely troublesome in autonomic rhinitis.

**Sodium Cromoglycate**

Sodium cromoglycate reduces the release of histamine. It can reduce nasal itching, sneezing and watery discharge but it has to be taken very regularly to be effective. It has to be used four times a day, so it can be difficult to remember to take it regularly compared to the once or twice a day nasal steroid sprays. It is not as effective as topical nasal steroids.

## ■ Sinus Infection

"Infective sinusitis" is a term used to describe any inflammation or swelling of the mucus-producing lining of a sinus or all of the sinuses (pansinusitis) when it is due to an infection.

### Associated Causes

The majority of problems follow a cold or viral upper respiratory tract infection. The infection causes the lining at the opening of the sinus to swell, and leads to a build-up of mucus in the sinuses. The mucus can then become infected with bacteria. Fungal infections are very rare and occur sporadically.

A dental extraction or dental root infections can occasionally cause problems as the roots of teeth are near the sinus in the cheek.

Some inflammation of the sinuses can occur after an infection even when there is no evidence of any bacteria present. The inflammation may be due to the after-effects of a bacterial infection when some inflammation continues. Infection may also be due to a virus. It is not known or understood why a small proportion of people have "chronic" problems and others do not. Some people's immunity (their body's ability to fight infection) is low and this means they are more prone to have problems.

### Symptoms

Acute sinusitis causes pain over the affected sinus, usually the cheek, or on one side of the forehead, a blocked nose and/or a discharge, feeling unwell, and a temperature. Facial pain alone *without* any nasal symptoms is rarely due to sinus disease and is often caused by other types of pain such as midfacial segment pain, tension-type headaches, migraine, dental pain, or trigeminal neuralgia.

Sinusitis is chronic when the symptoms have persisted for longer than three months. The features are mainly of nasal congestion, and there is a mucky nasal discharge that is often painless in a patient who feels quite well.

### Management

#### Medical Management

Antibiotics are important in the treatment of acute infective sinusitis and should be given for *at least seven days after* the symptoms have disappeared and often for 14 days altogether. It is important for the antibiotics to be given for this length of time because they do not get into the infected sinus very well. Pain relief is important as acute sinusitis is very painful. To help the drainage of pus from the sinus, a local nasal decongestant can be used. This is one of the few situations where a topical decongestant spray is a good idea, but it should only be used for a limited time (up to seven days—they can cause damage if used for longer). Steam inhalations can help to thin the thickened mucus.

#### Surgical Management

Surgery is used to help drainage of the involved sinus when antibiotics do not work.

### Complications

The complications of sinusitis are rare because of the use of antibiotics. As the sinuses surround the eye on three sides, inflammation and infection can spread to the eye socket. Swelling around the eye, the eye protruding, decreased vision, or a reduced range of eye movements with pain all require urgent consultation to prevent any permanent eye damage.

Osteomyelitis (infection of the bone), mainly of the frontal bone (that makes the forehead), is rare but if it is left it can lead to an abscess on the forehead. Extension of the infection into the brain is rare and usually occurs "out of the blue." It is associated with a progressive headache, drowsiness, and effortless vomiting. Urgent medical advice should be sought.

Swelling of the cheek, rather than around the eye, is rarely due to sinus disease and is usually due to a problem arising from the teeth.

## ■ Nasal Polyps

A polyp is a swelling of the lining of the nose, which is usually due to inflammation of the lining of the nose.

Nasal polyps come from the lining of the nose and often originate from the ethmoid sinuses (in the face, either side of the nose), which drain into the nasal cavity. Nasal polyps contain inflammatory fluid and while they can be associated with allergy and infection, the exact reason why some people get them and not others is unknown. Allergy is no more common in people with nasal polyps than in people who do not have polyps.

### Conditions Associated with Nasal Polyps

Nasal polyps can occur in association with more general diseases such as adult-onset asthma; an uncommon association is with aspirin intolerance, and very occasionally they occur in children with cystic fibrosis.

Adult-onset asthma rather than childhood asthma is associated with nasal polyps. 20–40% of patients with polyps will have asthma as well. Eight in every 100 patients with polyps also have asthma and aspirin sensitivity, and in these patients the polyps tend to recur more than in other people.

### Symptoms and Signs

Nasal polyps are overall four times more common in men than in women, but in people who have adult-onset asthma they occur equally in both sexes. The incidence is between 1 per 1000 and 20 per 1000, and after the age of 60 years the chance of developing polyps declines.

Polyps look like small grapes and they can appear singly or in clusters in the nasal cavity. They can cause
- Blocked nose
- Runny nose and/or sneezing
- Poor sense of smell and taste
- Catarrh

### Unilateral (One-sided) Polyps

One-sided nasal polyps are rare and are associated with a range of conditions that need further investigations both in adults and in children.

### Investigations

Endoscopy in the clinic using a small illuminated telescope may help to see up the nose to exclude infection or any unusual feature.

### Treatment

#### Medical Treatment

Most inflammatory nasal polyps are known to shrink when nasal sprays or drops containing topical nasal steroids are used. New local nasal steroid drops or sprays can be taken to control symptoms for many years as very little is absorbed into the body; they can work well, but it may take up to six weeks of treatment before their full benefit is felt. Steroids in tablet form can provide good relief, but the effects are short-lived and they are used sparingly because of concerns about side effects. If medicines don't work, then surgery can usually help.

#### Surgical Treatment

When the medical treatment has failed, polyps can be removed surgically and this often helps the patient to breathe better. In 3 out of 4 patients with polyps they come back after an average period of 6 years. If polyps repeatedly return, the sinuses can be cleaned out and opened up and it is thought that this gives a longer symptom-free period before they return. Even after surgery, local medical treatment is often still needed using anti-inflammatory sprays or drops to slow down the recurrence of polyps.

## ■ Advice for Patients after Endoscopic Surgery for Nasal Polyps

An endoscope is often used to help see the polyps and sinuses better and this type of surgery is called endoscopic sinus surgery.
1 Please rest for a few days.
2 Do not blow your nose hard for two days, even though your nose may feel blocked—sniff!
3 Nasal drops and/or steam inhalation may be advised for you by the doctors. Medical or nursing staff will give you instructions on how to do this if it is necessary.
4 It is normal to feel blocked for several days and, while this improves over one to two weeks, it may take 6 weeks before the maximum improvement is felt.
5 It is normal to have mucus that is blood-stained for a few days.
6 It is NOT normal to have discomfort that gets worse day by day; if this happens advice should be sought from the ward or your doctor.
7 If bleeding occurs, pinch the nose for 10 minutes while sitting upright with the head tilted forward. If bleeding persists, contact the ward, your doctor, or the nearest emergency room.

## ■ The Complications of Endoscopic Surgery for Nasal Polyps

- In rare cases the nose bleeds so much after the surgery that more nasal dressings have to be placed and very occasionally the patient has to return to the operating theater to have it stopped.
- A recent audit showed an overall complication rate of 9 per 1000 in endoscopic sinus surgery, which compares favorably with other techniques to remove nasal polyps.
- Adhesions—strands of tissue between the septum (the central partition of the nose) and the lateral wall of the nose—can form in the first few days after surgery and you can help prevent these by douching regularly and coming to the outpatient department for your nose to be checked in the week after surgery. If adhesions are starting to form, you may need some cleaning of the cavity of the nose when you are seen.
- The bone between the eye socket and the sinuses is thin and if the surgeon goes through this bone then the patient will get a black eye for a few days. This is not a problem in itself as long as the patient does not blow their nose or hold onto a sneeze during the four days after surgery, otherwise this can blow air into the tissues and cause swelling around the eye for a few days. If the surgeon goes deeper into the eye socket, the muscles of the eye may be damaged, causing double vision or even blindness, but these complications are very rare and the surgeon will do all they can do to avoid this.
- The roof of the nasal cavity is the floor of the brain. There is a sac containing fluid that goes around the brain and the fluidis called cerebrospinal fluid. If the surgeon goes through this sac it can cause a leak of the cerebrospinal fluid. If this is recognized, it is often possible to repair it at the time of surgery. This is an uncommon complication. If a cerebrospinal fluid leak is not recognized until later, it will need to be repaired, otherwise the patient can develop meningitis.
- The tear duct that drains tears from the eyes runs into the nose and occasionally this can be damaged by endoscopic sinus surgery; this can cause a watery eye. This is uncommon and it is possible to correct it with surgery to drain the tear system into the nose if necessary.
- Surgery for nasal polyps often helps restore the sense of smell if it was missing, although continued medical treatment with nasal sprays or nose drops is often needed to stop the polyps returning. However, approximately 1% of patients lose their sense of smell after this type of surgery.

# References

Adelroth E, Rak S, Haahtela T, Aasand G, Rosenhall L, Zetterstrom O, Byrne A, Champain K, Thirlwell J, Della C (2000) Recombinant humanised mAb-E25, an anti-IgE mAb, in birch pollen-induced seasonal allergic rhinitis. Journal of Allergy and Clinical Immunology 106(2): 253–259.

Albritton FD, Kingdom TT, DelGaudio JM (2001) Malleable registration mask: application of a novel registration method in image guided sinus surgery. American Journal of Rhinology 15(4): 219–224.

Anand VK, Kacker A (2000) Value of radiologic imaging and computer assisted surgery in surgical decisions of the anterior skull base lesions. Rhinology 38(1):17–22.

Anon JB, Lipman SP, Oppenheim D, Halt RA (1994) Computer-assisted endoscopic sinus surgery. Laryngoscope 104(7): 901–905.

Anon JB, Klimek L, Mosges R, Zinreich SJ (1997) Computer-assisted endoscopic sinus surgery. An international review. Otolaryngologic Clinics of North America 30(3): 389–401.

Bachert C, Gevaert P, Holtappels G, Johansson SG, van Cauwenberge P (2001) Total and specific IgE in nasal polyps is related to local eosinophilic inflammation. Journal of Allergy and Clinical Immunology 107(4): 607–614.

Barki S, Carney, SA, Jones NS, Downes RN (1998) Endonasal laser assisted dacryocystorhinostomy. Hospital Medicine 59(3): 210–215.

Bateman N, Jones NS (2000) Rhinorrhoea feigning CSF leak: nine illustrative cases. Journal of Laryngology and Otology 114: 462–464.

Bateman N, Mason J, Jones NS (1999) Use of fluorescein for detecting cerebrospinal fluid rhinorrhoea: A safe technique for intrathecal injection. ORL J Otorhinolaryngol Relat Spec. 61: 131–2.

Beasley N, Jones NS (1995a) The brow incision for access to the anterior skull base and paranasal sinuses. Journal of Laryngology and Otology 109: 134–136.

Beasley N, Jones NS (1995b)The role of endoscopy in the management of mucocoeles. American Journal of Rhinology 9(5): 251–256.

Beasley NJ, Jones NS, Downes RN (1995) Enophthalmos secondary to maxillary sinus disease: single-stage operative management. J Laryngol Otol. 109: 868–70.

Benninger MS (1997) Nasal endoscopy: its role in office diagnosis. American Journal of Rhinology 11(2): 177–180.

Bent P, Cuilty-Siller C, Kuhn FA (1994) The frontal cell as a cause of frontal sinus obstruction. American Journal of Rhinology 8(4): 185–191.

Berger A (2000) Science Commentary: Th1 and Th2 responses: what are they? BMJ 321: 424.

Bolger MWE and Kennedy DW (1992) Nasal endoscopy in the outpatient clinic. Otolaryngologic Clinics of North America 25(4): 791–801.

Bolger WE, Mawn CB (2001) Analysis of the suprabullar and retrobullar recesses for endoscopic sinus surgery. Annals of Otology, Rhinology and Laryngology Supplement 186 110(5 part 2): 3–14.

Bolger WE, Butzin CA, Parsons DS (1991) Paranasal sinus bony anatomic variations and mucosal abnormalities: CT analysis for endoscopic sinus surgery. Laryngoscope 101(1 part 1): 56–64.

Borish LC, Nelson HS, Corren J, Bensch G, Busse WW, Whitmore JB, Agosti JM (2001) Efficacy of soluble IL-4 receptor for the treatment of adults with asthma. Journal of Allergy and Clinical Immunology 107(6): 963–970.

Bradley PJ, Jones NS, Robertson I (2003) Diagnosis and management of esthesioneuroblastoma. Curr Opin Otolaryngol Head Neck Surg. 11: 112–118.

Briner HR, Simmen D (1999) Smell diskettes as screening test of olfaction. Rhinology 37: 145–148.

Briner HR, Simmen D, Jones N (2003) Impaired sense of smell in patients with nasal surgery. Clin Otolaryngol. 28: 417–419.

Carney S, Jones NS (1996) Idiopathic rhinitis: idiopathic or not? Clinical Otolaryngology 21: 198–202.

Cartellieri M, Vorbeck F (2000) Endoscopic sinus surgery using intraoperative computed tomography imaging for updating a three-dimensional navigation system. Laryngoscope 110(2 part 1): 292–296.

Cartellieri M, Vorbeck F, Kremser J (2001) Comparison of six three-dimensional navigation systems during sinus surgery. Acta Otolaryngologica 121(4):500–504.

Casiano RR, Numa WA, Falquez AM (2000) Endoscopic resection of olfactory esthesioneuroblastoma. American Journal of Rhinology 15: 271–279.

Caversaccio M, Bachler R, Ladrach K, Schroth G, Nolte LP, Hausler R (1999) The "Bernese" frameless optical computer-aided surgery system. Computer Aided Surgery 4(6): 328–334.

Chee LWJ, Sethi DS (1999) The endoscopic management of sinonasal inverted papillomas. Clinical Otolaryngology 24: 61–66.

Conboy N, Jones NS (2000) NO and the paranasal sinuses: a review. Clinical Otolaryngology 25: 337–341.

Conboy PJ, Jones NS (2003) The place of endoscopic sinus surgery in the treatment of paranasal sinus mucoceles. Clin Otolaryngol. 28: 207–210.

Cooke LD, Hadley DM (1991) MRI of the paranasal sinuses: incidental abnormalities and their relationship to symptoms. Journal of Laryngology and Otology 105: 278–281.

Cooney T, Jones NS (2001) Investigation for immunodeficiency in patients with recurrent infections. Clinical Otolaryngology 26: 184–188.

Cousin JN, Har-El G, Li J (2000) Is there a correlation between radiographic and histologic findings in chronic sinusitis? Journal of Otolaryngology 29(3): 170–173.

Cumberworth VL, Djazaeri B, Mackay IS (1995) Endoscopic fenestration of choanal atresia. Journal of Laryngology and Otology 109: 31–35.

Dammann F, Bode A, Heuschmid M, et al. (2000) Multislice spiral CT of the paranasal sinuses: first experiences using various parameters of radiation dosage. Rofo. 172: 701–706.

Davis WE, Templer JW, Lamear WR, Davis WE, Craig SB (1991) Middle meatal antrostomy: patency rates and risk factors. Otolaryngology – Head and Neck Surgery104: 467–472.

Diamantopopolous I, Jones NS (2000) All nasal polyps need histological examination: an audit based appraisal of clinical practice. Journal of Laryngology and Otology 114: 755–759.

Donald PJ (1982) Frontal sinus ablation by cranialisation: a report of 21 cases. Archives of Otolaryngology 108: 560–565.

Draf W, Weber R, Keerl R, Constantinidis J (1995) Aspekte zur Stirnhöhlenchirurgie. Teil I: Die endonasale Stirnhöhlendrainage bei entzundlichen Erkrankungen der Nasennebenhöhlen. HNO 43: 352–357.

Drake-Lee AB (1987) Nasal polyps. In: Kerr AG, Groves J, eds. Scott-Brown's Otolaryngology. London: Butterworths, pp. 142–153.

Droste JHJ, Kerhof M, de Monchy JGR, Schouten JP, Rijcken B (1996) Dutch ECRHS Group. Association of skin test reactivity, specific IgE, total IgE, and eosinophils with nasal symptoms in a community-based population study. Journal of Allergy and Clinical Immunology 97: 922–923.

Durham SR, Walker SM, Varga E-M, Jacobson MR, O'Brien F, Noble W, Till SJ, Hamid QA, Nouri-Aria KT (1999) Long-term clinical efficacy of grass-pollen immunotherapy. New England Journal of Medicine 341: 468–475.

Earwacker J (1993) Paranasal sinus osteomas: a review of 46 cases. Skeletal Radiology 22: 417–423.

Eljamel MSM (1993) The role of surgery and beta-2-transferrin in the management of cerebrospinal fluid fistula. MD thesis, University of Liverpool.

Enepekides DJ (2004) Recent advances in the treatment of juvenile angiofibroma. Curr Opin Otolaryngol Head Neck Surg. 12: 495–499.

Ezekowitz RAB, Mulliken JB, Folkman J (1992) Interferon alfa-2 a therapy for life-threatening haemangiomas of infancy. New England Journal of Medicine 326: 1456–1463.

Fahy C, Jones NS (2001) Nasal polyposis and facial pain. Clinical Otolaryngology 26: 510–513.

Fergie, N, Jones NS, Halvat MF (1999) Nasal sarcoidosis. Journal of Laryngology and Otology 113: 893–898.

Ferguson BJ (2000) Eosinophilic mucin rhinosinusitis: a distinct clinicopathological entity. Laryngoscope 110: 799–813.

Flynn JT, Mitchell KB, Fuller OG (1979) Ocular motility complications following intranasal surgery. Archives of Ophthalmology 97: 453–458.

Fried MP, Morrison PR (1998) Computer-augmented endoscopic sinus surgery. Otolaryngologic Clinics of North America 31(2): 331–340.

Gawandee AA (2001) Creating the educated surgeon in the 21 st century. American Journal of Surgery 181(6): 551–556.

Gibbons MD, Gunn CG, Niwas S, Sillers MJ (2001) Cost analysis of computer-aided endoscopic sinus surgery. American Journal of Rhinology 15(2): 71–75.

Gliklich RE, Metson R (1995) The health impact of chronic sinusitis in patients seeking otolaryngologic care. Otolaryngology – Head and Neck Surgery Laryngoscope 105: 387–390.

Goldwyn BG, Sakr W, Marks SC (1995) Histopathologic analysis of chronic sinusitis. American Journal of Rhinology 9: 27–30.

Gormley P, Bowyer J, Downes R, Jones NS (1997) Endoscopic orbital decompression. Eye 11: 723–726.

Groscurth P, Eggli P, Kapfhammer J, Rager G, Hornung J-P, Fasel J (2001) Gross anatomy in the surgical curriculum in Switzerland: improved cadaver preservation, anatomical models, and course development. The Anatomical Record (New Anat) 265: 254–256.

Harrison D, Lund VJ (1993) Nonepidermoid epithelial neoplasms. Tumours of the Upper Jaw, Chapter 7. Edinburgh: Churchill Livingston, pp. 105–108.

Havas TE, Motbey JA, Gullane PJ (1988) Prevalence of incidental abnormalities on computerised tomographic scans of the paranasal sinuses. Archives of Otolaryngology – Head and Neck Surgery 114: 856–859.

Heatley DG, McConnell KE, Kille TL, Leverson GE (2001) Nasal irrigation for the alleviation of sinonasal symptoms. Otolaryngology – Head and Neck Surgery 125: 44–48.

Hegazy HM, Carrau RL, Snyderman CH, Kassau A, Zweig J (2000) Transnasal endoscopic repair of cerebrospinal fluid rhinorrhoea: a meta-analysis. Laryngoscope 110: 1166–1172.

Hehar SS, Jones NS (1997) Fronto-ethmoidal osteoma: the place of surgery. Journal of Laryngology and Otology 111: 372–375.

Hemmi H, Takeuchi O, Kawai T, Kaisho T, Sato S, Sanjo H, Matsumoto M, Hoshino K, Wagner H, Takeda K, Akira S (2000) Toll-like receptor recognizes bacterial DNA Nature 408: 740–745.

Homer J, Jones NS, Bradley PJ (1997) The role of endoscopy in the management of nasal neoplasms. American Journal of Rhinology 11(1): 41–47.

Homer J, Jones NS, Sheard C, Herbert M (2000) Cognitive dissonance, the placebo effect and the evaluation of surgical results. Clinical Otolaryngology 25: 195–199.

Howard DJ, Lund VJ (1993) Surgical options in the management of nose and sinus neoplasia. In: Harrison D, Lund VJ, eds. Tumours of the Upper Jaw. Edinburgh: Churchill Livingstone, pp. 329–336.

Howe L, Jones NS (2004) Guidelines for the management of periorbital cellulitis/abscess. Clin Otolaryngol. 29: 725–8.

Huggins K, Brostoff J (1975) Local production of specific IgE antibodies in allergic rhinitis patients with negative skin tests. Lancet 2: 148–150.

Hughes R, Jones NS (1998)The role of endoscopy in outpatient management. Clinical Otolaryngology 23: 224–226.

Ikeda K, Tanno N, Tamura G, Suzuki HI, Oshima T, Shimomura A, Nakabayashi S, Takasaka T (1999) Endoscopic sinus surgery improves pulmonary function in patients with asthma associated with chronic sinusitis. Annals of Otology, Rhinology and Laryngology 108: 355–359.

Irving RM, McMahon R, Clark R, Jones NS (1997) Cystic fibrosis transmembrane conductance regulator gene mutations in severe nasal polyposis. Clinical Otolaryngology 22: 519–521.

Jahnsen FL, Haye R, Gran E, Brandtzaeg P, Johansen FE (1999) Glucocorticosteroids inhibit mRNA expression of eotaxin, eotaxin-2, and monocyte-chemotactic protein-4 in human airway inflammation with eosinophilia. Journal of Immunology 163: 1545–1551.

Janecka IP, Chandranath S, Laligam S, Curtin H (1994) Treatment of paranasal sinus cancer with cranial base surgery: results. Laryngoscope 104: 553–555.

Jeffery Modell Foundation. The Jeffrey Modell Foundation and the National Primary Immunodeficiency Resource Center (NPI) is the central resource and clearing house on Primary Immunodeficiency (PI). Available at: http://www.jmfworld.com/ or http://www.info4pi.org/

Jennings C, Dugar J, Jones NS, Powell R, Lowe J (1998) The rhinological features of Wegener's granulomatosis. Rhinology 36: 188–191.

Jianetto DP, Pratt MP (1995) Correlation between preoperative computed tomography and operative findings in functional endoscopic sinus surgery. Laryngoscope 105: 924–927.

Jiang R-S, Hsu C-Y, Shan B-H (2001) Endoscopic optic nerve decompression for the treatment of traumatic optic neuropathy. Rhinology 39: 71–74.

Johnson M, Jones NS (2002) The complications of endoscopic sinus surgery. Clinical Risk 8: 133–136.

Jones NS (1997) Visual evoked potentials in endoscopic and anterior skull base surgery. Journal of Laryngology and Otology 111: 513–516.

Jones NS (1998 a) Microendoscopy in Rhinology. Minimally Invasive Therapy and Allied Technologies 7: 149–154.

Jones NS (1998 b) Endoscopic sinus surgery. In: Jones AS, Phillips DE, Hilgers FJ, eds. Diseases of the Head & Neck, Nose & Throat. London: Arnold, pp. 846–867.

Jones NS (1999 a) Current concepts in the management of paediatric rhinosinusitis. Journal of Laryngology and Otology 113: 1–9.

Jones NS (1999 b) The ENT manifestations of rheumatological diseases. Annals of Rheumatology 58: 589–590.

Jones NS (1999 c) Current best treatment in children with allergic rhinitis. Current Medical Literature – Allergy 7(3): 49–56.

Jones NS (2001 a) The classification and diagnosis of facial pain. Hospital Medicine. 62(10): 598–606.

Jones NS (2001 b) Unilateral clear discharge: advances in the management of CSF leaks. BMJ 322: 122–123.

Jones NS (2002) CT of the paranasal sinuses: a review of the correlation with clinical, surgical and histopathological findings. Clin Otolaryngol. 27: 11–7.

Jones NS (2004) Midfacial segment pain: implications for rhinitis and sinusitis. Curr Allergy Asthma Rep. 4: 187–92.

Jones NS, Cooney TR (2003) Facial pain and sinonasal surgery. Rhinology 41: 193–200.

Jones NS, Rog D (1998) Olfaction: a review. Journal of Laryngology and Otology 112: 11–24.

Jones NS, Strobl A, Holland I (1997 a) CT findings in 100 patients with rhinosinusitis and 100 controls. Clinical Otolaryngology 22: 47–51.

Jones NS, Bullock P, Hewitt S et al. (1997 b) Head injuries and the priciples of craniofacial repair. In: Jones NS, ed. Craniofacial Trauma: An Interdisciplinary Approach. Oxford: Oxford University Press, pp. 18–60.

Jones NS, Carney AS, Davis A (1998) The prevalence of allergic rhinosinusitis: a review. Journal of Laryngology and Otology 112: 1019–1030.

Khan OA, Majumdar S, Jones NS (2002) Facial pain following sinonasal surgery or facial trauma. Clinical Otolaryngology 27: 171–174.

Kennedy DW, Josephson JS, Zinreich SJ, Mattox DE, Goldsmith MM (1989) Endoscopic sinus surgery for mucoceles. Laryngoscope 99: 885–895.

Kennedy DW (1992) Prognostic factors, outcomes and staging in ethmoid sinus surgery. Laryngoscope 102(57S): 1–18.

Kimelman CP (1994) The risk to olfaction from nasal surgery. Laryngoscope 104: 981–988.

Kleinjan AJK, Vinke JG, Severijnen LW, Fokkens WJ (2000) Local production and detection of (specific) IgE in nasal B-cell and plasma cells of allergic rhinitis patients. European Respiratory Journal 15: 491–497.

Klimek L, Mosges R, Schlondorff G, Mann W (1998) Development of computer-aided surgery for otorhinolaryngology. Computer Aided Surgery 3(4): 194–201.

Kraft M, Simmen D, Kaufmann T, Holzmann D (2003) Long-term results of endonasal sinus surgery in sinonasal papillomas Laryngoscope. 113: 1541–7.

Kramer MF, Ostertag P, Pfrogner E, Rasp G (2000) Nasal interleukin-5, immunoglobulin E eosinophilic cationic protein, and soluble intercellular adhesion molecule-1 in chronic sinusitis, allergic rhinitis, and nasal polyposis. Laryngoscope 110: 1056–1062.

Lale A, Mason JDT, Jones NS (1998) Mucociliary transport and its assessment. Clinical Otolaryngology 23(5): 388–396.

Lang J (1989) Clinical Anatomy of the Nose, Nasal Cavity and Paranasal Sinuses. Stuttgart: Georg Thieme Verlag.

Lawson W, LeBenger J, Som P (1989) Inverted papilloma: an analysis of 87 cases. Laryngoscope 99: 1117–1124.

Leckie MJ, ten Brinke A, Khan J, Diamant Z, O'Connor BJ, Walls CM, Marthur AK, Cowley HC, Chung KF, Djukanovic R (2000) Effects of an interleukin-5 blocking monoclonal antibody on eosinophils, airway hyper-responsiveness, and the late asthmatic response. Lancet 356(9248): 2144–2148.

Lee SH, Park JH, Oh BH, Jung KY, Lee HM, Choi JO, Lim HH (2001) Analysis of proteoglycan gene messages in human nasal mucosa and nasal polyp using dot blot hybridization. Acta Otolaryngologica 121(3): 398–402.

Levine PA, Gallagher R, Cantrell RW (1999) Esthesioneuroblastoma: reflections on a 21-year experience. Laryngoscope 109: 1539–1543.

Lloyd,GA (1990) CT of the paranasal sinuses: study of a control series in relation to endoscopic sinus surgery. Journal of Laryngology and Otology 104(6): 477–481.

Lloyd GAS, Lund VJ, Scadding GK (1991) CT of the paranasal sinuses and functional endoscopic sinus urgery: a critical analysis of 100 asymptomatic patient. Journal of Laryngology and Otology 105(3): 181–185.

Lloyd MNH, Kimber PM, Burrows EH (1994) Post traumatic cerebrospinal fluid rhinorrhoea: modern high definition computed tomography is all that is needed for the effective demonstration of the site of leakage. Clinical Radiology 49: 100–103.

Lund VJ (1994) Allergic and infective rhinosinusitis: differential diagnosis and interrelationship. Otolaryngology – Head and Neck Surgery 111: 335–339.

Lund VJ and Mackay IS (1993) Staging in rhinosinusitis. Rhinology 31: 183–184.

Maclennan A, MacGarry GW (1995) Diagnosis and management of chronic sinusitis. BMJ 310(6978): 529.

Majumdar S, Raghavan U, Jones NS (2002) Solitary plasmacytoma and extramedullary plasmacytoma of the paranasal sinuses and soft palate. J Laryngol Otol. 116: 962–965.

Mansell NJ, Bates GJ (2000) The inverted Schneiderian papilloma: a review and literature report of 43 new cases. Rhinology38: 97–101.

Marshall AH, Jones NS (2003) The Utility of Radiologic Studies in the Diagnosis and Management of Rhinosinusitis. Curr Infect Dis Rep. 5: 199–204.

Marshall A, Jones NS, Robertson I (2001 a) CSF rhinorrhoea: a multidisciplinary approach to minimise patient morbidity. British Journal of Neurosurgery 15(1): 8–13.

Marshall A, Jones NS, Robertson IJA (2001 b) The endoscopic management of nasal encephalocoeles. Journal of Laryngology and Otology 115: 545–547.

Mason JDT, Haynes RJ, Jones NS (1998 a) Interpretation of the dilated pupil during endoscopic sinus surgery. Journal of Laryngology and Otology 112: 622–627.

Mason JDT, Jones NS, Hughes RJ, Holland IM (1998 b) A systematic approach to the interpretation of computed tomography scans prior to endoscopic sinus surgery. Journal of Laryngology and Otology. 112: 986–990.

McCoombe A, Lund VJ, Howard D (1990) Recurrence in juvenile angiofibroma. Rhinology 28: 1–6.

Metson RB, Cosenza MJ, Cunningham MJ, Randolph GW (2000) Physician experience with an optical image guidance system for sinus surgery. Laryngoscope 110(6): 972–976.

Moffat MF, Hill MR, Cornelis F, Schou C, Faux JA, Young RP, James AL, Ryan G, le Souef P, Musk AW, Hopkin JM (1994) Genetic linkage of T-cell receptor $\alpha/\delta$ complex to specific IgE responses. Lancet 343: 1597–1599.

Muneer A, Jones NS, Bradley PJ, Downes R (1998) ENT pathology and diplopia. Eye 12: 672–678.

Murdoch C, Finn A (2000) Chemokine receptors and their role in inflammation and infectious diseases. Blood 95(10): 3032–3043.

Murphy J, Jones NS (2004) Frontal sinus obliteration. J Laryngol Otol. 118: 637–639.

Myers EN, Carrau, RL (1993) Neoplasms of the nose and paranasal sinuses. In: Bailey BJ, ed. Head and Neck Surgery – Otolaryngology. Philadelphia: JB Lipincott, pp. 1091–1109.

Newlands SD, Weymuller EA (1999) Endoscopic treatment of juvenile nasopharyngeal angiofibroma. American Journal of Rhinology 13: 213–219.

Olson G, Citardi MJ (2000) Image-guided functional endoscopic sinus surgery. Otolaryngology – Head and Neck Surgery 123(3): 188–194.

Openshaw PJM, Hewitt C (2000) Protective and harmful effects of viral infections in childhood on wheezing disorders and asthma. American Journal of Respiratory and Critical Care Medicine 162: S40-S43.

Openshaw P, Walzl G (1999) Infections prevent the development of asthma- true, false or both? Journal of the Royal Society of Medecine 92: 495–498.

Panzani RC, Mercier P, Delord Y (1993) Prevalence of patent and latent atopy among a general normal adult population in the south of France by RAST investigation and correlation with circulating total IgE levels. Allergology and Immunopathology (Madrid) 21(6): 211–219.

Perelmurrer L, Potvin L, Phipps S (1979) Immunoglobin E response during viral infections. Journal of Allergy and Clinical Immunology 64(2): 127–130.

Ponikau JU, Sherris DA, Kern EB, Homburger HA, Frigas E, Gaffey TA, Roberts GD (1999) The diagnosis and incidence of allergic fungal sinusitis. Mayo Clinic Proceedings 74(9): 87–874.

Powe D, Huskisson R, Carney A, Jenkins D, Jones NS (2001) Evidence for an inflammatory pathophysiology in idiopathic rhinitis. Clinical and Experimental Allergy 31: 864–872.

Powe DG, Jagger C, Kleinjan A, Carney AS, Jenkins D, Jones NS (2003) "Entopy": localized mucosal allergic disease in the absence of systemic responses for atopy. Clin Exp Allergy 33: 1374–9.

Price JC, Holliday MJ, Johns ME (1998) The versatile midfacial degloving approach. Laryngoscope 98: 291–295.

Quraishi MS, Jones NS, Mason J (1998) The rheology of nasal mucus: a review. Clinical Otolaryngology 23: 403–413.

Quraishi MS, Bessell EM, Clark D, Jones NS, Bradley PJ (2000) Non-Hodgkin's lymphoma of the sinonasal tract. Laryngoscope 110: 1489–92.

Raghavan U, Jones NS (2004) The place of Riedel's procedure in contemporary sinus surgery. J Laryngol Otol. 118: 700–705.

Robson AK, Woolons AC (1996) Validation of the combined olfactory test. Clinical Otolaryngology 21: 512–518.

Romer HC (2001) Medical management of facial pain. Hospital Medicine 62(10): 607–610.

Rudert H, Maune S (1997) Endonasal coagulation of the sphenopalatine artery in severe posterior epistaxis. Laryngorhinootologie. 76: 77–82.

Rudman DT, Stredney D, Sessanna D, Yagel R, Crawfis R, Heskamp D, Edmond CV, Wiet GJ (1998) Functional endoscopic sinus surgery training simulator. Laryngoscope 108: 1643–1647.

Schick B, Steigerwald C, Rhaman el Tahan AE, Draf W (2001) The role of endonasal surgery in the management of frontoethmoid osteomas. Rhinology 39: 66–70.

Schuknecht B, Simmen D (2002) State of the Art. Diagnostic imaging of paranasal sinus diseases. Laryngorhinootologie. 81: 126–146.

Sessions RB, Lerner DN, Harrison LB (1993) A pivot-shifting palate flap for enhanced exposure of the posterior choanae and nasopharynx. Otolaryngology – Head and Neck Surgery 109: 96–100.

Sessle BJ (2000) Acute and chronic craniofacial pain: brainstem mechanisms of nocioceptive transmission and neuroplasticity, and other clinical correlates.Critical Reviews in Oral Biology and Medicine 11(1): 57–91.

Shaw CL, Dymock RB, Cowin A, Wormald PJ (2000) Effect of packing on nasal mucosa of sheep. Journal of Laryngology and Otology 114(7): 506–509.

Shaw CW, Cowin A, Wormald PJ (2001) A study of the normal temporal healing pattern and the mucociliary transport after endoscopic and partial and full thickness removal of nasal mucosa in sheep. Immunology and Cell Biology 79(2): 145–148.

Simmen D (1997) Endonasale, mikroskopisch kontrollierte Stirnhohlenchirurgie. Laryngo -Rhino- Otologie 76: 131–136.

Simmen D (2000) Fortschritte der endonasalen Mikrochirurgie der Nasennebenholen. Laryngo -Rhino- Otologie 79: 645–647.

Simmen D, Bischoff Th. (1998) Rhinochirurgisches Konzept zur Versorgung von Frontobasisdefekten mit Rhinoliquorrhoe. Laryngo -Rhino- Otologie 77: 264–271.

Simmen D, Heinz B (1998) Epitaxis-Stratergie-Erfahrungen der letzten 360 Hospitaisationen. Laryngo -Rhino- Otologie 77: 100–106.

Simmen D, Schuknecht B (1997) Computertomographie der Nasennebenhohlem-eine praoperative Checkliste. Laryngo -Rhino- Otologie 76: 8–13.

Simmen D, Bischoff Th., Schuknecht B (1997) Erfahrungen mit der Abklarung von Frontobasisdefekten, ein diagnstisches Konzept. Laryngo -Rhino- Otologie 76: 583–587.

Simmen D, Briner HR, Schar G, Schuknecht B (1998) Chronische Mycosen der Nasennebenholen-Stellenwert der endonasalen Nasennebenhohlenchirurgie. Laryngo -Rhino- Otologie 77: 444–453.

Simmen D, Briner HR, Hess K (1999) Screeningtest des Geruchssinnes mit Riechdisketten. Laryngo -Rhino- Otologie 78: 125–130.

Sissons GA, Toriumi DM, Atiyah RA (1989) Paranasal sinus malignancy: a comprehensive update. Laryngoscope 99: 143–150.

Slavin RG (1997) Nasal polyps and sinusitis. JAMA. 278: 1849–54.

Sofferman RA (1995) The recovery potential of the optic nerve. Laryngoscope, Supplement No. 72 105(7 part 3): 1–38.

Sohaib SA, Peppercorn PD, Horrocks JA, et al. (2001) The effect of decreasing mAs on image quality and patient dose in sinus CT. Br J Radiol. 74: 157–61.

Stafford Johnson DB, Brennan P, Toland J, O'Dwyer AJ (1996) Magnetic resonance imaging in the evaluation of cerebrospinal fluid fistula. Clinical Radiology 51: 837–841.

Stammberger H (1986) Endoscopic endonasal surgery—concepts in treatment of recurring rhinosinusitis. Anatomic and pathophysiologic considerations. Otolaryngology – Head and Neck Surgery 94: 143–147.

Stammberger H (1991) Functional Endoscopic Sinus Surgery. Philadelphia: Decker.

Stankiewicz JA (1987) Complications of endonasal intranasal ethmoidectomy. Laryngoscope 97: 1270–1273.

Stankiewicz JA (1989) Complications in endoscopic intranasal ethmoidectomy: an update. Laryngoscope 99: 686–90.

Strachan D, Wickens K, Crane J, Pearce N, Beasley R (2000) Family size, infection and atopy: the first decade of the "hygiene hypothesis". Thorax 55: S2–S10.

Taccariello M, Parikh A, Darby Y, Scadding G (1999) Nasal douching as a valuble adjunct in the management of chronic rhinosinusitis. Rhinology 37: 29–32.

Tevaearai T, Mueller XM, von Segesser LK (2000) 3-D vision omproves performance in a pelvic trainer. Endoscopy 32(6): 464–468.

Thaler ER, Kotapka M, Lanza DC, Kennedy DW (1999) Endoscopically assisted anterior cranial skull base resection of sinonasal tumours. American Journal of Rhinology 13: 303–310.

Trimas JT, Stringer SP (1994) The use of nasal endoscopes in the diagnosis of nasal and paranasal sinus masses. American Journal of Rhinology 8: 1–5.

Tufano RP, Thaler ER, Lanza DC, Goldberg AN, Kennedy DW (1999) Endoscopic management of inverted papilloma. American Journal of Rhinology 13: 423–429.

Uddin FJ, Sama A, Jones NS (2003) Three-dimensional computer-aided endoscopic sinus surgery. J Laryngol Otol. 117: 333–339.

Van Benton I, Kleinjan A, Neijens HJ, Osterhaus AD, Fokkens WJ (2001) Prolonged nasal eosinophilia in allergic patients after common cold. Allergy 56(10): 949–956.

Voynow JA, Selby DM, Rose MC (1998) Mucin gene expressio (MUC1, MUC2, and MUC5/5AC) in nasal epithelial cells of cystic fibrosis, allergic rhinitis, and normal individuals. Lung 179(5): 345–354.

Waitz G, Wigand ME (1992) Results of endoscopic sinus surgery for the treatment of inverted papillomas. Laryngoscope 102(8): 917–922.

Wareing MJ, Padgham ND (1998) Osteologic classification of the sphenopalatine foramen. Laryngoscope 108(1 part 1): 125–127.

Weber R, Draf W, Kahle G, Kind M (1999) Obliteration of the frontal sinus—state of the art and reflections on new materials. Rhinology 37: 1–15.

West B, Jones NS (2001) Endoscopy negative, CT negative facial pain in a nasal clinic. Laryngoscope 111: 581–586.

Winstead W, Barnett SN (1998) Impact of endoscopic sinus surgery on global health perception: an outcome study. Otolaryngology – Head and Neck Surgery 119: 486–491.

Wolfensberger M, Schnieper I, Welge-Lussen A (2000) Sniffin'Sticks: a new olfactory test battery. Acta Otolaryngologica 120: 303–306.

Woolford TJ, Jones NS (2000) Endoscopic ligation of anterior ethmoidal artery in treatment of epistaxis. Journal of Laryngology and Otology 114: 858–860.

World Health Organization (2001) WHO Initiative Allergic Rhinitis and its Impact on Asthma. ARIA. 1–214. Presented at the 2nd International Symposium on Allergy Management, Cannes. December 2000.

Wormald PJ, McDonagh M (1997) Bath plug technique for the endoscopic management of cerebrospinal fluid leaks. Journal of Laryngology and Otology 111: 1042–1046.

Yung MW, Harman-Lea S (1998) Endoscopic inferior dacryocystorhinostomy. Clinical Otolaryngology 23: 152–157.

# Index

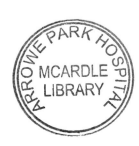